Boh's Pharmacy Practice Manual: A Guide to the Clinical Experience

Boh's Pharmacy Practice Manual: A Guide to the Clinical Experience

THIRD EDITION

EDITOR

Susan M. Stein, MS, RPh
Dean
School of Pharmacy
Pacific University
Hillsboro, Oregon

Wolters Kluwer | Lippincott Williams & Wilkins
Health

Philadelphia • Baltimore • New York • London
Buenos Aires • Hong Kong • Sydney • Tokyo

Acquisitions Editor: John Goucher
Managing Editor: Meredith Brittain
Director of Nursing Production: Helen Ewan
Senior Managing Editor / Production: Erika Kors
Senior Production Editor: Tom Gibbons
Art Director, Design: Stephen Druding
Art Director, Illustration: Brett MacNaughton
Manufacturing Coordinator: Margie Orzech
Production Services / Compositor: Aptara, Inc.

Third Edition
Copyright © 2010 Wolters Kluwer Health | Lippincott Williams & Wilkins.

351 West Camden Street   530 Walnut Street
Baltimore, MD 21201   Philadelphia, PA 19106

9   8   7   6   5   4   3   2   1

Printed in China

Library of Congress Cataloging-in-Publication Data

Boh's pharmacy practice manual : a guide to the clinical experience. –
3rd ed. / editor, Susan M. Stein.
    p. ; cm.
  Rev. ed. of: Pharmacy practice manual / editor, Larry E. Boh. 2nd ed. 2001.
  Includes bibliographical references and index.
  ISBN 978-0-7817-9764-1
  1. Pharmacy–Practice–Handbooks, manuals, etc. 2. Hospital pharmacies–Handbooks,
manuals, etc. I. Boh, Larry E. II. Stein, Susan M. (Susan Marie), 1966- III. Title:
Pharmacy practice manual.
  [DNLM: 1. Pharmacy Service, Hospital–Handbooks. 2. Clinical Clerkship–Handbooks.
3. Pharmacy–Handbooks.   QV 735 B676 2009]
    RS122.5.P483 2009
    615′.1068–dc22

                                                                    2008045473

DISCLAIMER

Care has been taken to confirm the accuracy of the information present and to describe generally accepted practices. However, the authors, editors, and publisher are not responsible for errors or omissions or for any consequences from application of the information in this book and make no warranty, expressed or implied, with respect to the currency, completeness, or accuracy of the contents of the publication. Application of this information in a particular situation remains the professional responsibility of the practitioner; the clinical treatments described and recommended may not be considered absolute and universal recommendations.

The authors, editors, and publisher have exerted every effort to ensure that drug selection and dosage set forth in this text are in accordance with the current recommendations and practice at the time of publication. However, in view of ongoing research, changes in government regulations, and the constant flow of information relating to drug therapy and drug reactions, the reader is urged to check the package insert for each drug for any change in indications and dosage and for added warnings and precautions. This is particularly important when the recommended agent is a new or infrequently employed drug.

Some drugs and medical devices presented in this publication have Food and Drug Administration (FDA) clearance for limited use in restricted research settings. It is the responsibility of the health care provider to ascertain the FDA status of each drug or device planned for use in his or her clinical practice.

To purchase additional copies of this book, call our customer service department at (**800**) **638-3030** or fax orders to (**301**) 223-2320. International customers should call (**301**) **223-2300**.

Preface

Pharmacy practice and our health care system continue to evolve with blistering speed. Pharmacy education also continues to develop, incorporating clinical experience throughout the curriculum. Pharmacists are drawn to their field because of an inherent desire to care for patients, a fascination with pharmacokinetics and pharmacotherapy, and a passion to help. We have a wonderful profession, and each of us carries a responsibility to nurture and support the next generation of pharmacists.

We proudly bring you the third edition of *Pharmacy Practice Manual: A Guide to the Clinical Experience*, which we have renamed *Boh's Pharmacy Practice Manual: A Guide to the Clinical Experience* to honor an inspiring, brilliant mentor: Larry Boh. Larry had a powerful, lasting impact on many successful clinical pharmacists practicing today. As editor of the first edition (*Clinical Clerkship Manual*) and the second edition (*Pharmacy Practice Manual: A Guide to the Clinical Experience*), he motivated knowledgeable, talented contributing editors to create an anthology that provided practitioners a valuable reference throughout their career. It has been called "a preceptor in your pocket."

This third edition carries the tradition forward, expanding and restructuring to include additional talented clinicians and valuable topics. Antibiotics, Antiviral, and Infections (Chapter 15), Pain Management (Chapter 16), Preventative Health and Immunization (Chapter 19), and Patient Safety (Chapter 20), are new chapters which have been added. The pharmacy profession provides us a unique opportunity to improve the quality and value of our patients' lives. We hope you find this book an indispensable tool in that endeavor and encourage you to never stop learning, questioning, or striving to expand your knowledge and impact on patient care.

Susan M. Stein

Acknowledgments

I wish to acknowledge and thank the contributing authors and colleagues from the previous editions of "the Boh book." Many of you are dear friends of mine from Madison and share my experience in being inspired and motivated by Larry Boh. Thank you for paving the way for the third edition.

To the talented contributing authors of the third edition, thank you so very much for your dedication and for sharing your expertise and valuable resources (time, energy, and patience) in creating this indispensable resource. Through this compilation, your knowledge, insight, and experience will support clinicians far beyond your spheres of influence. We will all gain from your excellence as clinical practitioners.

To the publishing staff at Lippincott Williams & Wilkins, especially Anne Stewart Seitz, thank you for your endless persistence, guidance, and insight in bringing this book to press in our vision.

Finally, I wish to thank Danny, my husband, honey bunny, and spirit guide. Without his support and wisdom, this book would not be in your hands.

This book is in memory of Larry E. Boh and Martin F. Stein, my mentors in pharmacy and life.

Contributors

Roberta A. Aulie, PharmD
Pharmacy Resident
Department of Pharmacy
St. Mary's Hospital
Madison, Wisconsin

David T. Bearden, PharmD
Clinical Associate Professor
Department of Pharmacy
    Practice
Oregon State University
College of Pharmacy
Portland, Oregon

Joseph K. Bonnarens, PhD
Assistant Dean for Student
    Affairs
School of Pharmacy
Pacific University
Hillsboro, Oregon

**Robert M. Breslow, BS Pharm,
    BCPS**
Clinical Associate Professor
School of Pharmacy
University of Wisconsin
Madison, Wisconsin

**Kristina L. Butler, PharmD,
    BCPS**
Assistant Professor of Medicine
Department of Medicine
Oregon Health and Science
    University
Portland, Oregon

Kam L. Capoccia, PharmD, BCPS
Clinical Assistant Professor
School of Pharmacy
Department of Family Medicine
University of Washington
Seattle, Washington

Pauline A. Cawley, PharmD
Assistant Professor
School of Pharmacy
Pacific University
Hillsboro, Oregon

**Shelley L. Chambers-Fox,
    BS Pharm, PhD**
Washington State University
Clinical Associate Professor
Department of Pharmaceutical
    Sciences
Pullman, Washington

Sandra B. Earle, PharmD
Adjunct Faculty
School of Pharmacy
University of Findlay
Findlay, Ohio

Kate Farthing, PharmD, BCPS
Drug Information/Drug Policy
    Pharmacist
Department of Pharmacy Services
Oregon Health and Science
    University
Portland, Oregon

William E. Fassett, PhD, RPh
Professor of Pharmacy Law and
  Ethics
Department of Pharmacotherapy
Washington State University
Spokane, Washington

Devon Flynn, PharmD
Clinical Adjunct Professor
School of Pharmacy
Pacific University
Hillsboro, Oregon

Jeffery Fortner, PharmD
Assistant Professor
School of Pharmacy
Pacific University
Hillsboro, Oregon

Brad S. Fujisaki, PharmD, BCPS
Assistant Professor
School of Pharmacy
Pacific University
Hillsboro, Oregon

Molly B. Gates
Pharmacy Student
School of Pharmacy
University of Finlay
Finlay, Ohio

Amy Hodgin, PharmD
Clinical Instructor
School of Pharmacy
University of Wisconsin-Madison
Wisconsin and Nutrition Support/
  Clinical Care Pharmacy
  Resident
Department of Pharmacy
University of Wisconsin Hospital
  and Clinics
Madison, Wisconsin

Kenneth C. Jackson II, PharmD
Assistant Dean for Program
  Development
School of Pharmacy
Pacific University
Hillsboro, Oregon

**Jennifer M. Jordan, PharmD,
  BCPS**
Assistant Professor
School of Pharmacy
Pacific University
Hillsboro, Oregon

**Linda Garrelts MacLean,
  BS Pharm, CDE**
Chair and Clinical Associate
  Professor of Pharmacotherapy
Washington State University
Spokane, Washington

**Kristine B. Marcus, BS Pharm,
  BCPS**
Assistant Professor
School of Pharmacy
Pacific University
Hillsboro, Oregon

**Patricia M. Mossbrucker,
BS Pharm**
Kaiser Permanente
Medication Management Program
Portland, Oregon

**Teresa A. O'Sullivan, PharmD,
BCPS**
Director of Experiential Education
Lecturer, Department of Pharmacy
School of Pharmacy
University of Washington
Seattle, Washington

**Katherine E. Rotzenberg,
PharmD**
Pharmacy Resident
Department of Pharmacy
St. Mary's Hospital
Madison, Wisconsin

Gordon Sacks, PharmD, BCNSP
Clinical Professor and Chair
School of Pharmacy
University of Wisconsin-Madison
Madison, Wisconsin

**Kathleen A. Skibinski, MS,
BS Pharm**
Clinical Pharmacy Supervisor
St. Mary's Hospital
Department of Pharmacy
Madison, Wisconsin

Susan M. Stein, MS, RPh
Dean
School of Pharmacy
Pacific University
Hillsboro, Oregon

Ty Vo, PharmD, BCPS
Assistant Professor
School of Pharmacy
Pacific University
Hillsboro, Oregon

**Ann K. Wittkowsky, PharmD,
CACP, FASHP, FCCP**
Clinical Professor
School of Pharmacy
University of Washington
Director
Anticoagulation Services
University of Washington Medical
Center
Seattle, Washington

Contents

Professionalism in Pharmacy

Susan M. Stein, William E. Fassett, and Jeffery Fortner

Professionalism plays a vital role in the practice of pharmacy. It is an all-encompassing concept that conjures images of how to make a positive impression on patients, other health care professionals, and the public. It includes how to dress, how to communicate, how to behave, how to treat others with respect, how to acknowledge and accept cultural diversity, and how to express empathy to others. Developing professionalism, or professional socialization, begins with taking pride in the profession and growing this pride throughout the didactic and clinical components of education and beyond.[1] Maintaining professionalism provides the gateway to successful delivery and acceptance of clinical pharmacy practice.

Professionalism and Trust

Imagine yourself boarding an airplane for a flight in the middle of a stormy day. What will be the impact on your confidence in the pilot if he or she is not in a sharply pressed uniform, is unshaven or unkempt, or acts as if he or she doesn't care about the business at hand? On the other hand, when the pilots and flight attendants look sharp and act sharp, isn't the quality of your trip improved? Aren't you more likely to trust them and follow their directions when your life may depend on it?

Now, consider what it is like to be sick. Your illness impairs your ability to function, to work, to enjoy life, perhaps to keep on living. Patients with grave or potentially disabling illnesses must rely on strangers—physicians, nurses, laboratory technicians, pharmacists, and others—to do for them things they cannot do for themselves. As retold by Zaner, "A man with lung cancer emphasized: 'When the doctor told me I had this tumor, frankly, it alarmed me, but he did it in such a way that it left me with a feeling of confidence.' A diabetic underscored the point: 'if you can't communicate and you can't understand your disease, then you don't have confidence in the medical help you are getting [citations omitted].'"[2]

So much of success in health care depends on patient trust in his or her health care provider that establishing a trusting relationship is the very first principle in the Code of Ethics for Pharmacists (see Box 1.1). The critical first step to earn patient trust is to act professionally.

▦ Professionalism and Performance

Many philosophers, Aristotle prime among them, have noted that to become a person whose actions are worthy of respect, including self-respect, it is important at the outset to behave in a respectable manner. But this is much more than merely acting the part. Behaving consistently in the way you wish to become forms good habits and reinforces the desired behavior. Professionalism describes in part the way you act to create in others an image of you as a "pro." But being professional is in and of itself a desirable way to act. People who behave professionally are significantly more likely to deliver high quality care. Perhaps as important, you will find that when patients and other professionals trust you, their confidence in you helps build your own self-assurance.

A recent popular phrase describes well how a person behaves professionally to become professional: he or she "talks the talk and walks the walk."

▦ Positive First Impressions

One's outward physical appearance greatly influences his or her effectiveness. Presenting yourself as awake, alert, and well-groomed (clean-shaven, no body odor, clean hair, etc.) to your patients creates a positive impression. Companies and institutions have dress codes, and professional associations use statements such as "business casual," "business dress," and "casual" to describe appropriate and acceptable dress at their meetings. These recommendations prepare the individual to meet expectations and be accepted professionally. What you wear creates an immediate impression and the goal is to be professional. Remember to know the dress code of each facility or event to confirm expectations. Also, it is advised to overdress if unsure. By the way, no one expects young health care

---

Box 1.1 **Code of Ethics for Pharmacists**

Preamble

Pharmacists are health professionals who assist individuals in making the best use of medications. This Code, prepared and supported by pharmacists, is intended to state publicly the principles that form the fundamental basis of the roles and responsibilities of pharmacists. These principles, based on moral obligations and virtues, are established to guide pharmacists in relationships with patients, health professionals, and society.

I. A pharmacist respects the covenantal relationship between the patient and pharmacist.

Considering the patient-pharmacist relationship as a covenant means that a pharmacist has moral obligations in response to the gift of trust received from society. In return for this gift, a pharmacist promises to help individuals achieve optimum benefit from their medications, to be committed to their welfare, and to maintain their trust.

II. A pharmacist promotes the good of every patient in a caring, compassionate, and confidential manner.

A pharmacist places concern for the well-being of the patient at the center of professional practice. In doing so, a pharmacist considers needs stated by the patient as well as those defined by health science. A pharmacist is dedicated to protecting the dignity of the patient. With a caring attitude and a compassionate spirit, a pharmacist focuses on serving the patient in a private and confidential manner.

III. A pharmacist respects the autonomy and dignity of each patient.

A pharmacist promotes the right of self-determination and recognizes individual self-worth by encouraging patients to participate in decisions about their health. A pharmacist communicates with patients in terms that are understandable. In all cases, a pharmacist respects personal and cultural differences among patients.

(continued)

Box 1.1 **Code of Ethics for Pharmacists** (*continued*)

IV. A pharmacist acts with honesty and integrity in professional relationships.

A pharmacist has a duty to tell the truth and to act with conviction of conscience. A pharmacist avoids discriminatory practices, behavior or work conditions that impair professional judgment, and actions that compromise dedication to the best interests of patients.

V. A pharmacist maintains professional competence.

A pharmacist has a duty to maintain knowledge and abilities as new medications, devices, and technologies become available and as health information advances.

VI. A pharmacist respects the values and abilities of colleagues and other health professionals.

When appropriate, a pharmacist asks for the consultation of colleagues or other health professionals or refers the patient. A pharmacist acknowledges that colleagues and other health professionals may differ in the beliefs and values they apply to the care of the patient.

VII. A pharmacist serves individual, community, and societal needs.

The primary obligation of a pharmacist is to individual patients. However, the obligations of a pharmacist may at times extend beyond the individual to the community and society. In these situations, the pharmacist recognizes the responsibilities that accompany these obligations and acts accordingly.

VIII. A pharmacist seeks justice in the distribution of health resources.

When health resources are allocated, a pharmacist is fair and equitable, balancing the needs of patients and society.

Adopted by the membership of the
American Pharmaceutical Association
October 27, 1994

professionals to spend a lot of money on business attire; you can "dress for success" and stay within your budget. An online Google search for the phrase "dress for success for less" will provide you with several sources of useful information. See Table 1.1 for some specific suggestions.

Professional Behavior

Impressions are also created based on an individual's behavior and attitude. When you arrive at work, how you interact with others, or how you shake hands are behaviors that can influence how others perceive you. See Table 1.2 for examples of appropriate and inappropriate behavior. Seek clarification if there is a misunderstanding. If you find that some of your habits fall in the "inappropriate" category—figure out how to change, and do it as soon as you can.

Communication

Effective communication is the ability to share ideas and receive information using verbal, written, and visual skills. The importance of effective communication in health care also influences first impressions and cannot be overemphasized. It involves patients, caregivers, and other health care providers. Miscommunication can be fatal. Frequent use of good communication skills improves effectiveness. Tables 1.3 and 1.4 provide examples of effective communication styles and techniques to improve effectiveness.

Particular types of patients may require different communication techniques. See Table 1.4 for techniques to improve communication effectiveness with these patient groups.

Confidentiality

Respecting patient confidentiality and that of others is an integral part of professionalism. Confidential information may be shared or discussed only in appropriate environments and only with appropriate individuals. The federal Health Insurance Portability and Accountability Act (HIPAA) specifies appropriate confidentiality guidelines. Use the following online link for more information: http://www.cms.hhs.gov/HIPAAGenInfo/. Understand this also: Those confidential conversations you have with

Table 1.1 DRESS CODE SUGGESTIONS

Dress Code	Men	Women	Avoid
Academic clinical experiences	White lab coat and name tag (unless otherwise directed by preceptor), professional dress	White lab coat and name tag (unless otherwise directed by preceptor), professional dress	Anything worn or torn Anything unclean or wrinkled Anything interpreted as revealing or suggestive Blue jeans, sweatshirts Athletic shoes, sandals
Professional dress	Dress pants, buttoned shirt, tie, suits	Dress pants or skirts, blouse, suits	Anything worn or torn Anything unclean or wrinkled Anything interpreted as revealing or suggestive Blue jeans, sweatshirts Athletic shoes, sandals
Business casual	Dress pants, buttoned shirt, collared shirt	Dress pants, blouse	Anything worn or torn Anything unclean or wrinkled Anything interpreted as revealing or suggestive Blue jeans, sweatshirts Athletic shoes, sandals
Business dress	Suit or sport coat with pressed slacks	Suit or skirt with dressy top, dress	Too casual Anything worn or torn Anything unclean or wrinkled Anything interpreted as revealing or suggestive Blue jeans, sweatshirts Athletic shoes, sandals
Casual	Casual pants, collared shirt	Casual pants, collared shirt or casual top	Anything worn or torn Anything unclean or wrinkled Anything interpreted as revealing or suggestive

Table 1.2 APPROPRIATE AND INAPPROPRIATE BEHAVIOR EXAMPLES

Appropriate	Inappropriate
Prompt: on time or even early; call if delayed and provide estimated time of arrival	Late or inconsistent about being on time; not calling if late, just not showing up
Identify and introduce yourself when interacting with others: "Hello, my name is Jill and I am the pharmacy resident"	Crashing into a conversation: "Why aren't they on ampicillin?"
Strong, crisp handshake	Not offering your hand for handshake greeting, "wet and wimpy" handshake
Consistent in actions and communication	Inconsistency in actions and communication
Attitude: positive, willing to try new things, willing to participate	Negative attitude, unwilling to try new things or participate
Confidence and willingness to learn more: "I would like to learn more about that"	Overconfidence, arrogance: "I already know that"
Respectful: nonjudgmental and respectfully agree or disagree: "I can see your point; thanks for the clarification"	Disrespectful: "You are wrong"; "That's not what the book says"
Empathetic: "This must be hard for you"	Not concerned: "It's not my problem"
Involved, self-directed, and proactive	Stand around and wait for someone to tell you what to do next, reactive
Time management: schedule meetings, study time, rest, etc., to maximize efficiency	Late for meetings, cram-study style, little or no sleep, etc
Prioritize time conflicts, projects, requests, presentations; maintain focus	Double-booked meetings at same time, late projects, most important item forgotten
Character: • Honesty—your own words, your own work, confidentiality • Accountability—to yourself, patients, other health care professionals • Responsibility—for you, your actions, your time, your knowledge	• Plagiarize, gossip, use someone else's work and claim as your own • Blame others for your lack of: completing a task, knowledge, promptness, etc. • Claim it's not your responsibility

Table 1.3 EFFECTIVE AND INEFFECTIVE COMMUNICATION EXAMPLES

Effective	Ineffective
Verbal: • Enunciate • Project your voice • Avoid colloquialisms, idioms, clichés • Speak slowly, regular cadence • Ask open-ended questions (which require an answer other than yes/no) • Ask direct questions to gather detailed information and descriptions rather than generalizations: "How does your pain feel today?"	• Mumble • Talk softly or away from the audience • Example of a colloquialism: "burning fever" or "dead as a doornail" • Speak too quickly or in irregular cadence • Ask only yes or no type questions • Ask generalizations: "How is it going?"
Nonverbal: • Eye contact when being spoken to or when asking a question • Proxemics (spatial relationships): lean toward but not too close • Ask permission to touch a patient • Body language: open posture, warm smile, alert eyes	• Looking away or not paying attention visibly when being spoken to • Crowding or too far away, barrier between the individual and you • Touching without being given permission • Crossed arms, furrowed brow, repeatedly clearing throat, sleepy eyes
Active listening: • Use ears, eyes, other senses to absorb information • Focus, document information acquired • Listen, not just hearing • Retain and remember • Respond with reflection and clarifications • Stay with one topic • Don't interrupt • Don't complete sentences • "Gate" yourself to listen more effectively • Sympathy (pity/compassion) vs. empathy (identify with what patient feels) • Respect others' thoughts and ideas	• Not paying attention to information shared • Not documenting information obtained • Forget details or, worse, improvise information • Respond with what you want to hear • Introduce multiple topics and confuse issues • Interrupt and rush information retrieval • Finish others' sentences and project/assume • Close off to interaction, projecting lack of interest • Pity the situation and disregard feelings of the other; not care, not interested, not involved • Disrespectful: "It wouldn't be possible to have that side effect with that drug. . . you are wrong"

(continued)

Table 1.3 EFFECTIVE AND INEFFECTIVE COMMUNICATION EXAMPLES *(continued)*

Effective	Ineffective
Oral presentation to an audience: • Relax, prepare, practice • Organize your thoughts • Come to the point promptly	 • Rush, last-minute creation, don't practice • Disorganized, confused information • Wander, talk in circles, repeat issues
Writing for notes or a paper: • Organized • Appropriate spelling, grammar, punctuation • Referenced correctly • Efficiently written	• Disorganized, inconsistent • Don't proofread, poor grammar, typos • Poorly referenced, plagiarized, referenced wrongly • Poorly written, too long, too short, disjointed
Interaction with patient or health care professional:[6] • Environment—appropriate location and time to discuss confidential information • Preparation—plan what to say, how to say it, what the goal of the interaction is, how to close the discussion • Greeting—introduce self and describe intent of the interaction • Present your statement and discuss—state purpose, provide information, encourage discussion, provide recommendation, obtain answer • Closure and documentation—summarize and address need for follow-up or monitoring if necessary	 • Too loud, not private, in the middle of the hallway, too busy • Disorganized, not planned out earlier, no goal for interaction • Forget to introduce self, forget to describe intent of interaction • Blurt recommendation with no background information, demand answer with no discussion, forget to obtain answer • No closure or fail to document

Adapted from Hosley JH, Molle E. *A Practical Guide to Therapeutic Communication for Health Professionals.* St. Louis, MO: Saunders Elsevier; 2006[3]; and Herrier RN, Boyce RW. Communicating more effectively with physicians, Part 2. *J Am Pharm Assoc.* 1996;NS36(9):547–548.[4]

colleagues concerning their personal issues or workplace concerns must be treated with great care. You should reveal to others the private matters you discuss with friends or colleagues only when patient care or safety, or equally important legal or ethical issues, require. In most cases, more damage is done to otherwise effective teams by gossip than by any other interpersonal factors.

Table 1.4   PATIENT-DEPENDENT COMMUNICATION TECHNIQUES

Patient Population	Technique
Geriatric	• Treat with respect, avoid condescending • Use surname and title (Mr., Ms., etc.) • Maintain eye contact throughout interaction • Increase font size of instructions and labels if possible • Speak clearly and directly, don't rush, and avoid mumbling • Provide medication adherence tools when appropriate (medication box, reminder timer, calendar/time chart for marking doses taken, etc.) • Provide opportunities to sit if waiting for interaction to occur
Pediatric	• Direct interaction to parent/guardian if child appears in distress, uninterested, too young to interact • Ideally address both parent/guardian and child • If speaking to child, speak calmly, avoid quick movements, avoid condescending statements, maintain eye contact at child's eye level if possible, keep it simple
Deaf	• Make eye contact prior to beginning conversation; if needed touch their hand to gain attention • Position directly in front of individual with clear eye contact as much as possible during interaction • Avoid turning away from patient until interaction completed • Speak clearly, calmly, without exaggerated facial expressions • Use short words and phrases • Use visual aids to emphasize important points or instructions (inhaler, diagram, instruction sheet, label instructions, etc.) • Learn sign language to improve trust and rapport
Language barrier	• Use an interpreter if necessary • Provide written information, labeled instructions, posted signs in appropriate language • Use normal tone of voice and slower speed, not louder and faster • Use shorter, more basic words ("pain" rather than "discomfort") and phrases, repeat as needed, staying with one topic until receptive • Use more yes/no questions for ease of translation • Avoid slang and idioms • Learn greetings and other phrases in other languages to improve trust and rapport ("Please," "Thank you," "Good day")

(continued)

Table 1.4 PATIENT-DEPENDENT COMMUNICATION TECHNIQUES *(continued)*	
Patient Population	**Technique**
Cultural barrier	• Watch for verbal signs of misunderstanding or anxiety; repeat information or explain in a different style • Need for confidentiality may vary regarding comfort in discussing certain medical issues in public • Matriarchal or patriarchal society may determine who makes the decisions in the family regarding care • Time sensitivity may vary (within 30 minutes of intended appointment may be culturally acceptable) • Eye contact may be offensive; decrease eye contact to decrease anxiety • Diet may vary; confirm before making recommendations
Cognitive issue	• Interact with caregiver if possible • Keep phrases short, increase yes/no questions • Avoid correcting the individual or creating conflict • Avoid distractions and keep length of interaction short • Obtain information through observation and listening as much as possible
Hostility	• Remain calm, focus on intent of interaction • Avoid arguing or further escalating the interaction • Obtain information through observation and listening as much as possible • Attempt to redirect to complete interaction effectively • Set limits to what is appropriate and what will not be tolerated • Know policies and procedures of the facility, access to security or backup • Document when interaction completed
Other (financial, male/female)	• Avoid judging patient based on financial status, ability to afford health care or medication • Avoid berating obvious value of prevention and provide care and education respectfully • Provide support and access if possible (medication assistance programs, medication adherence tools, etc.) • Recognize potential conflict in perceived weakness of illness, avoid emphasizing, focus on providing information

Adapted with permission from Hosley JH, Molle E. *A Practical Guide to Therapeutic Communication for Health Professionals.* St. Louis, MO: Saunders Elsevier; 2006.[3]

Table 1.5 CULTURAL DIVERSITY RECOMMENDATIONS

Cultural Diversity Recommendations

- Learning about cultural diversity is a lifelong process
- Be genuinely respectful in your interactions with others
- Look inside, look outside, and recognize the differences
- Unfamiliar behavior is an opportunity for learning
- Assumptions provide recognition but should not be acted on
- Accept that values may be entrenched; therefore, modify tools to be effective
- Promote culturally diverse educational techniques
- Learn a language's common phrases to build trust and rapport
- Refer patients to community cultural resources
- If needed, use an interpreter or bilingual family member
- Visual aids will likely improve communication

From Zweber A. Cultural competence in pharmacy practice. *Am J Pharm Educ.* 2002;66:172–176.[5]

 ## Cultural Diversity

The concept of cultural diversity is discussed frequently, generally focusing on recognizing and accepting differences between individuals deriving from cultural influences. Differences can include knowledge, values, beliefs, and behaviors. Recommendations for appropriately and effectively working with culturally diverse patients and health care professionals are listed in Table 1.5.

 ## Professional or Academic Misconduct

Inappropriate or illegal behavior is the opposite of professionalism. Depending on the degree of the infringement or action, a student or resident may be penalized with failure of a course or clinical experience or even expulsion from an academic program. A licensed professional may receive a fine, license suspension, license revocation, or be banned from the profession. To avoid the possibility of losing the privilege to practice pharmacy, educate yourself. Be aware of and follow policies and procedures and laws. See Table 1.6 for additional information regarding misconduct.

Plagiarizing, most commonly defined as using another author's original material and claiming it as your own, should be avoided. Be diligent and reference sources appropriately. See Table 1.7 for types of plagiarism and Chapter 8 for additional information.

Table 1.6 MISCONDUCT EXAMPLES

Misrepresenting, falsifying, or altering data	Falsifying records (i.e., to steal controlled substances)
Plagiarizing a report or article	Abusing controlled substances
Cheating on an examination	Using illicit drugs
Stealing supplies, medication, journals, etc.	Breaking the law (civil, criminal, or administrative) in any way
Selling products in violation of policy	Compromising ethics or integrity
Sharing confidential information (patient, financial, contractual, etc.)	

Sexual Harassment and Discrimination

Sexual harassment has broad interpretations and can occur in many different environments. Academia, organizations, and corporations have extensive policies and procedures describing sexual harassment and guidance regarding an incident. Federal and state laws also address this issue. An example of the definition of sexual harassment is listed in Table 1.8.

This behavior is unacceptable and illegal. The key to the definition is the victim's interpretation of an individual's actions. Examples may include the following:

- Offensive sexual comments directed at particular individuals.
- Offensive comments about another person's body.
- Any offensive sexual advances.

Table 1.7 TIPS TO AVOID PLAGIARISM

Four common types of plagiarism:
- Direct: lifting passages in their entirety without quotations
- Mosaic: intertwining ideas of original author with own without giving credit
- Paraphrase: using different words to provide the same idea without giving credit to the original author
- Insufficient: providing credit to the original author for only a portion of the material used

Source: Iverson C, Flanagin A, Fontanarosa PB, et al. *American Medical Association Manual of Style. A Guide for Authors and Editors.* 9th ed. Philadelphia: Williams & Wilkins; 1998.[6]

Table 1.8 DEFINITION OF SEXUAL HARASSMENT

Sexual harassment is defined as any offensive sexual advances, requests for sexual favors, and other conduct of a sexual nature when:
1. Submission to the conduct is made a term or condition of employment or education;
2. Submission to or rejection of the conduct is used as the basis for a decision affecting an individual's employment or education, including, but not limited to, employment or academic evaluation; or
3. The conduct has the purpose or effect of unreasonably interfering with the individual's work performance or education, or creating an intimidating, hostile or offensive employment or educational environment

Source: *Pacific University 2007–2008 Student Handbook*. Forest Grove, OR: Pacific University; 2007.[7]

- Engaging in offensive touching of another person.
- Engaging in or attempting to develop a romantic or sexual relationship with an individual who is a supervisor or who is in a less powerful position.

If an incident of sexual harassment is suspected or does occur, it should be reported promptly to the proper administrator with documentation and details. Ideally, report the information to the preceptor, Assistant/Associate Dean, manager, or supervisor outlined in the policy. If this individual is involved in the harassment, report to the next individual in rank. The allegation will be investigated thoroughly and possibly break a cycle of unacceptable and illegal behavior.

It is also unprofessional and illegal in virtually all health care settings to discriminate against others based on factors such as race, color, creed, religion, nationality, disability, ancestry, age, socioeconomic status, or sexual orientation. In the opinion of the authors, if this concept is not inherently sensible to you, you probably shouldn't be seeking to become a pharmacist.

Code of Ethics for Pharmacists and Oath of a Pharmacist

Two documents exist that reinforce the commitment pharmacists have to their patients and the health care community. The American Pharmacists Association created the Code of Ethics for Pharmacists (Box 1.1). It is updated regularly to reflect current practice. The American Pharmaceutical Association Academy of Students of Pharmacy/American Association

Box 1.2   **Pledge of Professionalism**

As a student of pharmacy, I believe there is a need to build and reinforce a professional identity founded on integrity, ethical behavior, and honor. This development, a vital process in my education, will help ensure that I am true to the professional relationship I establish between myself and society as I become a member of the pharmacy community. Integrity must be an essential part of my everyday life and I must practice pharmacy with honesty and commitment to service.

To accomplish this goal of professional development, I as a student of pharmacy should:

DEVELOP a sense of loyalty and duty to the profession of pharmacy by being a builder of community, one able and willing to contribute to the well-being of others and one who enthusiastically accepts the responsibility and accountability for membership in the profession.

FOSTER professional competency through life-long learning. I must strive for high ideals, teamwork and unity within the profession in order to provide optimal patient care.

SUPPORT my colleagues by actively encouraging personal commitment to the Oath of Maimonides and a Code of Ethics as set forth by the profession

INCORPORATE into my life and practice, dedication to excellence. This will require an ongoing reassessment of personal and professional values.

MAINTAIN the highest ideals and professional attributes to ensure and facilitate the covenantal relationship required of the pharmaceutical care giver.

The profession of pharmacy is one that demands adherence to a set of rigid ethical standards. These high ideals are necessary to ensure the quality of care extended to the patients I serve. As a student of pharmacy, I believe this does not start with graduation; rather, it begins with my membership in this professional college community. Therefore, I must strive to uphold these standards as I advance toward full membership in the profession of pharmacy.

(continued)

Box 1.2   Pledge of Professionalism *(continued)*

Developed by the American Pharmaceutical Association Academy of Students of Pharmacy/American Association of Colleges of Pharmacy Council of Deans (APhA-ASP/AACP-COD) Task Force on Professionalism; June 26, 1994,

Reprinted from http://www.aacp.org/site/page.asp?TRACKID=&VID= 1&CID=735&DID=5020. With permission from the American Pharmacists Association. Accessed 04/01/2008.

Box 1.3   Oath of a Pharmacist

"I promise to devote myself to a lifetime of service to others through the profession of pharmacy. In fulfilling this vow:

I will consider the welfare of humanity and relief of suffering my primary concerns.

I will apply my knowledge, experience, and skills to the best of my ability to assure optimal outcomes for my patients.

I will respect and protect all personal and health information entrusted to me.

I will accept the lifelong obligation to improve my professional knowledge and competence.

I will hold myself and my colleagues to the highest principles of moral, ethical, and legal conduct.

I will embrace and advocate changes that improve patient care.

I will utilize my knowledge, skills, experiences, and values to fulfill my obligation to educate and train the next generation of pharmacists.

I take these vows voluntarily with the full realization of the responsibility with which I am entrusted by the public."

The revised Oath was adopted by the AACP House of Delegates in July 2007. The revised Oath will be considered by the American

(continued)

> **Box 1.3**   **Oath of a Pharmacist**
> **(*continued*)**
>
> Pharmaceutical Association Academy of Students of Pharmacy
> in spring 2008. AACP should plan to use the revised Oath of a
> Pharmacist during the 2008–2009 academic year and with spring
> 2009 graduates.
>
> *Reprinted with permission from http://www.aacp.org/site/page.asp?*
> *TRACKID=&VID=1&CID=735&DID=5020. Accessed 04/01/2008.*

of Colleges of Pharmacy Council of Deans (APhA-ASP/AACP-COD) Task
Force on Professionalism created the Pledge of Professionalism (Box 1.2)
and Oath of a Pharmacist (Box 1.3) through a joint effort. Although students often recite this statement on graduation, it should be followed and
practiced throughout their training to further emphasize their commitment to the profession of pharmacy.

 Summary

Being a professional and acting professionally are characteristics that develop over time. The examples and recommendations in this chapter are
just the beginning of resources available to help improve and polish a
pharmacist. If you observe and emulate those around you whom you ad-
mire, commit yourself to continuous personal improvement, and treat
others with respect, you will succeed as a pharmacy professional.

References

1. American Pharmacists Association. White Paper on Pharmacy Student Professionalism. APhA-Academy of Students of Pharmacy-American Association of Colleges
   of Pharmacy Council of Deans Task Force on Professionalism. *J Am Pharm Assoc.*
   2000;40(1):96–102.
2. Zaner RM. Trust and the patient-physician relationship. In: Pellegrino ED, Veatch
   RM, Langan JP, eds. *Ethics, Trust, and the Professions.* Washington, DC: Georgetown
   University Press; 1991;49.
3. Hosley JH, Molle E. *A Practical Guide to Therapeutic Communication for Health Professionals.* St. Louis, MO: Saunders Elsevier; 2006.
4. Herrier RN, Boyce RW. Communicating more effectively with physicians, Part 2. *J Am
   Pharm Assoc.* 1996;NS36(9):547–548.

5. Zweber A. Cultural competence in pharmacy practice. *Am J Pharm Educ*. Summer 2002;66:172–176.

6. Iverson C, Flanagin A, Fontanarosa PB, et al. *American Medical Association Manual of Style. A Guide for Authors and Editors*. 9th ed. Philadelphia: Williams & Wilkins; 1998.

7. *Pacific University 2007–2008 Student Handbook*. Forest Grove, OR: Pacific University; 2007.

Other Suggested Readings and Resources

American Association of Colleges of Pharmacy (AACP). Professionalism: pharmacy student professionalism resources: http://www.aacp.org/site/page.asp?TRACKID=& VID=1&CID=735&DID=5020
Pharmacy Professionalism Toolkit for Students and Faculty

American Pharmacists Association (APhA). Leadership and Professionalism: http:// www.pharmacist.com/AM/Template.cfm?Section=Leadership_and_Professionalism1 &Template=/TaggedPage/TaggedPageDisplay.cfm&TPLID=78&ContentID=6087.

Hammer DP, Berger BA, Beardsley RS, et al. Student professionalism. *Am J Pharm Educ*. 2003:67:Article 96.

Hosley J, Molle JH. *A Practical Guide to Therapeutic Communication for Health Professionals*. St. Louis, MO: Saunders Elsevier; 2006.

Rantucci MJ. *Pharmacists Talking with Patients: A Guide to Patient Counseling*. 2nd ed. Philadelphia: Lippincott Williams & Wilkins; 2007.

2 Professional Experiential Education—Why, How, and What to Expect

Joseph K. Bonnarens

The profession of pharmacy, as with any other vocation, changes over time—making momentous leaps through innovation and discovery, steady growth through hard work and dedication, and the occasional slip or stagnation that can appear when a professional doesn't learn from past mistakes or becomes too preoccupied with itself and gets passed by in the ever-changing flow of progress. As a student, you are moving into your own professional time line. You are currently receiving the most advanced training ever provided to students wanting to become pharmacists. You will be entering a profession that offers, some might say, too many opportunities for new graduates to navigate—postgraduate opportunities ranging from residency experience to advance degrees, seemingly limitless job opportunities, and career opportunities that offer challenges and financial security. So, your time line begins with entering the profession as a professional in training through pharmacy school, learning about all of your options. The next point is when you become a licensed pharmacist and you are now ready to go out and join the profession: get paid for your work, begin to have a life, and for most, not have to worry about any exams.

Now, allow me to present an example of a professional time line that you may have seen exhibited by a pharmacist. Within 5 years after graduation, the pharmacist will look at the new graduates and say, "What has happened to pharmacy education—do these students learn anything in pharmacy school?" Within 10 years, "Great, now I have to train these know-it-alls!" Within 15 years, "Wow, I'm glad I am not applying for pharmacy school now. I would never get in!" So, what is a major contributor to the change in this particular pharmacist along the time line? *Experience!*

This chapter will discuss experiential pharmacy education; featuring a brief review of the past, an update of the present, and a discussion of the immediate future that you are facing, and why the future of the profession depends on your current actions.

■ The Past—The Only Constant Is Change

Oh, no—a history lesson! Yes—but it is brief and is meant to show why things are the way they are, as well as to plant seeds within your professional psyche that over time, when these seeds have been exposed to enough fertilizer, they will sprout forth and help remind you to also not repeat the mistakes that have been previously made but to be innovative and examine the opportunities for creativity and positive growth.

Experiential education has long been a part of pharmacy education. The early education of pharmacists was primarily an apprenticeship (i.e., experiential) with some didactic (i.e., classroom) education. As the profession grew and pharmacy education evolved, the amount of didactic education increased as the amount of experiential education decreased. Your current preceptors have experienced a wide variety of experiential requirements during their education. Most pharmacists graduating between 1960 and 1990 received a Bachelor of Science degree in pharmacy, and in most cases, the experiential component of their education consisted of one quarter or semester of rotations in a few practice sites. However, most experiential hours were earned outside of class/school. In the 1990s, the long-time debate regarding the establishment of the Doctor of Pharmacy (PharmD) as the single entry-level professional practice degree reached its peak and culminated with the adoption of the 1997 revision of the Accreditation Council for Pharmacy Education (ACPE) accreditation standards for professional pharmacy education.[1] These new standards required that all baccalaureate pharmacy programs would end in the 2004–2005 academic year, completing the transition of pharmacy education to the single entry-level PharmD.[2]

Your preceptors from this time frame (1990 to current) experienced an increase in focused experiential education. With the PharmD transition, students saw more required experiential education. Most students were spending the entire final year of their professional program in the field on rotation. The number of experiential sites and preceptors increased. In addition, students received greater exposure to professional practice opportunities with schools offering 4-, 5-, or 6-week rotations during the final year in the program.

◼ The Present (at Least, When This Chapter Was Written)

Led by the latest revision to the accreditation standards, all colleges and schools of pharmacy are facing additional challenges in regard to experiential education. You might be asking yourself, "Why did the standards change again?" As noted in the background discussion regarding the revision of standards, ACPE identified a number of factors that contributed to the reassessment and revision of the current standards.[2] One of the key external factors included the Institute of Medicine reports addressing the need to improve patient care and safety, while also focusing on expansion of interdisciplinary training programs. Many interprofessional factors were also identified, including but not limited to the revision of the American Association of Colleges of Pharmacy's (AACP) Center for the Advancement of Pharmaceutical Education (CAPE) Educational Outcomes in 2004, the 2005 AACP APPI Summit to Advance Experiential Education in Pharmacy, and the Joint Commission of Pharmacy Practitioners' *Vision of Pharmacy Practice 2015* released in 2005. One of the largest changes to the standard and supported by the factors was in the area of experiential education.

The new standards, which went into effect July 2007, actually have a specific section dedicated to experiential education. Each college and school of pharmacy is required to provide a continuum of required and elective experiences throughout the curriculum, from introductory to advanced.[2]

Introductory Pharmacy Practice Experience (IPPE)

ACPE defines IPPEs as:[2]

> ...[IPPEs] must involve actual practice experiences in community and institutional settings and permit students, under appropriate supervision and as permitted by practice regulations, to assume direct patient care responsibilities.

In addition, this type of experience should begin early in the curriculum, in conjunction with the didactic course work, and should ultimately prepare the student for the advanced experiential rotations. This area of experiential expansion is the newest addition to the accreditation standards and has become one of the more difficult standards for colleges and schools of pharmacy to achieve. Although all programs have always needed to identify advanced experiential sites and preceptors, IPPEs have now increased the need for preceptors and practice sites.

Advanced Pharmacy Practice Experience (APPE)

The new standards also outline and detail APPEs.[2] APPEs consist of required and elective experiences for students in their final year. The standards identify four required experiences in the following settings: community pharmacy, hospital/health system pharmacy, ambulatory care, and inpatient/acute care general medicine. All students are to receive a balanced experience and "must include primary, acute, chronic, and preventive care among patients of all ages and develop pharmacist-delivered patient care competencies" in the previously mentioned settings.[2] The standard is very specific, stating all required APPEs must be conducted in the United States or its territories and possessions. In contrast, elective APPEs may be offered outside the United States and its territories and possessions as long as competencies are required of the student and the quality of the experience can be verified. Although the standards might support these experiences, it will be important for all students to ensure that their respective boards of pharmacy recognize out-of-country earned hours. Elective APPEs offer students a unique opportunity to experience pharmacy in other settings; such as academia, long-term care, research, nuclear pharmacy, and administration/management.

The number of APPEs will vary for each program due to the length of each rotation. It has been reported that the most common rotation length for schools is 4 weeks, followed by 6 weeks, and then 5 weeks.[3]

Experiential Education and Boards of Pharmacy

While the accreditation standards provide guidance to the colleges and schools of pharmacy, another group provides guidance about the practice of pharmacy: state boards of pharmacy. Each individual board oversees the pharmacy practice in its respective state. Colleges and schools of pharmacy all work closely with their state boards on various issues, specifically in areas such as defining intern status, licensing issues, and practical experience hours.

While students learn about the state boards in the state where their program is located, here are a couple of recommendations regarding learning about other states. If you are planning to obtain your license in another state, contact that state's board to determine their practice experience hours and documentation requirements. The same goes for the state in which you are receiving your pharmacy degree. You must know how each state deals with the other regarding documentation of hours. Each board of pharmacy has its own Web site that should provide you with the necessary information. If you have difficulties in finding the information, contact the board directly. Another valuable resource is the National Association of Boards of Pharmacy (NABP). NABP works with all boards of pharmacy and produces an annual document entitled the *Survey of Pharmacy Law*. In most cases, the graduating students from colleges and schools of pharmacy receive a copy of this valuable reference. It compiles various details about specific aspects of the law and how each state addresses each aspect. Please remember—each state is a little different regarding the laws related to pharmacy practice, so become informed. As each state board will remind you, ignorance is no excuse. Access NABP via the Web (www.nabp.net/) and find the *Survey of Pharmacy Law* under the Publications header.

Experiential Glossary

Colleges and schools of pharmacy are attempting to meet the challenging standards set forth by ACPE in regard to experiential education. Some programs have been more successful than others with the expansion of this aspect in pharmacy education. With the differences between state boards, as well as curriculum nuances, we offer a glossary of terms in Table 2.1 to set the stage for the discussion of your upcoming and/or current experiences with this aspect of your training.

General Recommendations Regarding Experiential Education

So, the changes in accreditation standards have been discussed, the general experiential requirements for colleges and schools of pharmacy reviewed, the important relationship between experiential education and state boards of pharmacy examined, and an experiential glossary has been provided—what is left to discuss? This section will offer comments and suggestions to any student regarding the unique opportunity experiential education provides to all future pharmacists.

Table 2.1 EXPERIENTIAL GLOSSARY

Advanced pharmacy practice experience (APPE)	Also referred to as rotations and clerkships; APPEs should provide a balanced series of required (the majority) and elective experiences that cumulatively provide sustained experiences of adequate intensity, duration, and breadth (in terms of patients and disease states that pharmacists are likely to encounter when providing care) to enable achievement of stated competencies as demonstrated by assessment of outcome expectations
	Additional key point—students cannot receive compensation for their time at the site[2]
Assessment	The formalized evaluation of the objectives, as well as of the preceptor, and general feelings of each experience. The assessment activities must use various valid and reliable measures systematically and sequentially throughout the professional degree program. The college or school must use the analysis of assessment measures to improve student learning and the achievement of the professional competencies
Assistant Dean for Clinical Education	One of many possible references to the individual responsible for overseeing the organization and coordination of all experiential education
Background check	A process, usually conducted by an outside contracted firm, of checking the background of each student for any past criminal infractions
	A growing human resource technique being used in health care facilities for all employees
Clerkships	An older, yet common, reference for APPE
Director of Advanced Experiential Education	One of many possible references to the individual responsible for overseeing the organization and coordination of the APPEs
Drug testing	A human resource process that more health care–related businesses are beginning to implement to identify any potential problems for their newly hired staff with illicit or prescription drugs
Electives	Those APPEs that are not part of the required rotations
Introductory pharmacy practice experience (IPPE)	Experiences must involve actual practice experiences in community and institutional settings and permit students, under appropriate supervision and as permitted by practice regulations, to assume direct patient care responsibilities[2]

(continued)

Table 2.1   EXPERIENTIAL GLOSSARY (continued)

Objectives	Identified criteria, achieved through task/duty/assignment, that are created for each experience and must be achieved by each student
Pharmacy intern	Defined by each state board of pharmacy—each definition usually includes (i) a currently enrolled student in an accredited (or recognized by the Accreditation Council for Pharmacy Education [ACPE]) college or school of pharmacy, (ii) in good academic standing, and (iii) who has completed some portion of his or her professional degree program (ranges from 0–2 years in the program). Check with your school and state board of pharmacy
Pharmacy student	An individual enrolled in an accredited college or school of pharmacy or college or school of pharmacy in the process of accreditation and is recognized by ACPE
Practice site	The actual pharmacy or pharmacy-related site identified as hosting a student for any type of experiential opportunity
Preceptor	A licensed pharmacist who helps guide and oversee a pharmacy student through experiential rotation at the particular practice site. Requirements vary by state
"Requireds"	Those APPEs that are required practice settings that each student must experience (complete)
Rotations	Refers to the APPEs
Shadow (shadowing)	A form of experience that a student may participate in that features a student shadowing a licensed pharmacist at a practice site to experience the work flow and daily routine of the site. Usually set for a short period of time (8-16 hours) and often used to introduce students to institutional practice settings prior to APPEs

"Try It, You Might Like It"

Let us attempt some creativity. Take a moment to relax, take a deep breath, clear your mind, and then read the following statement:

> There you sit. Before you an ominous site…
> a giant bowl of *green stuff*!
> (Note to reader: If you like green stuff, please insert another ominous color.)

You are 4 years old and your parents are explaining to you that this *stuff* is good and you should try it. The arsenal of motivational techniques is unleashed:

"Just try a bite, you will like it!"
"Take two bites and you get a special treat!"
"You don't know what you are missing!"
"No dessert if you don't try it!"

Whether we are 4 or it was yesterday, people are hardwired regarding trying new things. Some thrive on trying new things (foods, clothes, books, activities, etc.), whereas others are perfectly happy with their established choices and do not want to change. Where do you fit on the trying new things scale?

As many of you have already learned, experiential education is a lot like the previous scenario; however, there is very little control available to the student. Although many might argue that the motivational technique used in professional education is more of a forced feeding approach, the ultimate goal for experiential education is to expose a student to various practice settings and professional experiences from which the student will grow and cultivate a deeper understanding and interest in the profession. Trying things provides you with the experiences to begin to make informed decisions rather than holding loose assumptions based on limited information. The following are some points to consider as you go through pharmacy school and begin your experiential education:

- When handed a rotation site, go into the experience open minded, no matter what you hear from your peers or others. Remember, after it has been assigned, the likelihood of your changing sites is small. Make the most of it!
- When selecting an elective rotation site, try something different. Experiential education is one of the few times an individual has the opportunity to try a different job. If home infusion always sounded interesting, try to do a rotation.
- Work with the experiential people at your school. They are very busy people and want to find the best experience for each student, preceptor, and practice site. If you have an interest in an area of pharmacy practice, speak with your experiential people to begin learning about opportunities during your program.

"Little in Life is Guaranteed"

As a pharmacy student, you will have various practical experiences leading up to your graduation and licensure. How does all of this happen? Each college and school of pharmacy has individuals responsible for experiential education. Although the size of each program's experiential staffs vary greatly, the job they have is the same. Their job is to ensure that the students in each program achieve their experiential rotations required to graduate. Here are some friendly tips to remember when working with the individuals in experiential education in your program:

- Speak to the staff early about possible options, ranging from location to types of practice opportunities.
- Be professional in these interactions—respectful and helpful, not demanding.
- Follow the policies and procedures, instructions, and time lines provided by the staff as closely as possible (especially in the area of contacting preceptors and sites).

"You Get Out What You Put In"

Your experiences will be varied; some you will love, some you may classify as okay, some you may classify as not so good. How you ultimately view your experiences has a great deal to do with you. Although in most cases, you have little influence regarding where your rotation is, you do have a lot to do with how the experience progresses for you and your preceptor/practice site. Once you know where your rotations will be, it is human nature to learn about the site. No matter what you hear from others, approach your first day at any rotation with an open mind and be prepared to learn about this site. Here is a very important point: You are an invited guest at the site, and it is a privilege for you to be there. You are training to become a professional, and this experience will help you down that road. Use the objectives and assignments provided to you from the program to help you learn about the site. Work with your preceptor and begin to establish a good professional relationship with the preceptor and staff at each rotation. While on your rotation, always strive to work hard to complete all assignments, follow the rules of the practice site as well as those of the program, and continue to set a good example as a future professional. Finally, in any rotation or experience outside of your program, you are representing your program as well as yourself. If you can strive to follow this simple advice on any rotation, you will be successful and learn a great deal from the experience.

"Nothing Is Set in Stone"

Before you set foot in your first rotation site of your final year of pharmacy school, you may already know what your career will consist of:

- A postgraduate year one (PGY1) residency at X Hospital, a postgraduate year two (PGY2) pediatrics specialty at Y Health System, and then clinical coordinator for pediatrics at Z Medical Center; or
- Staff pharmacist with Joe's Pharmacy with responsibility for MTM services; or
- Staff pharmacist with Super Club Pharmacy in a neighboring state with a chance to get into the management training program within 6 months.

You may also be one of those individuals who isn't sure what aspect of pharmacy practice to pursue because there are just too many options to choose. In any case, your rotations can help you in your initial decision making.

First and foremost, your rotations should reinforce the fact that you should never believe that you have only one option for a job or career in pharmacy. The career opportunities that you have with your Doctor of Pharmacy in hand will be limited only by your imagination. Your rotations will introduce you to some experiences that you never knew existed, as well as reinforcing your interest in particular areas.

With each of your rotations, you are establishing your professional network—meeting pharmacists and learning about their career paths. This network will continue to grow and develop, while also providing you with additional future opportunities, all because of your rotation. From this network, you may develop mentors who will help provide guidance and support when making future decisions related to your professional career. In addition, this network that you are creating will not be made up of only pharmacists. Your network has the opportunity to grow to be as varied as your rotation site options—other soon-to-be professionals (students in all health care arenas), administrators, legislators, federal and state agency personnel, attorneys, and so on.

◼ The Future—It's Just Around the Corner

I know that you love to hear this from everyone you work with: "You are going to be a pharmacist before you know it!" In many ways, these individuals are correct. During pharmacy school, time is measured only by exams and breaks. When you near graduation, you will be amazed by how fast things seemed to pass. Your final year of rotations contributes to this perception greatly. The structure of your rotations provides you with an opportunity to use all of that knowledge that you have hidden away during the previous years of classroom experience.

So, graduation arrives, you prepare and successfully complete your licensure exams, and you are now a pharmacist. You have moved to the next spot on your professional time line. Now what? Do you just get on with life—focus on family, work, fun, career, and so on? Don't forget your professional responsibility.

Give Back

Don't worry, this is not a plea from the alumni association of your college or school to donate generously to the scholarship fund (although it is important to do that when you get the chance, plus, it will give you a needed tax write-off). Part of being a professional is being involved in the development of new professionals. This involvement may come in many forms; however, one of the most important forms is time—giving your time as a preceptor, a speaker, a volunteer, and as a mentor to these future professionals.

All colleges and schools of pharmacy depend a great deal on the professionals (including their alumni) to help with experiential education, as well as other areas of the program. How can you get involved? Here are a few examples:

- Become a preceptor.
- Begin a new rotation site at your practice setting.
- Offer to guest lecture at the college or school of pharmacy that you are near (alumnus/alumna or not).
- Volunteer to help at a college or school of pharmacy for such things as admissions interviews or clinical skills testing.
- Sponsor students at your state or national pharmacy association meetings.

This is certainly not a complete list. However, if every pharmacist chose to do any one of the listed examples, the profession would benefit greatly.

You have now entered your professional time line and begun your career journey in pharmacy. This is an amazing profession that has great opportunities, where one can be bored only if he or she chooses to be—job options and career choices abound. As you gain experience, your time line will collect interesting remarks about the new graduates from colleges and schools of pharmacy. Just make sure that you do have those comments in your time line because that means that you are truly a part of the profession, gaining and providing experience.

References

1. Accreditation Standards and Guidelines for the Professional Program in Pharmacy Leading to the Doctor of Pharmacy Degree, Adopted: June 14, 1997; Effective through June 30, 2007. Web document (www.acpe-accredit.org/shared_info/standards1_view.htm): Accessed May 6, 2008.
2. Accreditation Standards and Guidelines for the Professional Program in Pharmacy Leading to the Doctor of Pharmacy Degree, Adopted: January 15, 2006; Released: February 17, 2006; Effective: July 1, 2007. Word document accessible from following Web address: www.acpe-accredit.org/deans/standards.asp—under Revised PharmD Standards: Accessed May 6, 2008.
3. O'Sullivan T, Hammer DP, Gasdek Manolakis P, Skelton JB, Weber SS, Dawson KN, Flynn AA. Pharmacy Experiential Education Present and Future: Realizing the Janus Vision – A Background Paper for the AACP APPI Summit to Advance Experiential Education in Pharmacy, AACP Experiential Education Section Library, Web site: www.peplibrary.vcu.edu/result.asp?id=104_document Web site_www.pubinfo.vcu.edu/pharmacy/peplibrary/resources/AACP_SummitBackground Paper.pdf

3 Providing Drug Information

Brad S. Fujisaki, Kristine B. Marcus, and Kate Farthing

Preparing to Provide Drug Information

Regardless of which experiential rotation you are scheduled for, it is common for all pharmacy students to provide drug information as part of their patient care and non–patient care activities. When orienting to your experiential rotation, gain a clear understanding of your preceptor's expectations concerning your role as a provider of drug information. To get at the information you need quickly, you need to learn what resources are available to you through your experiential site, as well as any library access and resources available to you remotely through your pharmacy program. Spending 30 minutes with your preceptor, reference librarian, or drug information specialist at your site at the beginning of your rotation will pay off in efficiency later. Be sure to note any passwords or constraints to the use of that resource (e.g., single-user license, on campus only). If you are unfamiliar with an available reference, spend some time learning to use it so you are comfortable with its contents and organization.

To assist you in orienting to your available drug information holdings, we have created a Providing Drug Information Questionnaire in Appendix 3A. Identifying your available resources ahead of time will allow you to use our drug information question tables to find your answer more quickly.

Improvements in technology have allowed many drug information references to become available in various media formats. Within the last decade, content from traditional print resources have become available as e-books or electronic databases. Also, companies such as Lexi-Comp have partnered with American Society of Health System Pharmacists (ASHP) to have American Hospital Formulary Service (AHFS) Drug Information incorporated into the Lexi-Comp Online suite of products. Similarly, some monograph content from Clinical Pharmacology (Gold Standard) can be found in other vendor's products such as MDConsult (Elsevier) and McGraw-Hill's AccessMedicine and AccessPharmacy online sites. What this means is that you may have access to content from a traditional source of drug information via a nontraditional route that your school or site has subscribed to (e.g., Mosby's Drug Consult via STAT!Ref electronic book collection). Refer to the crosswalk of print and electronic resources in Appendix 3B to help you navigate to these alternative resources.

Finding Useful Drug Information

Traditionally, drug information questions are answered using a systematic approach. An example of a stepwise approach is outlined in Table 3.1.[1] The goal of using a systematic approach is to consistently provide drug information to the requestor that is useful.

The usefulness of medical information has been described as a function of validity, relevance, and the time it takes to find the information.[2] With this in mind, pharmacy students can maximize the usefulness of drug information by the following:

1. Locating information that is valid
2. Locating information that is relevant to the posed question
3. Locating information efficiently in the least amount of time

Table 3.1	MODIFIED SYSTEMATIC APPROACH TO DRUG INFORMATION
Step I	Secure demographics of requestor
Step II	Obtain background information
Step III	Determine and categorize ultimate questions
Step IV	Develop strategy and conduct search
Step V	Perform evaluation, analysis, and synthesis
Step VI	Formulate and provide response
Step VII	Conduct follow-up and documentation

Table 3.2	LIST OF RESOURCES TO ASSIST IN LITERATURE EVALUATION

Resource in Print	**Resource on Internet**
The Evidence-Based Medicine Working Group. Users' Guide to the Medical Literature. American Medical Association (AMA) Press	Similar information available online at the Centre for Health Evidence website: www.cche.net/usersguides/main.asp
Greenhalgh T. How to read a paper—the basics of evidence based medicine. BMJ Books	Similar information available online at British Medical Journal (BMJ) website: www.bmj.com/collections/read.dtl

Centre for Evidence Based Medicine. EMB Tools for literature evaluation. Available from www.cebm.net.
MedlinePLUS website. Evaluating internet health information: a tutorial from the national library of medicine. Available from www.nlm.nih.gov/medlineplus/webeval/webeval.html.

Locating Information That Is Valid and Relevant

Table 3.2 provides a list of resources to serve as a review in evaluating the validity and relevancy of literature in answering drug information questions. Finding valid and relevant information often requires a search of the primary literature. As the volume of published journal articles continues to increase, the utility of indexing and abstracting services (also known as secondary resources) has become that much more important. MEDLINE is the primary electronic indexing system for medical journals and is available as a free searchable database through the National Library of Medicine's PubMed. A comprehensive tutorial is available for PubMed: www.nlm.nih.gov/bsd/disted/pubmedtutorial/. In addition, a review of your Drug Information course notes or textbook on basic search techniques such as the use of Boolean operators (e.g., AND, OR, NOT) may be useful.

Locating Information Efficiently

Finding valid and relevant drug information is important; however, efficiently finding this information is equally critical—providing information after the point that it is needed clearly decreases its overall usefulness. Therefore, the remainder of this chapter is designed to assist you in efficiently locating the most likely resources that will answer a particular type of drug information question. We have focused our efforts on the types of questions that pharmacists often face in practice. Certain types of questions are best answered using specialized resources.

However, pharmacists do not always have easy access to these specialized resources, so we have taken into consideration the most common information resources that you will likely have access to. From there, we have recommended resources that are most likely to provide you, and subsequently the requestor, with useful information. In our tables we designate specific resources when needed or whether any General Drug Information Compendia is likely to answer your question. Familiarize yourself with the bibliographic list in Appendix 3C that is organized by the resource types referred to in our tables.

Published drug information resource matrices or pathfinders[3,4] are available by type of request. We have tried to improve on these excellent resources by incorporating the element of time and limiting the scope of our recommendations to the most common scenarios where pharmacy students are asked to provide drug information. Our time frames reflect both the usual expected turn-around-time for a given scenario and the amount of research time that is generally required to use the cited references and synthesize a response for that question type. We used the following standard time estimates in the tables:

- Minutes (e.g., question asked on rounds for an immediate patient need).
- Minutes to hours (e.g., question on a patient to be seen in clinic later that same day).
- Hours to days (e.g., preparing a 5-minute in-service for tomorrow).

Answering the Most Common Question Types

Knowing the frame of reference of your requestors and how they plan to use the drug information you give them is fundamental to providing a targeted response that will be put into action. Obtaining adequate background material and defining the ultimate question the requestor is asking requires practice, and your approach needs to vary for different question types. Until this skill is second nature, it is not uncommon to need to contact the requestor after the initial question is received to gain further clarification. Standard questions to elicit background information by question type can be found in Appendix 3D.

The remainder of this section of the chapter is organized by drug information question type so that you can quickly find the resources that are most likely to be useful in answering your question. Asking yourself, "What question type is this?" and "How much time do I have to answer this question?" will facilitate the use of the following tables. The tables are

Table 3.3 COMMON DRUG INFORMATION QUESTION TYPES ASKED OF PHARMACY STUDENTS

Frequency of Question Type Encountered by Students	Corresponding Table in this Chapter
Highest frequency	
• Adverse Drug Reactions	Table 3-4, page 37
• Dosing or Administration	Table 3-6, page 40
• Drug Interactions	Table 3-7, page 44
• Indication or Therapeutic Use	Table 3-8, page 47
• Product Information or Identification	Table 3-9, page 48
Moderate frequency	
• Safety in Pregnancy and Lactation	Table 3-10, page 51
• IV Compatibility Stability	Table 3-11, page 53
Lowest Frequency	
• Natural Products and Dietary Supplements	Table 3-12, page 56
• Nonsterile Compounded Formulations	Table 3-13, page 58

organized from the most common question type you are likely to encounter to the least common question type (Table 3.3). As part of your preparation for providing drug information you may find it helpful to practice using the references associated with the higher-frequency question types.

Adverse Drug Reactions

Requestors seeking information on side effects or adverse drugs reactions often have two basic questions:

1. Has this adverse reaction been previously associated with this drug?
2. How do you prevent or manage this adverse drug reaction?

Questions related to accidental or intentional ingestion of drugs or chemicals should be immediately triaged to a Poison Center (1-800-222-1222).

General tertiary resources will often provide information on adverse drug reactions that are common, serious, or classic. Information on the clinical presentation, time course, risk factors, and management of specific adverse drug reactions are often described in textbooks and review articles. There are also a handful of specialized tertiary references focused around drug-induced disease such as *Meyler's Side Effects of Drugs and Drug Induced Diseases*. Conversely, information in handbook-type drug compendia are less detailed, often limited to a list of adverse drug reactions with approximated frequency of occurrence. Therefore, a more comprehensive search of the primary literature is often required for finding information on reactions associated with drugs. Drug-focused secondary indexing references may be useful for finding information on adverse drug reactions. These include subscription indexing databases such as EMBASE, International Pharmaceutical Abstracts, and Iowa Drug Information Service.

Pharmacists, as health care providers in the United States, are not currently required to report adverse drug reactions to the Food and Drug Administration (FDA). However, voluntary reporting of adverse drug reactions via the MedWatch program is strongly encouraged, particularly for drugs that have been marketed for less than 3 years (www.fda.gov/medwatch/). Adverse reactions from vaccines are currently reported through the Vaccine Adverse Event Reporting System (VAERS) program (www.vaers.hhs.gov/). Many health care systems and hospitals use a centralized reporting system for adverse drug reactions or medication errors; therefore, it is prudent to determine the practice setting's standard procedure for reporting to minimize duplication of effort. Table 3.4 describes common adverse drug reactions questions with resources for information given an amount of time to research the response.

A slight variation on the adverse drug reaction question may be posed as, "Is this reaction associated with any of the medications my patient is taking?" Some electronic drug information databases allow you to query by a specific adverse reaction and provide results in the form of drug lists associated with that reaction—Micromedex DrugDex, Lexi-Comp Online, and Clinical Pharmacology allow you to search by reaction. Additionally, some niche textbooks are also designed in this way.

Dosing or Administration

The entire medical team and the patient rely on the pharmacist to be the expert on the dosing of medicines. One of the pharmacist's key functions is to review medication orders for appropriate dosing given the patient's age, weight, organ function, other medical conditions, and current treatments. When responding to questions regarding "What is the dose of drug X?," your recommendation must also consider the treatment indication and the route of administration.

Pharmacy students are often also consulted by nurses and prescribers regarding switching patients' medications from one route to another when there is a change in the patient's status (e.g., scheduled for surgery and now unable to take anything by mouth). Due to differences in bioavailability or drug release characteristics, dosing conversions may be necessary when a

Table 3.4 QUESTIONS ON ADVERSE DRUG REACTIONS

	How Much Time Do You Have?			
Question Type	Minutes	Minutes to Hours	Hours to Days	Comments
Has this adverse reaction been previously associated with this drug?	• General print DI compendia • General electronic DI compendia • Product information/package insert	• Therapeutics textbooks and databases • Gilman, Goodman and Gilman's Pharmacologic Basis of Therapeutics • Katzung, Basic and Clinical Pharmacology • MEDLINE	• Aronson, Meyler's Side Effects of Drugs • Davies, Textbook of Adverse Drug Reactions • Tilsdale, Drug-Induced Diseases • Pharmacy-focused primary literature indexing databases	–Information on common and classic adverse drug reactions are often covered in most General DI compendia. –Specialized resources and a search of the primary literature are usually required to find information on specifics such as time course, clinical presentation, proposed mechanism, risk factors, and management strategies of less common adverse drug reactions –General DI compendia provide variable depth of information with regard to adverse drug reactions

(continued)

Table 3.4 QUESTIONS ON ADVERSE DRUG REACTIONS *(continued)*

How Much Time Do You Have?

Question Type	Minutes	Minutes to Hours	Hours to Days	Comments

How do you prevent or manage this adverse drug reaction?	• Electronic resources
	  • Micromedex DrugDex
	  • Clinical Pharmacology
	• Print resources
	  • Drug Facts and Comparisons
	  • AHFS drug information
	  • Product information/package insert
		• Therapeutics textbooks and databases
		• MEDLINE
			• Aronson, Meyler's Side Effects of Drugs
			• Davies, Textbook of Adverse Drug Reactions
			• Tilsdale, Drug-Induced Diseases
			• Pharmacy-focused primary literature indexing databases
				–Package insert information may include specifics on the management of an adverse drug reaction in the cautions, warnings, or Black Box sections rather than the adverse reactions section

Is this reaction associated with any of the medications my patient is taking?	• Micromedex Drugdex • Clinical Pharmacology • Lexi-Comp Online • Facts and Comparisons 4.0	• General print DI compendia • General electronic DI compendia • Therapeutics textbooks and databases • Gilman, Goodman and Gilman's Pharmacologic Basis of Therapeutics • Katzung, Basic and Clinical Pharmacology • MEDLINE • Aronson, Meyler's Side Effects of Drugs • Davies, Textbook of Adverse Drug Reactions • Tilsdale, Drug Induced Diseases • Pharmacy-focused primary literature indexing databases		–Electronic databases that allow you to query by adverse reaction will be the most efficient means to evaluate a patient's medication list for likely offenders

DI, drug information.
• General print DI compendia: AHFS drug information; Lexi-Comp Drug Information Handbook; Drug Facts and Comparisons.
• General electronic DI com: Micromedex Healthcare Series; Clinical Pharmacology; Lexi-Comp Online; Facts and Comparisons 4.0 (eFacts)
• Therapeutics textbooks and database: DiPiro, Pharmacotherapy; Helms, Textbook of Therapeutics; Koda-Kimble, Applied Therapeutics; MDconsult or FIRSTConsult; UpToDate
• Pharmacy -focused primary literature indexing and abstracting databases: EMBASE, IDIS/Web, IPA.
See Appendix 3C for bibliography of cited resources.

Table 3.5 INTRAVENOUS (IV) ADMINISTRATION LANGUAGE

Phrase	Usual Meaning
Direct IV injection or infusion	May be administered as provided. Does not require further dilution
IV bolus or IV push	May be administered as fast as desired
Slow IV push	Should be administered no more quickly than over 3–5 minutes
Intermittent injection or infusion	Administered intermittently according to ordered schedule. During the time between administrations, no drug is given. Nurse should follow instructions for "Administer over X minutes or hours" as labeled
Continuous injection or infusion	Administered continuously over 24 hours

route of administration or dosage formulation is changed. Dose conversions are also common when interchanging patients from one formulary agent to another in the same therapeutic class.

For parenteral medications, nurses often also consult the pharmacy regarding how to prepare and administer a drug and how quickly it can be given. Pharmacy students need to be familiar with common language used by nurses and in drug administration texts (Table 3.5). Questions dealing with the compatibility of coadministering parenteral drugs are included elsewhere in this chapter.

Your general drug information compendia are initial resources for all of these types of questions but usually are most useful for adult patients. For pediatric patients, additional specialized references are frequently checked. Table 3.6 summarizes questions on dosing or administration while listing resources for information.

Drug Interactions

Medications on a patient's profile change frequently, especially during a hospital stay. To complicate this even further, drug interactions include not just drug–drug interactions, but drug–food, drug–lab, and drug–disease interactions. When a patient experiences a new side effect or unexpected change in laboratory value, the medical team frequently cites the patient's drug therapy as the cause for the change. Understanding the time course of drug interactions, along with the mechanism of the interaction, is important in providing helpful information in determining

Table 3.6 QUESTIONS ON DOSING OR ADMINISTRATION

	How Much Time Do You Have?		
Question Type	**Minutes**	**Minutes to Hours**	**Hours to Days**	**Comments**
What is the dose of drug X?	• General print DI compendia • General electronic DI compendia • Product information/package insert	• Therapeutics textbooks and databases • MEDLINE	• Pharmacy-focused primary literature indexing databases • Contact drug manufacturer	–It is important to know what indication the drug is intended for as most DI resources list dosing by specific indication –Certain indications such as oncology regimens will need specialized references or review of the primary literature
Do you need to taper drug X when discontinuing therapy?	• General print DI compendia • General electronic DI compendia • Product information/package insert	• Therapeutics textbooks and databases • MEDLINE	• Pharmacy-focused primary literature indexing databases • Contact drug manufacturer	–Dosing tapers for discontinuing therapy is often recommended to avoid a withdrawal syndrome with specific drugs. The dosing information may be listed in the adverse effects or warnings section under "withdrawal syndrome"

How do I adjust the dose for a patient with organ dysfunction (e.g., renal dysfunction; liver failure)?	• General print DI compendia (AHFS for liver dosing) • General electronic DI compendia • Product information/package insert • Institution-specific protocols or guidelines for dosage adjustment	• Aranoff, Drug Dosing in Renal Failure	• Pharmacy-focused primary literature indexing databases • Contact drug manufacturer	–When clinical data are not available, evaluation of pharmacokinetic parameters may be helpful in guiding dosing changes. Some of these data will be included in the pharmacokinetics section of drug monographs –Some institutions also have renal dosing protocols in place
What is the dose for patients in this special population (e.g., pediatrics, geriatrics, obesity)?	• General print DI compendia • General electronic DI compendia • Product information/package insert • Institution-specific dose standardization or dose rounding protocols or guidelines	• Semla, Geriatric Dosage Handbook • Taketomo, Pediatric Dosage Handbook • Robertson, Harriet Lane Handbook • Young, NeoFax • Phelps, Pediatric Injectable Drugs (teddy bear book) • MEDLINE	• Pharmacy-focused primary literature indexing databases • Contact drug manufacturer	–Many institutions that specialize in care of these populations often have drug dosing guidelines for commonly used medications. This guidance may be searchable via the internet or may be restricted to the site's intranet

(continued)

Table 3.6 QUESTIONS ON DOSING OR ADMINISTRATION *(continued)*

Question Type	How Much Time Do You Have?			Comments
	Minutes	Minutes to Hours	Hours to Days	
How do I adjust the dosage regimen for a patient receiving renal replacement therapy (e.g., hemodialysis, peritoneal dialysis, continuous venovenous hemodiafiltration)	• General print DI compendia • General electronic DI compendia • Product information/package insert	• Aranoff, Drug Dosing in Renal Failure • MEDLINE	• Pharmacy-focused primary literature indexing databases • Contact drug manufacturer	–Removal of drug via renal replacement therapy is related to many factors including the rate of filtration, the size of the molecule, the filter type, and other physiochemical properties of the drug
How do I administer this parenteral drug?	• Gahart, Intravenous Medications Handbook for Nurses • General print DI compendia • General electronic DI compendia • Product information/package insert • Institution-specific policies for IV administration	• Trissel, Handbook on Injectable Drugs • King, King Guide to Parenteral Admixture	• Pharmacy-focused primary literature indexing databases • CINAHL • Contact drug manufacturer	–Many institutions will have policies regarding administration of high-alert medications and required monitoring for certain IV medications. This guidance may be searchable via the internet or may be restricted to the site's intranet

DI, drug information; CINAHL, Cumulative Index to Nursing & Allied Health Literature; IV, intravenous.
• General print DI compendia: AHFS drug information; Lexi-Comp Drug Information Handbook; Drug Facts and Comparisons
• General electronic DI compendia: Micromedex Healthcare Series; Clinical Pharmacology; Lexi-Comp Online; Facts and Comparisons 4.0 (eFacts)
• Therapeutics textbooks and database: DiPiro, Pharmacotherapy; Helms, Textbook of Therapeutics; Koda-Kimble, Applied Therapeutics; MDconsult or FIRSTconsult; UpToDate
• Pharmacy-focused primary literature indexing and abstracting databases: EMBASE, IDIS/Web, IPA.
See Appendix 3C for bibliography of cited resources.

the patient's continued or change in drug therapy. For a comprehensive review of the principles of drug interactions, consider reading the introductory chapter of one of the major drug interactions textbooks (*Drug Interactions Analysis and Management* or *Drug Interaction Facts*). Other books also contain a review of the principles of drug interactions (Goodman & Gilman's The Pharmacological Basis of Therapeutics; Pharmacotherapy; Applied Therapeutics; Lexicomp). These references typically include lists of known CYP450 and P-glycoprotein inducers, inhibitors, and substrates. Similar lists or tables are available online (for CYP 450, www.medicine.iupui.edu/flockhart/table.htm; drugs known to prolong the QT interval, www.torsades.org/medical-pros/drug-lists/drug-lists.htm).

Indication for Therapeutic Use

Pharmacy students may need to research these types of questions either from the drug or disease perspective. When reviewing a patient's medication profile, your preceptor and medical team will expect you to be able to state the associated treatment indication for each drug the patient is currently receiving or has received recently. You may also be asked to recommend a therapy or review the available pharmacologic treatment options given a stated disease, treatment indication, or need for prophylaxis.

Although drugs are approved by the FDA based on evidence submitted with their New Drug Application (NDA), prescribers are not limited to prescribing marketed drugs in these doses, by these routes, or only for the tested indications. Although the FDA does not regulate the prescribing of drugs, the pharmacist still has the duty to assess the safety and likely effectiveness of the unlabeled use before recommending or dispensing it. Manufacturers may be pursuing obtaining a labeled use for a drug by conducting clinical trials to gather evidence to submit to the FDA. New drugs, new uses for old drugs, and new formulations of old drugs being studied in these ways are considered investigational new drugs (INDs). Until the manufacturer submits a NDA these data are proprietary and largely unavailable. Patients may be eligible to have access to these INDs before they receive market approval by enrolling in a clinical trial or through a Treatment IND (formerly called compassionate use). Treatment INDs are reserved for individual patients with no other treatment options. Navigating the pathways to these drugs in the pipeline will require the assistance of preceptors and their understanding of applicable rules and site policies and procedures. Table 3.7 lists drug interaction questions frequently received by pharmacists and pharmacy students.

Table 3.7 QUESTIONS ON DRUG INTERACTIONS

Question Type	How Much Time Do You Have?			
	Minutes	Minutes to Hours	Hours to Days	Comments
Do these drugs interact?	• Lexi-Comp online (Lexi-Interacts) • Facts and Comparisons 4.0 (Interactions checker) • Clinical Pharmacology • Hansten, Drug Interactions Analysis and Management • Tatro, Drug Interaction Facts • Lexi-Comp Drug Interactions Handbook	• Micromedex (Interactions tab to build a list of drugs to evaluate for interactions) • General electronic DI compendia • General print DI compendia	• MEDLINE • Pharmacy-focused primary literature indexing databases	–The general electronic DI compendia have drug interaction checking databases; create a list of products for the database to analyze and evaluate the potential or documented interactions –The general DI compendia have drug interaction listings in the individual drug monograph
Does this herb–herb or herb–drug combination interact?	• Facts & Comparisons 4.0 (Herbal Interaction Facts) • Jellin, Natural Medicines Comprehensive Review (Natural product/drug interaction checker)	• Micromedex (AltMedDex) • General DI compendia may be helpful for more common herbal products	• MEDLINE • Pharmacy-focused primary literature indexing databases • CINAHL	

44

Does this drug interact with foods my patient may be taking?	• Start in general drug–drug interaction references for specific foods • Tatro, Drug Interaction Facts: Herbal Supplements and Food • Drug–food interactions: GlobalRPh.com, www.globalrph.com/drugfoodrxn.htm • Beers, Merck Manual of Diagnosis and Therapy (Nutrient–drug interactions)	• MEDLINE • Pharmacy-focused primary literature indexing databases • CINAHL
Does this drug interact with or affect laboratory values?	• Young, Effects of Drugs on Clinical Laboratory Tests	• MEDLINE • Pharmacy-focused primary literature indexing databases • CINAHL
Is this drug impacted by my patient's disease state? Or, can this drug alter my patient's disease state?	• General electronic DI compendia • General print DI compendia • Tilsdale, Drug-Induced Diseases	• MEDLINE • Pharmacy-focused primary literature indexing databases • CINAHL

DI, drug information; CINAHL, Cumulative Index to Nursing & Allied Health Literature.
• General print DI compendia: AHFS drug information; Lexi-Comp Drug Information Handbook; Drug Facts and Comparisons
• General electronic DI compendia: Micromedex Healthcare Series; Clinical Pharmacology; Lexi-Comp Online; Facts and Comparisons 4.0 (eFacts)
• Pharmacy-focused primary literature indexing and abstracting databases: EMBASE, IDIS/Web, IPA.

See Appendix 3C for bibliography of cited resources.

Orphan drugs are FDA-approved drugs that came to market to serve patients with rare diseases. In exchange for pursuing licensing of these drugs that aren't likely to make the company a lot of money, manufacturers are rewarded with tax breaks and extended market exclusivity. Because these are unique drugs, they may be available only through specialty distributors and not through normal wholesale channels. Table 3.8 describes common questions on indications for therapeutic use with resources for information given an amount of time to research the response.

Product Information or Identification

Simply identifying a product (what it is and what it's used for) is possible with most of the readily available pharmacy references. Go to your favorite general drug information compendia and look up the information. With a few more steps or clicks, these same resources provide additional depth of product information to prepare you for the inevitable next questions (What's the dose? What else do I need to know before prescribing or dispensing this drug?). Accurate spelling of the drug in question is always a challenge when hearing the product name for the first time, especially from a patient or consumer. Ask the requestor to write it down, if possible, or to sound it out as he or she has interpreted the product name. Knowing its intended use or manufacturer can often help you to narrow the field of similar-sounding products.

If the product is a tablet or capsule to identify, collect the imprint code, shape, size, and color of the product. For foreign drug identification, request information on the country of origin, the indication or anticipated use of the product, and the dose of the product, if the patient has been using the drug while abroad. Be prepared that foreign drug identifications often become adverse reaction, dosing, or therapeutic use questions once the drug is identified. Table 3.9 summarizes questions on product information or identification while listing resources for information.

Safety in Pregnancy and Lactation

Drug information questions regarding safety of medication use in pregnancy and lactation typically fall into two categories: questions about the potential risk *before* exposure of the mother and fetus/infant to the drug, and questions about the potential risk to the fetus/infant *after* exposure to the drug. When assessing the potential risk to the fetus, it is important to determine the mother's stage or weeks of pregnancy since timing of the drug exposure is important when linking a defect with an exposure. The stages of fetal development and associated organogenesis are available at www.cerebralpalsychildren.com (click on Critical Periods of

Table 3.8 QUESTIONS ON INDICATION FOR THERAPEUTIC USE

Question Type	How Much Time Do You Have?			Comments
	Minutes	Minutes to Hours	Hours to Days	
Why was this drug prescribed? What can be used for prophylaxis or treatment of X?	• General print DI compendia • General electronic DI compendia • Product information/package insert	• Therapeutics textbooks and databases • Gilman, Goodman and Gilman's Pharmacologic Basis of Therapeutics • Katzung, Basic and Clinical Pharmacology	• MEDLINE • Pharmacy-focused primary literature indexing databases • All EBM Reviews • CINAHL • www.guidelines.gov	–General DI compendia often designate whether FDA approved or unlabeled use
Is the use of drug X for this purpose: • FDA approved? • Unlabeled use? • Investigational use? • Compassionate use? • Orphan drug designation?	• General electronic DI compendia • Facts & Comparisons 4.0 (unlabeled uses, orphan drugs)	• MEDLINE • Pharmacy-focused primary literature indexing • Government-funded clinical trials enrolling, in progress, or recently completed: www.clinicaltrials.gov • Orphan drug by drug: www.fda.gov/orphan/designat/list.htm • Orphan drug by disease: www.rarediseases.org/search/rdblist.html • Contact drug manufacturer		–Manufacturer's medical services divisions are often helpful in providing unlabeled use information and may have a standard letter on the topic if it is common. In contrast, medical product representatives are not allowed to discuss unlabeled uses –Manufacturers may be unable to provide detailed information on investigational drugs they are studying due to proprietary restrictions

DI, drug information; CINAHL, Cumulative Index to Nursing & Allied Health Literature.
• General print DI compendia: AHFS drug information; Lexi-Comp Drug Information Handbook; Drug Facts and Comparisons
• General electronic DI compendia: Micromedex Healthcare Series; Clinical Pharmacology; Lexi-Comp Online; Facts and Comparisons 4.0 (eFacts)
• Therapeutics textbooks and databases: DiPiro, Pharmacotherapy; Helms, Pharmacotherapeutics; Koda-Kimble, Applied Therapeutics; MDconsult or FIRSTconsult; UpToDate
• Pharmacy-focused primary literature indexing and abstracting databases: EMBASE, IDIS/Web, IPA.
See Appendix 3C for bibliography of cited resources.

Table 3.9 QUESTIONS ON PRODUCT INFORMATION OR IDENTIFICATION

How Much Time Do You Have?

Question Type	Minutes	Minutes to Hours	Hours to Days	Comments
What is this drug (assume commercially available in the United States)?	• General print DI compendia • General electronic DI compendia	• Product information/package insert • General internet search (Google or Dogpile) • Billups, American Drug Index • Fleeger, USP Dictionary of USAN and International Drug Names	• MEDLINE • Pharmacy-focused primary literature indexing databases	–Basic product information is covered in most general DI compendia. These provide variable depth of information with regard to the logical next questions –Searching the primary literature is the least efficient but may provide information on a little-used product
What is this drug (unknown origin or known foreign product)?	• Micromedex (integrated index to search Index Nominum, Martindale—the complete drug reference) • Facts & Comparisons 4.0 (Canadian drug index)	• Textbooks: foreign drug formularies or compendia; Fleeger, USP Dictionary of USAN and International Drug Names • Web sites: Farmamondo, international drug wholesaler: www.farmamondo.com • Pharmaceutical Journal, index of foreign third-party websites with lists of products available by country: www.pharmj.com/noticeboard/info/pip/foreign medicines.html • General internet search (Google, Dogpile)		–Both Index Nominum and Martindale have a synonym section, linking products with common generic names

| What is this drug (imprint code or product physical description)? | • Micromedex (drug identification)
• Facts & Comparisons 4.0 (drug identifier)
• Jellin, Ident-a-Drug
• Clinical Pharmacology | • Drugs.com Pill Identification Wizard: www.drugs.com/imprints.php | –Check with your preceptor prior to identifying tablets for consumers or the general public regarding site policies on doing this; other factors may need to be considered |

DI, drug information.
• General print DI compendia: AHFS drug information; Lexi-Comp Drug Information Handbook; Drug Facts and Comparisons
• General electronic DI compendia: Micromedex Healthcare Series; Clinical Pharmacology; Lexi-Comp Online; Facts and Comparisons 4.0 (eFacts)
• Pharmacy-focused primary literature indexing and abstracting databases: EMBASE, IDIS/Web, IPA.

See Appendix 3C for bibliography of cited resources

Fetal Development link). Also understanding the mother's indication for a medication or therapy along with the anticipated duration of therapy will be helpful in assessing the situation.

Useful information for questions about breast-feeding or lactation include the current age of the infant, the frequency of breast-feeding, the drugs or products the mother is taking (or considering taking), the indication for therapy, and the anticipated duration of therapy. Table 3.10 lists drug safety in pregnancy and lactation questions received by pharmacists and pharmacy students.

IV Compatibility/Stability

Pharmacists often have need to research information on the preparation and stability of intravenous (IV) admixtures that they provide for patients or that are administered at the bedside by other caregivers. To establish the institution's standard concentrations and policies on IV admixture production, pharmacies rely heavily on specialized textbooks and published literature. They also must consider applicable rules and standards of practice. Stability, sterility, preparation conditions, and anticipated storage must be considered when determining what fluid, drug concentration, and beyond-use dating will be assigned to a sterile compounded product. Chapter 797 in the United States Pharmacopeia (USP <797>) provides guidance for establishing acceptable beyond-use dating.[5]

Pharmacies often also receive questions from nurses administering these prepared doses. Nurses' questions often have to do with the practicality of administering the IV medication given how many IV administration ports the nurse has access to and the patient's other IV medications or maintenance fluids that are already running through those available ports. Pharmacy students need to be familiar with terms used in interpreting compatibility data in published references: additive syringe compatibility (drawn up in the same syringe), Y-site compatibility ("piggybacking" into the same administration line as a maintenance fluid or other IV medication that is already running), and in-solution compatibility (admixed in the same bag). Other common IV questions from nurses, especially in the intensive care setting, concern the ability to concentrate drips to deliver more medication in less volume or to change to another fluid based on the patient's clinical condition. Table 3.11 describes common questions on IV compatibility and stability with resources for information.

Natural Products and Dietary Supplements

Finding information on these products requires the use of specialized references. Students need to be aware that double-blind, placebo-controlled

Table 3.10 QUESTIONS ON SAFETY IN PREGNANCY AND LACTATION

Question Type	How Much Time Do You Have?			Comments
	Minutes	**Minutes to Hours**	**Hours to Days**	
What is the risk (or potential risk) to the fetus when exposed to this drug?	• Briggs GG, Drugs in Pregnancy and Lactation	• Micromedex (Drugdex and Reproductive Risk Databases: TERIS, Shepards, Reprotox and Reprotext) • Contact drug manufacturer	• MEDLINE • Pharmacy-focused primary literature indexing databases • CINAHL	–Briggs is the gold standard text reference; includes useful appendices with drugs grouped by use category and associated pregnancy risk categories –It is important to review the material in each of the Micromedex Reproductive Risk databases—each has a different style for presenting the information and with limited published information, reviewing all available material to generate an appropriate assessment of the patient's potential risk is important
What is the risk (or potential risk) to the fetus when exposed to this vaccine or biologic drug?	• Grabenstein, ImmunoFacts	• MEDLINE • Pharmacy-focused primary literature indexing databases • CINAHL • Contact product manufacturer		
For risk questions involving natural products, herbal or dietary supplements,	• Jellin, Natural Medicines Comprehensive Database	• Facts & Comparisons 4.0 (review of natural products) • Micromedex (AltMedDex) • MEDLINE • Pharmacy-focused primary literature indexing databases • CINAHL		

(continued)

Table 3.10 QUESTIONS ON SAFETY IN PREGNANCY AND LACTATION *(continued)*

Question Type	How Much Time Do You Have?			Comments
	Minutes	Minutes to Hours	Hours to Days	
What is the risk (or potential risk) to the breastfeeding infant when exposed to this drug (taken by mother)?	• Hale, Medications and Mothers Milk	• Micromedex (Drugdex and Reproductive Risk Databases: TERIS, Shepards, Reprotox and Reprotext) • American Academy of Pediatrics policy statement on transfer of drugs and other chemicals into human milk (aappolicy.aappublications.org), then search by title of article. • Lactation: Thomas Hale's Breastfeeding Pharmacology page, neonatal/ttuhsc.edu/lact • MEDLINE • Pharmacy-focused primary literature indexing databases • CINAHL • Contact drug manufacturer		–The Hale book is the best print reference available; the information in the front of the text is a helpful review of the pharmacokinetics of lactation
For lactation questions involving a vaccine or biologic drug	• Grabenstein, ImmunoFacts	• MEDLINE • Pharmacy-focused primary literature indexing databases • CINAHL • Contact product manufacturer		
For lactation questions involving natural products, herbal or dietary supplements	• Jellin, Natural Medicines Comprehensive Database	• Facts & Comparisons 4.0 (review of natural products) • MEDLINE • Pharmacy-focused primary literature indexing databases • CINAHL		

DI, drug information; CINAHL, Cumulative Index to Nursing & Allied Health Literature.
• General print DI compendia: AHFS drug information; Lexi-Comp Drug Information Handbook; Drug Facts and Comparisons
• General electronic DI compendia: Micromedex Healthcare Series; Clinical Pharmacology; Lexi-Comp Online; Facts and Comparisons 4.0 (eFacts)
• Pharmacy-focused primary literature indexing and abstracting databases: EMBASE, IDIS/Web, IPA.
See Appendix 3C for bibliography of cited resources.

Table 3.11 QUESTIONS ON INTRAVENOUS (IV) COMPATIBILITY/STABILITY

How Much Time Do You Have?

Question Type	Minutes	Minutes to Hours	Hours to Days	Comments
What concentration can an IV drug be admixed in?	• General electronic DI compendia • AHFS drug information • Product information/package insert • Institution-specific guidance on standard concentrations of IV admixtures	• Trissel, Handbook on Injectable Drugs • King, King Guide to Parenteral Admixture • Contact drug manufacturer • MEDLINE	• MEDLINE • Pharmacy-focused primary literature indexing databases • CINAHL	
What IV fluid can the drug be prepared in?	• General electronic DI compendia • AHFS drug information • Product information/package insert • Institution-specific guidance on standard concentrations of IV admixtures	• Trissel, Handbook on Injectable Drugs • King, King Guide to Parenteral Admixture • Contact drug manufacturer • MEDLINE	• MEDLINE • Pharmacy-focused primary literature indexing databases • CINAHL	–This information is sometimes located in the narrative section rather than the tables of the print resources

(continued)

Table 3.11 QUESTIONS ON INTRAVENOUS (IV) COMPATIBILITY/STABILITY *(continued)*

How Much Time Do You Have?

Question Type	Minutes	Minutes to Hours	Hours to Days	Comments
Can the following drugs be administered simultaneously in the same IV line? (Are these drugs y-site compatible?)	• Product information/package insert • Electronic IV compatibility checking • Micromedex (IV Index) • Lexi-Comp Online (King Guide)	• Trissel, Handbook on Injectable Drugs • King, King Guide to Parenteral Admixture • Gahart, Intravenous Medications A Handbook for Nurses • Contact drug manufacturer • MEDLINE	• Pharmacy-focused primary literature indexing databases • CINAHL	–Verify what each symbol/abbreviation/code means in the reference source you are using –It is also important to note the concentrations of drugs that are being used and how these compare to published compatibility data –Some references include compatibility as a sub-type of drug–drug interaction
What expiration date should be used on the prepared IV medication?	• General electronic DI compendia • AHFS drug information • Product information/package insert • Institution-specific policies for beyond-use dating of products	• Trissel, Handbook on Injectable Drugs • King, King Guide to Parenteral Admixture • Contact drug manufacturer • MEDLINE	• Pharmacy-focused primary literature indexing databases • CINAHL • USP Chapter 797	–Most studies evaluate stability of drug. Sterility is also a concern and largely dependent on the sterile technique of the person preparing the admixture and the conditions under which it was prepared –USP <797> specifies maximal beyond-use dating based on risk level of sterile preparation

DI, drug information; CINAHL, Cumulative Index to Nursing & Allied Health Literature.
• General print DI compendia: AHFS drug information; Lexi-Comp Drug Information Handbook; Drug Facts and Comparisons
• General electronic DI compendia: Micromedex Healthcare Series; Clinical Pharmacology; Lexi-Comp Online; Facts and Comparisons 4.0 (eFacts)
• Pharmacy-focused primary literature indexing and abstracting databases: EMBASE, IDIS/Web, IPA.

See Appendix 3C for bibliography of cited resources.

trials are not widely available to evaluate the safety and effectiveness of these agents. Even when clinical trials are found, dosing standardization remains an issue. A number of groups such as the National Center for Complementary and Alternative Medicine are continuing to add to the body of available literature for these products, which should improve our ability to apply evidence-based medicine principles to clinical decision making concerning these therapies.

Since these products are regulated under the Dietary Supplement Health and Education Act of 1994 (DSHEA), they are not required to meet the same burden of proof of efficacy as are drugs regulated by the FDA. Unsafe products are not allowed for human use, but premarketing safety testing is not required. The FDA must prove that a product is unsafe before its removal from the market can be mandated.[6] Even if adequate information on the clinical utility and potential harm of a product has satisfied the practitioner caring for the patient, the next issue that must be addressed is whether a reliable, quality product is available for patient use. Manufacturing standards for identity, strength, quality, purity, packaging, and labeling that are expected with drug therapies are not standardized or regulated by a single authority for products covered by the DSHEA. Voluntary good manufacturing practices (GMPs) are used by some manufacturers, but there is not a single GMP standard that is recognized industrywide. Products bearing a trade association (e.g., National Nutritional Foods Association), independent testing group (e.g., National Safety Foundation International, ConsumerLab), or quasi-public institution (e.g., U.S. Pharmacopeia, USP) Seal of Approval certify that the product has met that group's published standards. Certificates of Analysis may also be requested from reputable manufacturers detailing the assayed contents of their product.

The common question types asked of the pharmacy student concerning the use of these nondrug products are as follows:

- What is this product, what is it used for, and how is it used?
- Is there medical evidence to support the product's efficacy?
- Is the product safe for continued use in my patients given their medication regimens and disease states?
- What is the quality of the product?

Questions concerning interactions or safety in pregnancy and lactation of these products can be found under those question types published elsewhere in this chapter (see Table 3.10).

Your frontline specialty references are available in several formats and should be helpful in quickly answering the first three questions. All cover a

Table 3.12 QUESTIONS ON NATURAL PRODUCTS AND DIETARY SUPPLEMENTS

How Much Time Do You Have?

Question Type	Minutes	Minutes to Hours	Hours to Days	Comments
What is its use, pharmacologic action, dosing, safety, or efficacy?	• Jellin, Natural Medicines Comprehensive Database • Facts & Comparisons 4.0 (review of natural products) • Lexi-Comp Online (natural therapeutics pocket guide) • Micromedex (Allmedex)	• Blumental, Herbal Medicine Expanded Commission E Monographs • Brendler, PDR for Herbal Medicine	• MEDLINE • Pharmacy-focused primary literature indexing databases • All EBM reviews • CINAHL	–The Natural Medicines Comprehensive Database uses a safety and efficacy rating system and contains detailed summaries of available studies. Look up by natural product name, disease or condition –Lexicomp Natural Products has useful charts and lists, patient information leaflets on the top products, monographs, and disease decisions trees with incorporated product recommendations –The Review of Natural Products has particularly useful sections on botany, uses and pharmacology, chemistry, and toxicology
What is the quality of the product?	• Jellin, Natural Medicines Comprehensive Database • Look for Seal of Approval from reputable certifying body	• Natural Medicines Comprehensive Database • Look for Seal of Approval from reputable certifying body	• Request Certificate of Analysis from manufacturer	–Seals of Approval and Certificates of Analysis can be used to identify high-quality dietary supplements, but these do not ensure safety and effectiveness –The Natural Medicines Comprehensive Database has quick links to USP-verified products and will mention specific brands used in clinical trials in the Dosage/Administration section

DI, drug information; INAHL, Cumulative Index to Nursing & Allied Health Literature.
• Pharmacy-focused primary literature indexing and abstracting databases: EMBASE, IDIS/Web, IPA.
See Appendix 3C for bibliography of cited resources.

broad range of natural products, including herbs, nutritional supplements (vitamins, minerals, amino acids, essential fatty acids, antioxidants, and nutraceuticals), and glandular extracts. Information on Ayurvedic, Chinese, or homeopathic medicines are more difficult to find and may require you to first identify the active ingredients in the product and then proceed with looking up information on each component. Table 3.12 summarizes questions on natural products and dietary supplements with resources for information.

Compounded Formulations: Recipes and Stability

Certain patient populations such as children or those with enteral feeding tubes may require extemporaneously prepared pharmaceutical products. These scenarios often form the background for drug information questions regarding compounding recipes and stability/beyond-use dating (expiration dating) of these products. Lexi-Comp Online as well as the *Drug Information Handbook*, *Pediatric Dosage Handbook*, and Micromedex contain referenced information on common extemporaneous recipes and beyond-use dating. Specialized textbooks may also be available in the pharmacy. A search of specialized indexing systems such as IDIS (Iowa Drug Information Service) or IPA (International Pharmaceutical Abstracts) may also be necessary for more difficult-to-find recipes and stability data. Chapter 795 in the United States Pharmacopeia (USP <795>)[7] provides additional guidance for establishing beyond-use dating when published data are not available. Table 3.13 lists questions on recipes and stability of nonsterile compounded formulations with resources for obtaining information.

■ Citation Style and Resources

Referencing your written drug information response adds to its credibility and allows the requestor to identify and review the same source material you used to make your assessment or recommendation. In medical writing, the recognized standard format for reference citation is the National Library of Medicine's Style Guide:[8]

http://www.ncbi.nlm.nih.gov/books/bv.fcgi?rid=citmed.TOC&depth=2

These uniform requirements contain detailed explanations and examples of citing all of the various types of materials found in a physical or virtual medical library. A few referencing sources are often encountered in responding to drug information questions that are not covered in the

Table 3.13 QUESTIONS ON RECIPES AND STABILITY OF NONSTERILE COMPOUNDED FORMULATIONS

How Much Time Do You Have?

Question Type	Minutes	Minutes to Hours	Hours to Days	Comments
Is there a recipe and stability information for compounding this drug formulation?	• Lexi-Comp Online • Drug Information Handbook • Pediatric Dosage Handbook • Micromedex (Usually found under Dosage Forms section)	• Allen, Allen's Compounded Formulations • Jew, Children's Hospital of Philadelphia: Extemporaneous Formulations • Trissel, Trissel's Stability of Compounded Formulations • US Pharmacist Web site • Pharmacy Times Web site • Secundum Artem Web site • International Journal of Pharmaceutical Compounding (search by formulation—requires paid subscription)	• Pharmacy-focused primary literature indexing databases MEDLINE • Local compounding pharmacy • USP Chapter 795	–General DI compendia/resources do not contain compounding recipes –USP Chapter <795> provides guidance on beyond-use dating for situations where stability data cannot be obtained

DI, drug information.
• General print DI compendia: AHFS drug information; Lexi-Comp Drug Information Handbook; Drug Facts and Comparisons
• General electronic DI compendia: Micromedex Healthcare Series; Clinical Pharmacology; Lexi-Comp Online; Facts and Comparisons 4.0 (eFacts)
• Pharmacy-focused primary literature indexing and abstracting databases: EMBASE, IDIS/Web, IPA.

See Appendix 3C for bibliography of cited resources.

Table 3.14 REFERENCING SPECIAL SOURCES OF
DRUG INFORMATION

Type	Example
Package insert (Note: date is the date of publication of package insert and not the date cited)	Lexapro (escitalopram oxalate) tablets [product information]. St. Louis, MO: Forest Pharmaceuticals, May 2007
Personal communication	Personal communication with Jane Doe (Medical Services, Eisai, Inc., Woodcliff Lake, NJ), 2008 Feb 15

NLM's guidance: package inserts and personal communications with experts such as drug manufacturers or specialty practitioners (Table 3.14).

In providing drug information based on the question-type tables we have provided, the citation formats you will use repeatedly are more limited than the NLM's extensive list. We have cited our recommended resources in the NLM format in the Bibliography in Appendix 3C. If you need further guidance, the NLM's online style guide is very easy to navigate and allows you to quickly see the citation rules and examples for the type of material you are citing. Close attention must be paid to the use of capitalization, punctuation, spacing, and title source abbreviations to meet the NLM standards. According to NLM standards, all authors should be listed if there are six or fewer; otherwise the first three are listed followed by "et al."

References

1. Kirkwood CF, Kier KL. Modified systematic approach to answering questions. In: Malone PM, Kier KL, Stanovich JE, eds. *Drug Information: A Guide for Pharmacists.* 3rd ed. New York, NY: McGraw-Hill; 2006:29–37.
2. Slawson DC, Shaughnessy AF, Bennett JH. Becoming a medical information master: feeling good about not knowing everything. *J Fam Pract.* 1994;38:505–513.
3. Galt KA. Gathering drug information and evidence. In: *Developing Clinical Practice Skills for Pharmacists.* Bethesda, MD: American Society of Health-System Pharmacists; 2006:.114–162.
4. Shields KM, Lust E. Drug information resources. In: Malone PM, Kier KL, Stanovich JE, eds. *Drug Information: A Guide for Pharmacists.* 3rd ed. New York, NY: McGraw-Hill; 2006:61–101.
5. United States Pharmacopeial Convention. Revised general chapter <797> pharmaceutical compounding—sterile preparation [chapter on internet]. 2008 Jan (cited 2008 Mar). Available from www.usp.org/pdf/EN/USPNF/generalChapter797.pdf.

6. American Society of Health-System Pharmacists. ASHP statement on the use of dietary supplements. *Am J Health-Syst Pharm.* 2004; 61:1707–1711.

7. Allen LV. USP chapter <795> pharmaceutical compounding—non-sterile preparations. Secundum Artem [serial on the internet]. Date Unknown (cited 2008 Feb);13(4): [about 6 p.]. Available from www.paddocklabs.com/secundum_artem.html.

8. Patrias K. Citing medicine: the NLM style guide for authors, editors, and publishers [Internet]. 2nd ed. Wendling DL., technical ed. Bethesda, MD: National Library of Medicine (US); 2007 (cited 2008 Feb 29). Available from www.nlm.nih.gov/citingmedicine.

Appendix 3A

Providing Drug Information Questionnaire

- Discuss with your preceptor his or her expectation of your role in providing drug information.
  - Will both verbal and written drug information be provided?
  - May any type of drug information be provided to the requestor without prior approval of the preceptor?
  - What documentation format is to be followed for written drug information responses?
  - Is there an expectation of the number or types of questions that should be responded to during the learning experience?
- Discuss with your preceptor any resources that are available to students.
  - Is a medical library available on site or remotely? How is it accessed?
  - Build yourself a Drug Information Resource Finder (Table 3A.1) following the format below and note any constraints on use (e.g., on-site access only, log-in and password required, limited user access).

Appendix 3A.1

Examples of Drug Information Resource Finder

Resource	Format	Through Site (√)	Through School (√)	Access Constraints
General drug information compendia				
Example: Lexi-Comp Drug Information Handbook	Online and print	√	√	–Site: via UpToDate, on-site access only –School: access via Library page, student log-in/ password (PW) –Own: print 2006–2007 edition

(continued)

Examples of Drug Information Resource Finder *(continued)*

Resource	Format	Through Site (√)	Through School (√)	Access Constraints
Specialty references				
Example: Briggs Drugs in Pregnancy and Lactation	Print	√		–Site: copies in Drug Information and pharmacy satellites
Primary literature indexing services				
Example: All EBM reviews	Via Ovid		√	Ovid: on-site and off-site access with log-in and password
CINAHL	Via Ovid	√	√	
EMBASE	Via Ovid		√	
IDIS	Via Web	√		Site: Single-user license at Drug Info only
IPA	Via Ovid		√	Ovid: on-site and off-site access with log-in and password
MEDLINE	Via Ovid or PubMed	√	√	Ovid: on-site and off-site access with log-in and password; PubMed: on-site and off-site access via NLM website

- Use the bibliography of resources in Appendix 3C to check for on-site General DI Compendia and Specialty Reference titles that may be useful.
- Review the list again to see if you may have access remotely through your school if the resource is not available on site.
- Use the crosswalk in Appendix 3B for any unavailable resources to see if you may have access via an alternative pathway.

- Discuss with your preceptor any resources that he or she consults frequently and why the preceptor finds them useful.

Appendix 3B

Crosswalk to Locating Alternative Sources of Drug Information)

If you are looking for information from...	...the same content may also be available from these sources
A to Z Facts	Facts and Comparisons 4.0 www.drugs.com
AHFS Drug Information	STAT!Ref (e-book collection) Lexi-Comp Online AHFSFirst
Basic and Clinical Pharmacology (Katzung)	AccessPharmacy (McGraw-Hill) STAT!Ref (e-book collection) Books@OVID
Cecil Medicine (Textbook of Medicine)	MD Consult (Elsevier)
Clinical Pharmacology (Gold Standard/Elsevier)	MD Consult (Elsevier) AccessPharmacy (McGraw-Hill)
Drug Facts and Comparisons	Facts and Comparisons 4.0
Drug Information Handbook	Lexi-Comp Online UpToDate
Drug Interaction Facts	Facts and Comparisons 4.0
Drugs in Pregnancy and Lactation (Briggs)	Books@OVID
Geriatric Dosage Handbook	Lexi-Comp Online UpToDate
Goodman & Gilman's The Pharmacologic Basis of Therapeutics	AccessPharmacy (McGraw-Hill) STAT!Ref (e-book collection)
Handbook of Injectable Drugs (Trissel)	STAT!Ref (e-book collection) Some data available via Micromedex IV Index (Trissel's 2 Clinical Pharmaceutics Database)
Harrison's Principles of Internal Medicine	AccessPharmacy (McGraw-Hill) STAT!Ref (e-book collection)
Index Nominum: International Drug Directory	Micromedex
King Guide to Parenteral Admixture	Lexi-Comp Online

(continued)

Crosswalk to Locating Alternative Sources of Drug Information) *(continued)*

If you are looking for information from...	...the same content may also be available from these sources
Martindale: The Complete Drug Reference	Micromedex
Mosby's Drug Consult	STAT!Ref (e-book collection)
Pediatric Dosage Handbook	Lexi-Comp Online UpToDate
Pharmacotherapy: A Pathophysiologic Approach (Dipiro)	AccessPharmacy (McGraw-Hill)
Physicians' Desk Reference (PDR)	Micromedex
Review of Natural Products	Facts and Comparisons 4.0
Stedman's Medical Dictionary	STAT!Ref (e-book collection) www.drugs.com
The Harriet Lane Handbook	MD Consult (Elsevier)
The Merck Manual of Diagnosis and Therapy	STAT!Ref (e-book collection)
The Washington Manual of Therapeutics	Books@OVID
USP DI Volume 2—Advice for the Patient (Detailed Drug Information for the Consumer)	Micromedex STAT!Ref (e-book collection) www.drugs.com

Appendix 3C

Bibliography of Resources in Drug Information Question Tables

General print drug information compendia:

- American Society of Health-System Pharmacists. *AHFS Drug Information 2008* (AHFS Drug Information). Bethesda, MD: American Society of Health-System Pharmacists; 2008.
- Drug facts and comparisons [looseleaf]. 2008 ed. St. Louis, MO: Wolters Kluwer Health; updated monthly.
- Lacey CF, Armstrong LL, Goldman MP, et al. *Drug Information Handbook*. 15th ed. Hudson (OH): Lexi-Comp, Inc; 2007.

General electronic drug information compendia:

- Clinical Pharmacology [database online]. Tampa, FL: Gold Standard, Inc.; 2008. Available from www.clinicalpharmacology.com. Updated periodically.
  - Includes: Adverse Reactions Report, Drug Class Overviews, Drug Interactions Report, IV Compatibility Report, MedCounselor Patient Education, Monographs, Product identification.
  - May include: Global Drug Name Directory, FirstCONSULT, Krames Consumer Disease Information, MDConsult, Mosby's Nursing Consult, PIER, and ToxED.
- Lexi-Comp ONLINE [database online]. Hudson, OH: Lexi-Comp, Inc.; 2008. Available from online.lexi.com./crlonline. Updated periodically.
  - Includes: Lexi-Drugs, Lexi-Drugs International, Pediatric Lexi-Drugs, Geriatric Lexi-Drugs, Lexi-Natural Products, Lexi-Infectious Diseases, Lexi-Poisoning & Toxicology, Lab Tests & Diagnostic Procedures, Lexi-Interact, Lexi-Drug ID, Lexi-I.V. Compatibility.
- Facts & Comparisons 4.0 [database online]. St. Louis, MO: Wolters Kluwer Health, Inc; 2008. Available from online.factsandcomparisons.com./login.aspx?url=/index.aspx&qs=. Updated periodically.
  - Includes: Drug Identifier, Drug Interaction Facts, Herbal Interaction Facts, Investigational Drugs from DFC, Nonprescription Drug Therapy, Off-label Drug Facts, and Review of Natural Products.
  - May include: Cancer Chemotherapy Manual.
- Micromedex® Healthcare Series [database online]. Greenwood Village, CO: Thomson Healthcare. Updated periodically.
  - Includes: DRUGDEX System and POISINDEX System.
  - May include: AltMedDex System, DRUG-REAX System, PDR, REPRORISK System, and Martindale: the complete drug reference.

Therapeutics textbooks and databases:

- Dipiro JT, Talbert RL, Yee GC, et al., eds. *Pharmacotherapy: A Pathophysiologic Approach.* 6th ed. New York, NY: McGraw-Hill; 2005.
- Helms RA, Herfindal ET, Gourley DR, et al., eds. *Textbook of Therapeutics: Drug and Disease Management.* 8th ed. Philadelphia. PA: Lippincott Williams & Wilkins; 2006.
- Koda-Kimble M, Kradjan WA, Young LY, et al., eds. *Applied Therapeutics: The Clinical Use of Drugs.* 8th ed. Philadelph, PA: Lippincott Williams & Wilkins; 2005.
- MDconsult [database online]. St. Louis, MO: MD Consult LLC. 1997–2008 (cited 2008 Feb 29). Available from www.mdconsult.com.

- UpToDate online [database online]. Wellesley, MA: UpToDate. 2001–2008 (cited 2008 Feb 29). Available from www.uptodate.com.

  Other drug information references:

- Allen LV. *Allen's Compounded Formulations: The Complete US Pharmacist Collection*. Washington, DC: American Pharmaceutical Association; 2003.
- Allen LV. USP chapter <795> pharmaceutical compounding—non-sterile preparations. Secundum Artem [serial on the internet]. Date unknown (cited 2008 Feb);13(4):(about 6 p.]). Available from www.paddocklabs.com/secundum_artem.html.
- Aranoff GR, Bennett WM. Drug *Prescribing in Renal Failure: Dosing Guidelines for Adults and Children*. 5th ed. Philadelphia, PA: American College of Physicians; 2007.
- Aronson JK, ed. *Meyler's Side Effects of Drugs—The International Encyclopedia of Adverse Drug Reactions and Interactions*. 15th ed. Amsterdam, the Netherlands: Elsevier; 2006.
- Bachmann KA, Lewis JD, Fuller MA, et al., eds. *Lexi-Comp's Drug Interactions Handbook*. 2nd ed. Hudson, OH: Lexi-Comp, Inc; 2003.
- Beers MH, ed. *The Merck Manual of Diagnosis and Therapy* [electronic book]. 18th ed. Whitehouse Station, NJ: Merck Research Laboratories; 2006 (cited 2008 Feb 29). Available from www.merck.com.
- Billups NF, Billups SM. *American Drug Index*. 50th ed. St. Louis, MO: Wolters Kluwer Health; 2006.
- Blumental M, ed. Herbal medicine: expanded Commission E monographs. 1st ed. Newton, MA: Integrative Medicine Communications; 2000.
- Brendler T, Jaenicke C, eds. *PDR for Herbal Medicines*. 6th ed. Montvale, NJ: Thomson PDR; 2007.
- Briggs GG, Freeman, RK, Yaffe SJ. *Drugs in Pregnancy and Lactation*. 7th ed. Philadelphia, PA: Lippincott Williams & Wilkins; 2005.
- Davies DM, Ferner RE, de Glanville H, eds. Davies's Textbook of Adverse Drug Reactions. 5th ed. London: Lippincott-Raven; 1998.
- Department of Medicine, Washington University School of Medicine. *The Washington Manual of Medical Therapeutics*. 38th ed. Philadelphia, PA: Lippincott Williams & Wilkins; 2007.
- Fleeger CA, ed. *USP Dictionary of USAN and International Drug Names*. Rockville, MD: United States Pharmacopeial Convention; 1996.
- Gahart BL. *Intravenous Medications: A Handbook for Nurses and Other Allied Health Personnel*. 24th ed. St. Louis, MO: Mosby; 2008.

- Gilman AG, Rall TW, Nies AS, et al., eds. *Goodman and Gilman's The Pharmacological Basis of Therapeutics.* 8th ed. New York, NY: Pergamon Press; 1990.
- Goldman L, Ausiello DA, edis. *Cecil Medicine.* 23rd ed. Philadelphia, PA: Saunders Elsevier; 2008.
- Grabenstein JD. *Immunofacts: Vaccines and Immunologic Drugs.* 6th ed. St. Louis, MO: Wolters Kluwer Health; 2008.
- Hale TW. Medications and Mothers' Milk. 12th ed. Amarillo, TX: Hale Publishing; 2006.
- Hansten PD, Horn JR. Drug interactions analysis and management. St. Louis, MO: Wolters Kluwer Health; 2007.
- International Journal of Pharmaceutical Compounding [serial on the internet]. Available from www.ijpc.com.
- Jellin JM, ed. *Ident-a-Drug.* Stockton, CA: Therapeutic Research Center; 2008.
- Jellin JM, edr. Pharmacist's letter/prescriber's letter natural medicines comprehensive database. 9th ed. Stockton (CA): Therapeutic Research Faculty; 2007.
- Jew RK, Mullen RJ, Soo-Hoo W. *Children's Hospital of Philadelphia: Extemporaneous Formulations.* Bethesda, MD: American Society of Health-System Pharmacists; 2003.
- Kasper DL, Braunweld E, Fauci AS, et al. *Harrison's Principles of Internal Medicine.* 16th ed. New York, NY: McGraw-Hill, Medical Pub. Division; 2005.
- Katzung BG, ed. *Basic and Clinical Pharmacology.* 9th ed. New York, NY: Lange Medical Books/McGraw-Hill; 2004.
- King JC, Catania PN. *King Guide to Parenteral Admixtures.* 35th ed. Napa, CA: King Guide Publications, Inc; 2008.
- Pharmacy Times [serial on the internet]. Princeton, NJ: Ascend Media; c2001–2008 (updated 2008; cited 2008 Feb 29). Available from www.pharmacytimes.com.
- Phelps SJ, Hak EB, Crill CM. *Pediatric Injectable Drugs* (teddy bear book). 8th ed. Bethesda, MD: American Society of Health-System Pharmacists; 2007.
- Robertson J, Shilkofski N, The Johns Hopkins Hospital. *The Harriet Lane Handbook: A Manual for Pediatric House Officers.* 17th ed. Chicago, IL: Year Book Medical; 2005.
- Secundum Artem [homepage on the internet]. Minneapolis, MN: Paddock Laboratories; c1988–2008 (updated 2007; cited 2008 Feb 29). Available from www.paddocklabs.com/secundum_artem.html.

- Semla TP, Belzer JL, Higbee MD. *Geriatric Dosage Handbook*. 7th ed. Hudson, OH: Lexicomp, Inc; 2002.
- Taketomo CK, Hodding JH, Kraus DM. *Pediatric Dosage Handbook*. 14th ed. Hudson, OH: Lexicomp, Inc; 2007.
- Tatro DS, ed. Drug interaction facts: herbal supplements and food [looseleaf]. St. Louis, MO: Wolters Kluwer Health; updated quarterly.
- Tilsdale JE, Miller DA, eds. *Drug-induced Diseases: Prevention, Detection, and Management*. Bethesda, MD: American Society of Health-System Pharmacists; 2005.
- Trissel LA. *Handbook on Injectable Drugs*. 14th ed. Bethesda, MD: American Society of Health-System Pharmacists; 2007.
- Trissel LA. *Trissel's Stability of Compounded Formulations*. 3rd ed. Washington, DC: American Pharmacists Association; 2005.
- U.S. Pharmacist [serial on the internet]. East Rutherford, NJ: Jobson Medical Information LCC; c2000–2008 (updated 2008; cited 2008 Feb 29). Available from www.uspharmacist.com/.
- United States Pharmacopeial Convention. Revised general chapter <797> pharmaceutical compounding—sterile preparation [chapter on internet]. 2008 Jan (cited 2008 Mar); (about 61 p.). Available from www.usp.org/pdf/EN/USPNF/generalChapter797.pdf.
- Young DS. *Effects of Drugs on Clinical Laboratory Tests*. 5th ed. Washington, DC: American Association for Clinical Chemistry; 2000.
- Young TE, Mangum B. *Neofax*. 20th ed. Montvale, NJ: Thomson Healthcare; 2007.

  Primary literature indexing and abstracting services:
- All EBM Reviews—Cochrane DSR, ACP Journal Club, DARE, CCTR, CMR, HTA, and NHSEED [database on Ovid SP]. New York, NY: Ovid Technologies. Through 4th Quarter 2007 (cited 2008 Feb 29). Available from ovidsp.ovid.com/.
- CINAHL—Cumulative Index to Nursing & Allied Health Literature [database on Ovid SP]. New York, NY: Ovid Technologies. 1982 to February Week 4 2008 (cited 2008 Feb 29). Available from ovidsp.ovid.com/.
- Ovid MEDLINE? [database on Ovid SP]. New York, NY: Ovid Technologies. 1950 to February Week 3 2008 (cited 2008 Feb 29). Available from ovidsp.ovid.com/.
- PubMed [database on the Internet]. Bethesda, MD: National Library of Medicine. 2008 (cited 2008 Feb 29). Available from www.ncbi.nlm.nih.gov/PubMed/.

Pharmacy-focused primary literature indexing and abstracting services:

- EMBASE Drugs & Pharmacology [database on Ovid SP]. New York, NY: Ovid Technologies. 1991 to 4th Quarter 2007 (cited 2008 Feb 29). Available from ovidsp.ovid.com/.
- IDIS/Web [database on Internet]. Iowa City, IA: Iowa Drug Information Service. 1994 to February 2008 (cited 2008 Feb 29). Available from itsnt14.its.uiowa.edu/.
- International Pharmaceutical Abstracts [database on Ovid SP]. New York, NY: Ovid Technologies. 1970 to February 2008 (cited 2008 Feb 29). Available from ovidsp.ovid.com/.

Appendix 3D

Standard Questions for Obtaining Background Information from Requestors

General information to gather for all question types:

- Requestor's name, title/profession, contact information and affiliation.
- Resources already consulted by requestor.
- How will the requestor use the information provided (e.g., patient-specific decision, research, or presentation, academic interest)?
- If patient-specific, is information concerning an inpatient, outpatient, or private patient (gather patient identifiers, and location)?
- Urgency of the request (negotiate time of response).
- Format of response (verbal or written or both).

Adverse drug reactions:

- What are the names, dosages, and routes for all drugs currently and recently prescribed?
- What are the patient specifics (age, gender, height, weight, organ dysfunction, and indication for drug use)?
- What were the events/findings that characterize this adverse drug reaction (ADR) (include onset and duration)?
- What is the temporal relationship with the drug?
- Has the patient experienced this adverse relationship (or similar event) with this drug (or similar agent) previously?

- Was the suspected drug ever administered before? Why was it discontinued then?
- Has any intervention been initiated at this time?
- What is the patient's current condition?
- Does the patient have any food intolerance?
- Is there a family history for this ADR and/or drug allergy?

Dosing or administration:
- What disease is being treated? What is the extent/severity of the illness? What is the clinical status of the patient?
- What are the drugs being prescribed? What drugs has the patient received to date?
- What is the patient's age, gender, height, and weight?
- Does the patient have any insufficiency of the renal, hepatic, or cardiac system?
- For drugs with renal elimination, what are the serum creatinine/creatinine clearance, blood urea nitrogen (BUN), and/or urine output? Is the patient receiving a renal replacement therapy (peritoneal or hemodialysis, continuous venovenous hemofiltration [CVVH])?
- For drugs with hepatic elimination, what are the liver function tests (LFTs), bilirubin (direct and indirect), and/or albumin? Does the patient have liver disease?
- For drugs with serum level monitoring utility, characterize the most recent levels per timing relative to dose and results.
- Are these lab values recent? Is the patient's condition stable?
- Does this patient have a known factor that could affect drug absorption or metabolism?
- What dosage form or preparation is to be used?

Drug interactions:
- What event(s) suggest that an interaction occurred? Please describe.
- For the drugs in question, what are the doses, volumes, concentrations, rate of administration, administration schedule, indication, and length of therapies?
- What is the temporal relationship between the drugs in question?
- Has the patient received this combination or a similar combination in the past?
- Other than the drugs in question, what other drugs is the patient receiving currently? When were these started?

- What other disease states does the patient have?
- Has clinical chemistry (or the appropriate laboratory) been contacted about the abnormal result? Are they aware of any known interference similar to this event?
- Was this one isolated test abnormality or a trend in results?

Indication for therapeutic use:
- What medications, including doses and routes of administration, is the patient receiving? Has the patient been compliant?
- What are we treating and what is the severity of illness?
- What are the patient's other pathology(ies) and disease(s) severity?
- What are the patient's specifics: age, weight, height, gender, organ dysfunction?
- Has the patient received the drug previously? What was the prior response?
- What alternative approved or accepted therapies has the patient received? Was therapy maximized for each of these before discontinuation? What other therapies are being considered?
- What monitoring parameters have been followed (serum concentrations/levels, clinical status, other clinical lab results, objective measurements, and subjective assessment)?

Product information or identification:
- What is the generic or trade name of the product? What is the dosage form and strength?
- Who is the manufacturer? What is the country of origin?
- What is the suspected use of this product? How is the patient taking it?
- What is the dosage form, shape, color, markings, size, coating, and so on?
- What is the source of your information about the product?
- Is the patient just visiting or planning on staying?

Safety in pregnancy and lactation:
- What was the drug the patient received and what was the dose? What was the duration of therapy?
- Is the patient pregnant or planning to become pregnant?
- When during pregnancy was the exposure (trimester or weeks)?
- What are the patient's specifics (age, height, weight, organ dysfunction, other medical conditions)?

- What was the indication for prescribing the drug? Was this initial or alternate therapy?
- What is the source of the case information?
- Was the patient compliant?
- How long has the infant been breast-feeding?
- What is the frequency of breast-feeding? What is the milk volume consumed?
- How old is the infant and what is his or her health status?
- Has the infant ever received feedings other than breast milk? Is bottle or cup feeding a plausible alternative?
- Has the mother breast-fed previously while on the drug?

IV compatibility/stability:
- What are the routes for the patient's medications?
- What are the doses (in mg), concentrations, and volumes for all pertinent medications?
- What are the infusion times/rates expected or desired?
- What is the base solution or diluent used?
- Does the patient have water, sodium, dextrose, or volume restriction?
- Was the product stored in the refrigerator or at room temperature? For how long?
- Was the product exposed to sunlight? For how long?
- Was the product frozen? For how long?
- When was the product compounded/prepared?
- Under what conditions was the product compounded/prepared?

Natural products and dietary supplements:
- Is there a particular concern about this product?
- Why was the patient receiving the product or what is the intended use?
- What drugs is the patient currently receiving? What alternative therapies were tried before?
- What is the product's name and manufacturer?
- What is the dosage form, strength, and how does the patient use it?

Recipes and nonsterile compounded formulations:
- What is the dosage form desired?
- What administration routes are feasible with this patient?

- Does the patient have a feeding tube in place that will be used to administer the drug? What type of feeding tube is it?
- What other special factors regarding drug administration should be considered?

Adapted with permission from Kirkwood CF and Kier KL. Modified systematic approach to answering questions. In: Malone PM, Kier KL, Stanovich JE, eds. *Drug Information: A Guide for Pharmacists.* 3rd ed. New York, NY: McGraw-Hill; 2006:29–37. © The McGraw-Hill Companies, Inc.

4 Physical Examination

Kam L. Capoccia

Entire books are dedicated to the topic of physical examination. The goal of this chapter is not to provide a thorough explanation of how to perform an adult physical examination but rather to describe and highlight some common physical exam techniques and assessments that a pharmacist may perform when evaluating a patient's drug therapy. It is not comprehensive. Basic knowledge and understanding of anatomy and physiology is assumed. For further explanation and details, refer to Bates' *Guide to Physical Examination and History Taking*, 9th edition, 2007.[1]

Medical History

When a patient is admitted to the hospital or undergoes a detailed medical evaluation, the clinician typically obtains a thorough medical history before physically examining the patient. The history describes the events in the life of the patient that are relevant to the patient's mental and physical health. Although this chapter concentrates on physical examination, it should be noted that the history itself contributes the most to understanding a patient's problem or monitoring a drug's effects. The components of the medical history usually follow a standardized format (Table 4.1).

Subjective and objective information obtained from the history and physical examination are crucial to the assessment of drug efficacy and toxicity. Both positive and negative findings may be noted. Pertinent positive findings can rule-in a diagnosis while pertinent negative findings can rule-out a diagnosis.

Table 4.1 THE MEDICAL HISTORY

Section	Contents
Patient profile	Age, race, sex, date of birth, marital status
Chief complaint (CC)	The reason for seeking medical attention
Present illness (PI)	A chronologic account of events and symptoms of the chief complaints; laboratory/diagnostic procedures and negative findings
Past medical history (PMH)	General state of health Childhood illnesses Immunizations Medical illnesses Psychiatric illnesses Surgical procedures Hospitalizations Injuries Medications Allergies
Family history (FH)	Age and health of living relatives Age and cause of death of relatives Occurrence and relation of family members with diabetes mellitus, high blood pressure, cancer, mental illnesses, tuberculosis, and other serious or hereditary illnesses
Social history (SH)	Financial situation, health habits (sleeping, diet, recreation, use of tobacco, alcohol, or other drugs of abuse), education, religion, and family dynamics
Review of systems (ROS)	Common symptoms by body system; the body areas reviewed are skin, head, eyes, ears, nose, and sinuses, mouth and throat, neck, breasts, chest and lungs, heart, vascular, gastrointestinal, urinary, reproductive, musculoskeletal, neurologic, psychiatric, endocrine, and hematologic

Techniques of the Physical Exam

Physical examination uses four main techniques: inspection, palpation, percussion, and auscultation. Inspection is visual observation of the patient with unaided eyes (e.g., examination of the skin), although instruments (e.g., an ophthalmoscope) are often used. Palpation is the use of touch to detect normal and abnormal physical findings (e.g., palpating enlarged lymph nodes). Percussion is the tapping of a body surface with a fingertip to produce sounds that help determine whether underlying structures are air filled, fluid filled, or solid (e.g., percussion of the chest). During percussion, the examiner strikes the body surface to sense the vibrations and sounds generated with each tap. Pitch and tone of the generated sounds help categorize the status of the underlying structures (see Chest, General for a more detailed description of findings on percussion). Auscultation, with the aid of a stethoscope, is listening for normal and abnormal sounds (e.g., heart tones, breath sounds, blood pressure measurement).

Signs and Symptoms

When interpreting a history and physical examination, clinical signs and symptoms are often described. A sign refers to objective information gathered by the examiner during the physical examination (e.g., heart murmur, ankle edema, rales). Signs can be a result of any part of the physical exam (inspection, palpation, percussion, auscultation) but do not include anything reported by the patient.

A symptom refers to subjective information gathered from the patient while obtaining the history (e.g., nausea, pain). The patient's descriptions of symptoms may be scrutinized further, clarified, and quantified by the examiner's additional questioning.

Approach and Organization to Adult Physical Examination

An outline of a comprehensive physical exam is provided below. Following the outline is a description of each system with abbreviated physical examination instructions. For a more complete explanation and additional information, please see *Bates' Guide to Physical Examination and History Taking*, 9th edition, 2007.

- General survey.
- Vital signs.
- Skin (hair and nails).
- Head, eyes, ears, nose, throat (HEENT).
- Neck.
- Back.
- Chest (general, lungs, breasts, axillae).
- Cardiovascular system.
- Abdomen.

- Genitourinary and rectal system.
- Peripheral vascular system.
- Musculoskeletal system.
- Neurologic system.

General Survey

Observe the patient's general state of health (acute or chronically ill, frail, etc.) and overall appearance, paying particular attention to the following:

- Level of consciousness (awake, alert, unresponsive, etc.).
- Note orientation to person, place, and thing; if normal, it is often documented as A & O × 3 (alert and oriented to (i) person, (ii) place, and (iii) thing).
- Signs of distress (cardiac, respiratory, pain, anxiety, fear, shock, etc.).
- Height (tall or short), build (muscular, slender, stocky), weight (overweight, obese, emaciated, thin).
- Skin color (jaundice, cyanosis, rashes or bruises).
- Dress (appropriate for the temperature and weather, clean, dirty, fit properly).
- Grooming and personal hygiene (appropriate for age, lifestyle, etc.).
- Facial expression (eye contact, change or reaction to certain topics during physical exam, interaction with others, flat or sad affect, etc.).
- Odor of body or breath (fruity odor of diabetes, scent of alcohol, etc.).
- Posture (sitting up, leaning forward, etc.).
- Gait (walking smoothly, with or without assistance, etc.).
- Motor activity (tremor, involuntary movements, paralyses).

The above observations are typically made throughout the interview and physical exam. An observation example might include: "This is a thin, elderly man who looks jaundiced and chronically ill. He is leaning forward in the chair, alert, and making good eye contact."

Vital Signs

Vital signs are important because they are coarse objective measurements for a patient's physical state. The four vital signs are temperature, pulse, blood pressure, and respiratory rate.

Temperature

Body temperature can be measured orally, rectally, in the axilla, or by using an infrared beam aimed at the tympanic membrane. Documentation of the route is essential for interpretation of the measured result.

Normal adult body temperatures are as follows:

- Oral: 35.8–37.3°C (96.4–99.1°F).
- Axillary: 35.3–36.8°C (95.9–99.6°F).
- Rectal: 36.3–37.8°C (94.9–99.6°F).

Fever is an oral temperature >37.9°C (100.9°F). Hypothermia is a core body temperature (confirmed rectally) of <35.0°C (95°F).

Pulse

Pulse or heart rate is the number of palpable transmitted heartbeats in 1 minute.

- Palpate the radial pulse at the wrist (do not use your thumb).
- Count the beats for 15 seconds (or 30 seconds) and multiply by four (or two).
- Note the rhythm of the pulse during palpation: regular, irregular, regularly irregular, irregularly irregular.

Normal adult sinus rhythm is 60 to 100 beats per minute (bpm). Bradycardia is <60 bpm. Tachycardia is >100 bpm.

Atrial fibrillation is the most common adult arrhythmia. It produces an irregularly irregular rhythm. In this setting, palpating the radial pulse will underestimate the actual ventricular response rate. Auscultate the cardiac apex to determine the heart rate.

Blood Pressure (BP)

- The patient should be seated still for at least 5 minutes (when possible) with feet resting comfortably on the floor.
- The bare upper arm should be at heart level.
- The bladder of the BP cuff should encircle at least 80% of the upper arm.
- The middle of the cuff should align with the brachial artery that was palpated just proximal to the antecubital fossa.
- The cuff should fit snugly and firmly around the bare upper arm.
- The lower edge of the cuff should be 2 to 3 cm proximal to the antecubital fossa.

Palpate

- Determine the level for maximal inflation by observing the pressure at which the radial pulse is no longer palpable as the cuff is rapidly inflated.
- Add 30 mm Hg to the measurement when the radial pulse disappears.
- Rapidly and steadily deflate the cuff.
- Wait at least 15 to 30 seconds before reinflating.

Auscultate

- Position the diaphragm of the stethoscope over the palpated brachial artery distal to the BP cuff at the antecubital fossa, making sure it is not underneath the cuff to prevent any extraneous sounds.
- Apply light pressure to the stethoscope, ensuring skin contact at all points.
- Heavy pressure may distort sounds.
- Sound generated over the vessels is relatively low in frequency; use of the bell (instead of the diaphragm) may enhance sound detection.
- Rapidly and steadily inflate the cuff 20 to 30 mm Hg above the pressure determined by palpation.
- Release the air in the cuff so that the pressure falls at a rate of 2 to 3 mm per second while auscultating the Korotkoff sounds.
- The first appearance of two consecutive faint, repetitive, tapping sounds is the systolic BP (phase I Korotkoff sounds).
- Disappearance of repetitive sounds is the diastolic BP (phase V Korotkoff sounds).
- Measure and record to the nearest 2 mm Hg.
  - Normal adult BP is <120/80 mm Hg. Prehypertension is 120 to 139/80 to 89 mm Hg.
- Hypertension is ≥140/90 mm Hg.

Orthostatic blood pressure and pulse are defined as a systolic BP drop of >20 mm Hg or a pulse rise of >20 bpm when the patient changes from a sitting to a standing position (after waiting for at least 3 minutes on position change).

In some patients the Korotkoff sounds temporarily disappear and then reappear as the cuff is deflated to the level below phase I. The area of disappearance is called an auscultatory gap. This may occur in 10% to 20% of the elderly hypertensive population. The cause is unknown. To avoid underestimating the systolic BP, palpate the radial pulse for the level of maximal inflation.

If the bladder of the BP cuff is too small, the BP may be falsely elevated.

Respiratory Rate (RR)

Observe the patient breathing and count the respirations for 15 seconds (or 30 seconds) and multiply by four (or two).

Normal adult RR is 8 to 20 breaths per minute. Bradypnea is RR <8. Tachypnea is RR >20. Apnea is the cessation of breath for ≥20 seconds.

Height, Weight, BMI

Although not classic vital signs, height and weight are typically recorded in this section. Height and weight can be used together to calculate body surface area (BSA), ideal body weight (IBW), and adjusted body weight (ABW).

BSA

$$\text{BSA (m}^2) = (\text{height in in.} \times \text{weight in lb})/3, 131)^{1/2} \text{ or}$$
$$(\text{height in cm}) \times \text{weight in kg})/3, 600)^{1/2}$$

IBW

IBW is the estimated ideal body weight in kilograms (kg):

Males: IBW = 50 kg + 2.3 kg for each inch over 5 ft
Females: IBW = 45.5 kg + 2.3 kg for each inch over 5 ft

ABW

ABW is the estimated adjusted body weight (kg).
If the actual body weight is >30% of the calculated IBW, calculate the ABW as follows:

$$\text{ABW} = \text{IBW} + 0.4 (\text{actual weight} - \text{IBW})$$

BMI

Body mass index (BMI) is a calculation based on the height and weight of the patient.

$$\text{BMI} = \text{weight in kg/height in m}^2 \text{ or weight in lb/height in in.}^2 \times 703$$

BMI CATEGORIES

Healthy	$18.5–24.9 \text{ kg/m}^2$
Overweight	$25–29.9 \text{ kg/m}^2$
Obese	$\geq 30 \text{ kg/m}^2$

Pain

Assess the patient's level of pain or discomfort. Traditionally, a scale of 1 to 10 (10 being the worst imaginable pain) is used.

Skin

The integumentary system is perhaps one of the most assessable organ systems for examination. See Table 4.2 and Figure 4.1 for information on descriptive dermatologic terms and examples.

Table 4.2 DESCRIPTIVE DERMATOLOGIC TERMS AND EXAMPLES

Lesion	Description	Example
Acneiform	Erythematous pustules	Acne
Annular	Ring shaped	Ringworm
Confluent	Lesions run together	Viral exanthems
Discoid	Disc shaped without central clearing	Lupus erythematosus
Eczematoid	An inflammation with a tendency to vesiculate and crust	Eczema
Erythroderma	Diffuse red color	Sunburn
Exfoliative	Sloughing of skin layers	Toxic epidermal necrolysis
Grouped	Clustered lesions	Vesicles of herpes simplex
Iris	Bull's-eye or target-type lesions	Erythema multiform
Keratotic	Thickening	Psoriasis
Linear	In lines	Poison ivy
Papulosquamous	Raised papules or plaques with scaling	Psoriasis
Urticarial	Raised local edema of the skin (wheal)	Hives
Zosteriform	Linear arrangement along a dermatome	Herpes zoster

Inspect

- Color (e.g., brownness, cyanosis, yellowness or jaundice).
- Vascularity (including ecchymoses such as petechiae or purpura).
- Edema.
- Temperature (use the backs of the fingers to make this relative assessment).
- Texture (roughness or smoothness).
- Moisture (dryness, sweating, and oiliness).
- Mobility.
- Turgor (the speed with which the skin returns into place when a fold is lifted).
- Lesions.

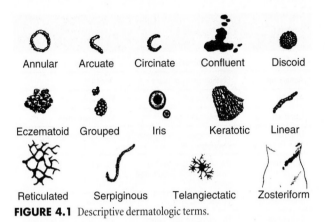

FIGURE 4.1 Descriptive dermatologic terms.

Skin lesions are described in terms of primary and secondary lesions (Fig. 4.2). Primary lesions may arise from previously normal skin and can be divided into three categories:

1. Circumscribed, flat, nonpalpable changes in skin color (macules and patches).
2. Palpable solid elevations in the skin (nodules, plaques, papules, cysts, and wheals).
3. Circumscribed superficial elevations of the skin formed by free fluid within the skin layers (vesicles, bulla, and pustules).

Secondary lesions result from changes in a primary lesion and include the development of erosions, ulcers, fissures, crusts, and scales.

Examples of skin lesions (with their potential drug culprits in parentheses) include the following:

- Acneiform or pustular (corticosteroids).
- Erythroderma (vancomycin-induced red man's syndrome).
- Exfoliation (Stevens-Johnson syndrome from sulfonamides).
- Maculopapular (beta-lactams).
- Lupuslike (procainamide, hydralazine).
- Photosensitivity (sulfonamides, fluoroquinolones, methotrexate).
- Urticaria (aspirin sensitivity).
- Hyperpigmentation (phenothiazines, hydroxychloroquine, amiodarone, oral contraceptives).

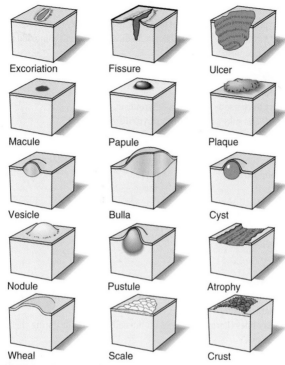

FIGURE 4.2 Basic types of skin lesions.

Hair
Hair is considered a skin appendage.

Inspect
- Quantity.
  - Alopecia or hair loss can be total, sparse, or patchy.
    - A result of drug therapy (during or after chemotherapy), infection (fungal such as tinea capitis or ringworm), or trichotillomania (pulling, plucking, or twisting ones' hair).
  - Hirsutism is the growth of hair in women in a characteristically male pattern.
    - A result of androgen excess syndromes, corticosteroids and Cushing syndrome, oral contraceptives, and androgenic medications.

- Distribution.
  - Hypertrichosis is increased hair growth, particularly on the face.
    - A result of an adverse effect of medications such as minoxidil and cyclosporine.

Palpate
- Texture.
  - Dry or coarse as seen in hypothyroidism.
  - Fine and silky as seen in hyperthyroidism.

Nails
Nails are considered a skin appendage. The fingernails and toenails should be examined.

Inspect
- Color.
- Shape.
- Lesions.

Palpate
- Nail beds.
  - Pitting and ridging of the nails is another common finding and is characteristic of psoriasis.
  - Beau lines (horizontal ridges on the nails) can occur during chemotherapy.

Clubbing of the fingers is the selective bullous enlargement of the distal segment of the digit due to an increase in soft tissue and is associated with flattening of the angle between the nail and nail base from 160 to 180 degrees or more (Fig. 4.3). The proximal nail bed feels spongy or

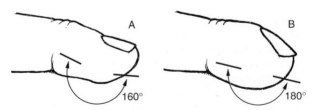

A. Normal angle of the nail.
B. Abnormal angle of the nail seen in late clubbing.
FIGURE 4.3 Clubbing of the finger.

floating. Clubbing can be hereditary or idiopathic and is associated with various conditions, including cyanotic heart disease and pulmonary disorders (such as chronic obstructive pulmonary disease, cystic fibrosis, tuberculosis, and lung cancer).

Head, Eyes, Ears, Nose, Throat (HEENT)

Head

Inspect

- Shape (normocephalic, hydrocephalic, or microcephalic).
- Hair (described above).
- Scalp (erythema, scales, lumps, evidence of trauma).
- Skull (size, contour, deformities, lumps, or tenderness).
- Face (expression, contour, asymmetry, involuntary movements, edema, masses).
- Skin (described above).

Several disorders have characteristic facial features, including the moon facies of Cushing syndrome (or corticosteroid use), exophthalmos of Grave disease, and the masked facies of scleroderma or parkinsonism. Several skin disorders and rashes affect the face, including acne vulgaris, acne rosacea, the butterfly-pattern malar rash over the cheeks in systemic lupus erythematosus (SLE), and the zosteriform rash of herpes zoster.

Eyes

The anatomy of the external and internal eye is depicted in Figures 4.4 and 4.5. Physical exam on the eye involves testing the vision, inspecting the eye, assessing the pupils and ocular motility, and an ophthalmoscopic exam.

Vision

- Visual acuity using the Snellen chart (commonly known as the "E" chart).
- Visual fields can be assessed via confrontation; if patient complains of blind spots, check each visual quadrant.

Inspection

- Eyebrows.
- Eyelids.
  - A stye (external hordeolum) is a painful tender nodule caused by a virus or bacteria; the gland/hair follicle of the eyelid margin is inflamed.

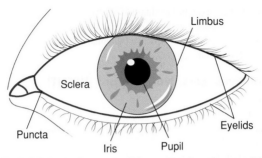

FIGURE 4.4 External anatomy of the eye. Note how the upper lid normally covers the upper rim of the iris and limbus. (Reprinted with permission from Longe RL, Calvert JC. In: Young LYY, ed. *Physical Assessment: A Guide for Evaluating Drug Therapy*. Vancouver, WA: Applied Therapeutics, Inc.; 1994.)

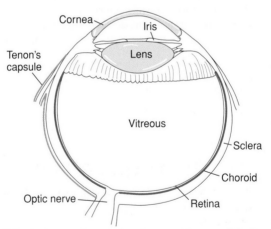

FIGURE 4.5 Internal eye and optic nerve. Diagram of the internal eye with its three layers (the retina, the choroids, and sclera) and the optic nerve, with its posterior chamber containing the lens and retina. (Reprinted with permission from Longe RL, Calvert JC. In: Young LYY, ed. *Physical Assessment: A Guide for Evaluating Drug Therapy*. Vancouver, WA: Applied Therapeutics, Inc.; 1994.)

- Lashes.
- Conjunctiva.
  - Inflammation, mattering or exudates (conjunctivitis or conjunctival infection).
  - Scleral icterus (a yellowish pigmentation of the sclera) signifies jaundice in a patient with a bilirubin serum concentration >2 to 3 mg/dL.
- Cornea.
- Interior chamber.
- Iris.

Pupillary Assessment
- Reactivity to light.
  - PERRLA (pupils equal, round, reactive to light and accommodation) is a typical mnemonic description.
- Pupil size.
  - Barbiturates may cause mydriasis or pupillary dilatation.
  - Opiates may cause miosis or pinpoint pupils.
- Pupil symmetry.
  - Anisocoria (a difference in the size of the pupils).
- Alignment of corneal light reflex with penlight.

Ocular Motility Assessment
- Cranial nerves III, IV, and VI and the muscles they innervate.
  - Muscle palsy or a cranial nerve problem could be detected if the patient is unable to follow the examiner's finger when directed up-down or left-right.
  - *Strabismus* is the lack of parallelism of the eyes' visual axes.
  - *Nystagmus* is an abnormal rapid rhythmic spontaneous movement of the eyes (i.e., under conditions of fixation, the eyes drift slowly vertically or horizontally and are corrected by a quick movement to the original position); can be a sign of drug toxicity (phenytoin, lithium).

Direct Ophthalmoscopy
- Red reflex.
- Optic cup/disc.
  - Papilledema is inflammation of the optic disc.
- Retinal blood vessels.
  - Hypertension can cause extensive changes in the eye including arteriovenous narrowing, hemorrhaging, exudates, papilledema.

- Diabetic retinopathy is characterized by early microaneurysm and exudates that can progress to proliferation of blood vessels, retinal detachment, and vitreal hemorrhage.
- Retinal background.
- Macula.
  - Macular edema (localized swelling or thickening of the macula) can be see in diabetes mellitus.

Ears

The normal anatomy of the external and middle ear is depicted in Figures 4.6 and 4.7.

Inspect for deformities, lumps, or skin lesions. Inspect the normal or noninfected ear first for easier comparison.

- External ear.
- Auricle.
- Surrounding tissue.

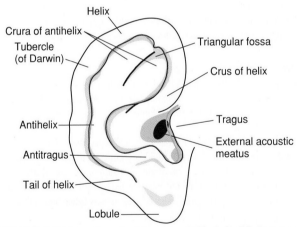

FIGURE 4.6 External ear (auricle or pinna). The helix, lobule, tragus, and external acoustic meatus (opening into the external auditory canal) are frequently used during physical examination to evaluate deeper structures. (Reprinted with permission from Longe RL, Calvert JC. In: Young LYY, ed. *Physical Assessment: A Guide for Evaluating Drug Therapy*. Vancouver, WA: Applied Therapeutics, Inc.; 1994.)

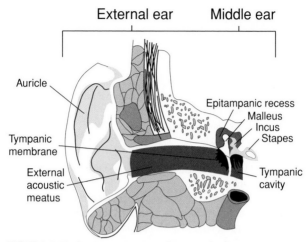

FIGURE 4.7 Three compartments of the ear. The three compartments of the ear include the external ear (auricle to tympanic membrane), middle ear (tympanic membrane to round window of inner ear), and inner ear. (Reprinted with permission from Longe RL, Calvert JC. In: Young LYY, ed. *Physical Assessment: A Guide for Evaluating Drug Therapy*. Vancouver, WA: Applied Therapeutics, Inc.; 1994.)

Palpate the pinna and tragus for tenderness:

- Suspect otitis externa (infection of the external ear) if pulling on the auricle or pressing on the tragus causes pain.
- Suspect otitis media (infection of the middle ear) if pressing firmly behind the ear causes pain or is tender.

Before inserting the otoscope, gently pull the auricle upward, backward, and away from the head so the ear canal is straightened. Holding the otoscope between the thumb and index finger, brace your hand against the patient's face to ensure your hand and instrument will move with the patient and any unexpected movements. Insert the speculum gently into the ear canal, moving it through any hair and in a downward and forward direction. Move the speculum so you can see as much of the drum as possible.

Inspect

- External auditory canal.
  - Redness.
  - Inflammation.
  - Discharge.
  - Cerumen or ear wax.
    - May obstruct the view of the eardrum or tympanic membrane.
    - Color (yellow to brown).
    - Consistency (flaky, sticky, hard).
  - Presence of foreign body.
- Tympanic membrane (TM).
  - Normal TM: a conical light reflex is observed due to the reflection of light from the otoscope.
  - Perforations or holes may be a result of middle ear infection.
  - Color (red in acute otitis media or amber if serous effusion).
  - Contour (bulging suggests fluid or pus in the middle ear).

By insufflating air using a pneumatic otoscope, the TM's ease of mobility can be assessed. Decreased mobility is seen in otitis media and eustachian tube dysfunction.

Hearing loss can affect one or both ears. To estimate hearing or auditory acuity, test one ear at a time. Occlude one ear at a time, stand 1 to 2 ft away from the patient and whisper a word or number of two equally accented syllables ("baseball" or "three-four") toward the unoccluded ear. You may need to increase the intensity of the whisper, possibly to a soft, medium, or loud voice. Cover your lips or ask the patient to close their eyes to avoid lip reading. If hearing is decreased, it is important to distinguish between conductive or sensorineural hearing loss. See Table 4.3 for an explanation of the differences and instructions on how to perform the physical exam to assess these patterns of hearing loss. A tuning fork (512 or 1,024 Hz) and a quiet room are needed.

Nose and Sinuses
Inspect

- Nose.
  - Asymmetry or deformities.
  - Swelling.
  - Septal defects.
  - Discharge.

Table 4.3 CONDUCTIVE HEARING LOSS VERSUS SENSORINEURAL HEARING LOSS

	Conductive Loss	Sensorineural Loss
	Tympanic membrane / Middle ear / Cochlear nerve	Tympanic membrane / Middle ear / Cochlear nerve
Pathophysiology	External or middle ear disorder impairs sound conduction to inner ear. Causes include foreign body, otitis media, perforated eardrum, and otosclerosis ossicles	Inner ear disorder involves cochlear nerve and neuronal impulse transmission to the brain. Causes include loud noise exposure, inner ear infections, trauma, tremors, congenital and familial disorders, and aging
Usual age of onset	Childhood and young adulthood, up to 40 years of age	Middle or later years
Ear canal and drum	Abnormality usually visible, except in otosclerosis	Problem not visible
Effects	• Little effect on sound • Hearing seems to improve in noisy environment • Voice becomes soft because inner ear and cochlear nerve are intact	• Higher registers are lost, so sound may be distorted • Hearing worsens in noisy environment • Voice may be loud because hearing is difficult
Weber test (in unilateral hearing loss)	• Tuning fork at vertex • Sound lateralizes to impaired ear—room noise not well heard, so detection of vibrations improves	• Tuning fork at vertex • Sound lateralizes to good ear—inner ear or cochlear nerve damage impairs transmission to affected ear
Rinne test	• Tuning fork at external auditory meatus then on mastoid bone • Bone conduction longer than or equal to air conduction (BC ≥AC). While air conduction through the external or middle ear is impaired, vibrations through bone bypass the problem to reach the cochlea	• Tuning fork at external auditory meatus then on mastoid bone • Air conduction longer than bone conduction (AC >BC). The inner ear or cochlear nerve is less able to transmit impulses regardless of how the vibrations reach the cochlea. The normal pattern prevails

Reprinted with permission from Bickley LS, Szilagyi PG. In: *Bates' Guide to Physical Examination and History Taking.* 9th ed. Philadelphia, PA: Lippincott Williams & Wilkins; 2007.

- Nasal mucosa: A penlight or an otoscope may be used to view inside the nostrils or nasal vestibules. The nasal mucosa is normally a bit redder than the oral mucosa.
  - Swelling.
  - Bleeding.
  - Exudates (clear, purulent, or mucopurulent).

In allergic rhinitis the mucosa may be pale, bluish, or red. In viral rhinitis the mucosa may be reddened and swollen. *Rhinitis medicamentosa*, a side effect of prolonged nasal vasoconstrictor therapy, may manifest as mucosal swelling and edema. *Epistaxis*, a nose bleed, may represent an adverse effect of anticoagulant therapy or steroid nasal spray.

Palpate for sinus tenderness by pressing on the frontal sinuses from under the bony brows and pressing on the maxillary sinuses. Tenderness, pain, fever, and nasal discharge suggest acute sinusitis involving the respective sinuses.

Throat (or Mouth and Pharynx)
Inspect
- Lips (color, moisture, ulcers, lumps, cracking).
- Oral mucosa (color, ulcers, white patches, nodules).
- Gums (color).
- Teeth (missing, discolored, loose).
- Roof of the mouth (color and architecture).
- Tongue (symmetry, color, texture, sides, undersides).
- Floor of the mouth (color, ulcerations).
- Pharynx (color, symmetry, exudates, swelling, ulcerations, and tonsillar enlargement).
  - Ask the patient to open the mouth very wide and say "ah." A tongue blade placed firmly down the midpoint of the tongue may help to see the pharynx better. Be careful not to place the tongue blade too far back or you may cause gagging.

Visual examination of the mouth and oropharynx can identify a number of diseases and adverse drug manifestations. Cyanosis of the lips might indicate hypoxemia. Gingival hyperplasia can be caused by phenytoin. *Stomatitis* (mouth sores) is a common complication of cytotoxic drugs. *Xerostomia* (dry mouth) is observed as a lack of saliva and can be caused by various connective tissue diseases (e.g., SLE, rheumatoid arthritis, Sjögren syndrome) and medications (e.g., anticholinergics). Infectious disease manifestations include pharyngitis, erythema (with or without exudates), oral thrush/candidiasis (e.g., in immunocompromised patients or infants), and herpetic lesions. Aphthous stomatitis is a common non-specific painful ulceration of the buccal mucosa. Hairy leukoplakia, a common manifestation of acquired immune deficiency syndrome, appears as a white, raised lesion on the lateral margins of the tongue.

Neck

Inspect

- Symmetry.
- Masses.
- Scars.
- Abnormal pulsations.
- Enlarged lymph nodes.
- Distention of the jugular veins (described below in Blood Vessels).
- Deviation of the trachea.
- Range of motion.
- Goiter.
  - › The normal neck should be soft, supple, and without masses or enlargement of the thyroid gland.

Lymph Nodes

There are many lymph nodes in the face and neck. To palpate the lymph nodes, use the pads on the index and middle fingers to move the skin over the underlying tissues in a gentle circular motion. The patient should be relaxed with the neck flexed slightly forward and toward the side being examined. Both sides can be examined at the same time when the examiner is standing in front of the patient. See Figure 4.8 for locations of the lymph nodes in the face and neck. The cervical, submandibular, and supraclavicular are most commonly examined.

Palpate the nodes and note the following:

- Discrete or matted together.
- Size.
- Shape (round, oblong, irregular or smooth).
- Mobility.
- Consistency (hard, soft, rubbery, fluid filled).
- Tenderness.

Normal nodes are nontender, discrete, mobile, and small. Tender nodes suggest inflammation, which may be a result of infection. Hard

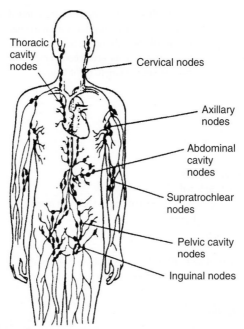

FIGURE 4.8 Location of lymph nodes in the body.

or fixed nodes suggest malignancy. If nodes are enlarged, it is important to determine between regional or generalized lymphadenopathy.

Blood Vessels

Before palpating the carotid artery, look for carotid pulsations medial to the sternomastoid muscles. Place your index and middle finger on the carotid artery in the lower third of the neck; pressing posteriorly, feel for pulsations. Do not palpate both carotid arteries simultaneously. To assess for amplitude and duration, the patient should be reclined at a 30-degree angle. A delayed upstroke is characteristic of aortic stenosis. A bounding pulse is characteristic of high-stroke volume states such as aortic regurgitation. Auscultation of the carotid arteries can detect bruits (a blowing or turbulent sound caused by blood flowing past an obstruction such as an atherosclerotic narrowing).

Jugular venous distention (JVD) reflects central venous pressure as seen in Figure 4.9. With the patient reclined at a 30-degree angle, apply

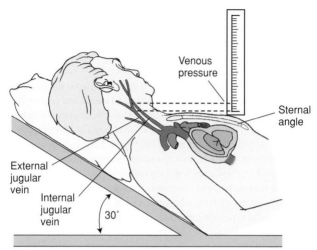

FIGURE 4.9 Assessment of jugular venous pressure. Place the patient supine in bed and gradually raise the head of the bed to 30, 45, 60 and 90 degrees. Using tangential lighting, note the highest level of venous pulsation. Measure the vertical distance between this point and the sternal angle. Record the distance in centimeters and the angle of the head of bed. (Reprinted with permission from Instructors Resource CD-ROM to Accompany *Critical Care Nursing: A Holistic Approach.* 8th ed. Philadelphia, PA: Lippincott Williams & Wilkins; 2005.)

pressure over the liver and observe subsequent neck vein distention. This is known as the hepatojugular reflux test and it assesses liver congestion and right ventricular function. The height of distention is measured in centimeters above the sternal angle. JVD >3 cm is considered positive for volume overload. JVD is decreased in patients who are hypovolemic. JVD is increased in patients with congestive heart failure (CHF), right ventricular dysfunction, cardiac tamponade, and cor pulmonale. In normal patients, JVD rises temporarily and returns to normal within a few seconds because the body can compensate for the shift in pressure and volume.

Thyroid Gland
The thyroid gland can be palpated from either the front or the back of the patient. With the patient seated comfortably, palpate down the midline of the neck to feel the hyoid bone, thyroid cartilage, cricoid cartilage, and

trachea. Diseases or masses in the neck or thorax (mediastinal mass, atelectasis, or pneumothorax) may push the trachea to one side. With the patient's head tilted back a bit, inspect the thyroid gland. Have the patient swallow and watch the thyroid gland, noting its contour and symmetry; thyroid cartilage and cricoid cartilage move upward with swallowing and then fall to their resting positions. Using these landmarks, displace the trachea to one side and feel for the thyroid gland medial and deep to the sternocleidomastoid muscle. If examining the left lobe, displace and stabilize the trachea to the left side with your left thumb and hand. Palpate the left lobe using your right index and middle fingers. Reverse the procedure to examine the other side. Note the size, shape (nodular or irregular), consistency (rubbery, hard, cystic), and any nodules or tenderness. A normal thyroid is smooth, soft, and nontender. If the thyroid gland is enlarged and tender, listen with the diaphragm of a stethoscope for a bruit, which may be heard in hyperthyroidism due to increased blood flow through the thyroid arteries.

Back

Examination of the back discloses any spinal deformities (e.g., scoliosis, kyphosis) or tenderness. Conditions of endogenous or exogenous corticosteroid excess can produce a "buffalo hump" over the upper back. Kyphosis in the elderly can occur due to osteoporosis.

The costovertebral angle (the angle formed by the lower border of the 12th rib and the transverse process of the upper lumbar vertebrae) defines the area to assess for kidney tenderness. Tenderness in the posterior flank is a classic sign of pyelonephritis.

Chest (General, Lungs, Breasts, Axillae)

General

Examination of the chest necessitates inspection, percussion, palpation, and auscultation. Because pulmonary and cardiac diseases are commonly associated, it is critical to do a thorough evaluation of both systems (see Cardiovascular System on page 99).

Inspection

- Look for any signs of respiratory difficulty.
  - Assess color of patient for cyanosis.
  - Listen to the patient breathing.
  - Inspect the neck for use of accessory muscles to help the patient breath.
  - Check for symmetry with respiratory efforts.

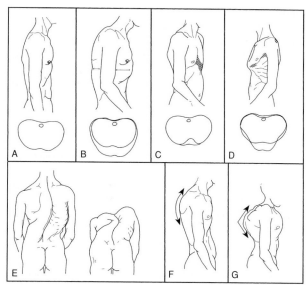

FIGURE 4.10 Chest wall contours. **A:** Normal. **B:** Barrel chest associated with emphysema. **C:** Pectus excavatum (i.e., funnel chest). **D:** Pectus carinatum (i.e., pigeon breast). **E:** Scoliosis. **F:** Kyphosis. **G:** Gibbus (i.e., extreme kyphosis). (Reprinted with permission from Longe RL, Calvert JC. In: Young LYY, ed. *Physical Assessment: A Guide for Evaluating Drug Therapy.* Vancouver, WA: Applied Therapeutics, Inc.; 1994.)

Note the shape of the chest and any deformities (Fig. 4.10).

Palpation

- Areas of tenderness (pain, lesions, or bruises).
- Masses.
- Tactile fremitus (normal vibration that can be felt on the thoracic wall during phonation).

Percussion

Percussion helps to determine whether tissue is air filled, fluid filled, or solid.

- Right and left sides, spine and costovertebral angles for tenderness.
  - Resonant (normal).
  - Flat or dull (consolidation, pleural effusion, atelectasis).
  - Hyperresonant or tympanitic (pneumothorax or emphysema).

Lungs

Auscultate the anterior and posterior lung fields using the diaphragm of a stethoscope on the skin of the chest wall (not over clothing). Auscultation involves listening to the sounds generated by breathing and for any added (adventitious) sounds. If abnormalities are detected, listen to the sounds of the patient's spoken or whispered words as they are transmitted through the chest wall.

Lung Sounds

- Vesicular—normal lung sounds; soft, low-pitched, noted with inhalation.
- Bronchial—abnormal lung sounds; hard, loud, high-pitched, suggestive of dense lung tissue or consolidated.
- Adventitious—abnormal lung sounds that are superimposed on normal vesicular breath sounds in the presence of disease.
  - Crackles are intermittent, brief, and not musical (once more commonly referred to as rales).
    - Coarse crackles are low-pitched rattles heard during early and mid inspiration. They are produced from rapid airflow in large central airways that cause the rupture of fluid films and bubbles along air-filled walls (acute or chronic bronchitis).
    - Fine crackles are soft and high-pitched like fine Velcro being pulled apart or like hairs being rubbed together. They occur in late inspiration when small partially collapsed airways suddenly reopen and pop (pneumonia, pulmonary edema).
  - Wheezes are high-pitched, hissing, continuous sounds produced by air movement through narrowed airways as in an asthma exacerbation or chronic obstructive pulmonary disease (COPD).
  - Rhonchi are low-pitched, snoring, continuous sounds that are suggestive of secretions in the airways.
  - Rubs are loud and creaky sounds caused by two inflamed pleural areas rubbing together.
- Transmitted voice—normally the sounds transmitted through the chest wall are muffled and indistinct.
  - Bronchophony is an increase in the clarity of spoken voice sounds.
  - Whispered pectoriloquy is an increase in clarity of whispered voice sounds (indicative of lung consolidation).
  - Egophony is a nasal bleating sound detected when the spoken letter "E" sounds more like "A" (indicative of lung consolidation).

Breasts

Breast examination is an important component of the physical examination and involves inspection and palpation of the breasts and nipples in women and men. Examination of the breasts in women should be completed in four views—arms at sides, arms over head, arms pressed against hips, and leaning forward. These views may reveal dimpling or retraction which suggests an underlying cancer.

Inspection

- Skin—color; large pores or thickening.
- Breasts—size, symmetry, contour (masses, dimpling, or flattening).
- Nipples—size, symmetry, direction in which they point, rashes, ulcerations, discharge.

Palpation

- Breast tissue—consistency, tenderness, nodules.
- Nipple—elasticity, nodules, swelling, ulcerations.

Axillae

Inspection and palpation of the axillae should be performed with the patient in a sitting position.

Inspection

- Skin of each axilla (rash, infection, unusual pigmentation).

Palpation

- Axillary nodes—the central nodes are most often palpable; if the central nodes are tender, large, or hard, palpate the other groups of axillary lymph nodes (pectoral, lateral, and subscapular nodes).

Cardiovascular System

It is best to have the patient supine and examine from the right of the patient.

Inspect and Palpate

- The point of maximal impulse (PMI) is palpable in only 30% of adults (Fig. 4.11).
  - Palpate at or medial to the midclavicular line between the 4th and 5th intercostal space (ICS).
  - Normal PMI is <2 cm diameter in the supine position and <4 cm in the partial left lateral decubitus position.

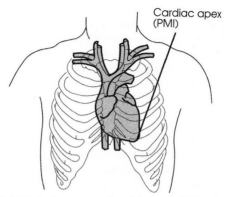

FIGURE 4.11 Surface topography of the heart. PMI, point of maximal impulse. (Reprinted with permission from Longe RL, Calvert JC. In: Young LYY, ed. *Physical Assessment: A Guide for Evaluating Drug Therapy.* Vancouver, WA: Applied Therapeutics, Inc.; 1994.)

- A *heave* or *lift* is a sustained, systolic outward movement of the precordium associated with heart failure.
- A *thrill* is a palpable vibration (like a cat purring) felt when a cardiac murmur is grade IV to VI/VI.

Auscultate

- Listen for several cardiac cycles to determine if there are additional sounds other than S1 and S2 ("lub-dub"). Focus on systole for a few cycles and then on diastole, listening for extra sounds or murmurs.
  - S1 is heard the loudest at the apex. It occurs with closure of the mitral and tricuspid valves at the onset of ventricular systole.
  - S2 is heard loudest between the 2nd and 3rd ICS. It occurs with closure of the aortic and pulmonic valves at the end of systole.
  - S3 is best heard with the bell of the stethoscope at the apex. It occurs during early diastole when blood is flowing into an overfilled noncompliant ventricle and suddenly decelerates. It is normal in young adults; age older than 40 years suggests severe systolic heart failure or valvular regurgitation. S3 occurs after S2 and sounds like "lub-dub-dah."
  - S4 is best heard with the bell of the stethoscope at the apex. It occurs in late diastole when the atrial contraction pushes blood into the left ventricle that is stiff as seen in hypertrophy. S4 precedes S1 and sounds like "luh-lub-dub."

- If a murmur is heard (use diaphragm of stethoscope), it should be graded and described:
  - Grades I–III (thrill absent).
    - I: hard to hear, faint.
    - II: quiet, but heard immediately with stethoscope.
    - III: moderately loud.
  - Grades IV–VI (thrill present).
    - IV: loud, heard with stethoscope on chest.
    - V: very loud, heard with edge of stethoscope on chest.
    - VI: very loud, heard with stethoscope off the chest.
  - Pitch of murmur: high, medium, or low.
  - Quality of murmur: blowing, harsh, rumbling, musical.
- Using the diaphragm of the stethoscope, press firmly on bare skin in a quiet room in four areas (Fig. 4.12).
  - Cardiac apex (mitral valve area, 5th ICS).
  - Tricuspid area (left lower sternal border (LLSB)).
  - Pulmonic area (left 2nd ICS).
  - Aortic area (right 2nd ICS).

Abdomen

The sequence of an abdominal exam is to look (inspection), listen (auscultation), and feel (percussion and palpation). The abdomen is divided

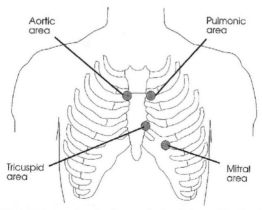

FIGURE 4.12 Location sites for auscultating the heart. (Reprinted with permission from Longe RL, Calvert JC. In: Young LYY, ed. *Physical Assessment: A Guide for Evaluating Drug Therapy*. Vancouver, WA: Applied Therapeutics, Inc.; 1994.)

into four quadrants based on two perpendicular planes drawn through the umbilicus. Noted tenderness or pain in a specific quadrant or location within a quadrant suggests involvement of the various organs as outlined in Figure 4.13.

Inspection

- Presence and level of patient distress (does it hurt the patient to move or cough?).
- Contour (flat, rounded, scaphoid, distension—localized or generalized).
- Skin (scars, striae [stretch marks], dilated veins, rashes, or lesions).
- Masses.
- Pulsations (normal aortic pulsation is visible in the epigastrium).

Auscultation

Auscultate to listen for bowel sounds and for bruits.

- Listen in one place until bowel sounds are heard (normal rate 5–34/minute):
  - Normal bowel sounds (borborygmi) are generally gurgling and relatively low pitched.
  - In bowel obstruction, sounds can be high pitched and tinkling.
  - In complete obstruction, no bowel sounds will be heard (listen for at least 2 minutes).
- Bruits can occur with pathologic arterial stenosis but are also common in normal adults:
  - Midabdominal bruit may suggest atherosclerotic disease in abdominal aorta.
  - Flank bruit may suggest atherosclerotic disease in renal arteries.
  - Hepatic bruit may suggest carcinoma of the liver or alcoholic hepatitis.

Percussion

Percuss all four quadrants and over any suspicious areas of abdominal asymmetry or swelling.

- General.
  - Normal abdomen should have tympanitic areas (gas-filled bowel) and dull areas (fluid-filled bowel).
  - Normal pattern is more tympanitic than dull.
- Liver.
  - Determine liver span, which is directly correlated to liver size.
  - Palpate in all four quadrants once, then again more deeply.

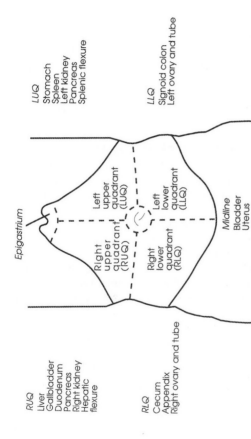

FIGURE 4.13 Location of physical findings in the abdomen are described in terms of the four-quadrant scheme as shown. (Reprinted with permission from Longe RL, Calvert JC. In: Young LYY, ed. *Physical Assessment: A Guide for Evaluating Drug Therapy*. Vancouver, WA: Applied Therapeutics, Inc.; 1994.)

RUQ
Liver
Gallbladder
Duodenum
Pancreas
Right kidney
Hepatic
flexure

RLQ
Cecum
Appendix
Right ovary and tube

LUQ
Stomach
Spleen
Left kidney
Pancreas
Splenic flexure

LLQ
Sigmoid colon
Left ovary and tube

Epigastrium

Left
upper
quadrant
(LUQ)

Left
lower
quadrant
(LLQ)

Right
upper
quadrant
(RUQ)

Right
lower
quadrant
(RLQ)

Midline
Bladder
Uterus

- Abdominal tenderness.
  - *Guarding* is voluntary contraction of the abdominal musculature due to fear, the patient's anxiety, the examiner's cold hands, or tenderness.
  - Rebound is abdominal tenderness that is worse when the palpating fingers are quickly removed from the area being palpated.
  - Rigidity is involuntary contraction of the abdominal musculature in response to peritonitis.
- Abdominal mass.
- Liver. A normal-sized liver generally does not distend more than 1–2 cm below the right costal margin.
- Spleen.
- Descending aorta.
  - Assess for enlargement in people older than 50 years or in those with risk factors for vascular disease.

Genitourinary (GU) and Rectal System

Male

The male GU examination is performed with the patient in the upright position. The penis is examined for skin lesions (e.g., syphilitic ulcers, chancroid, herpetic lesions, condyloma) and urethral discharge (suggesting a sexually transmitted disease). If the foreskin is present, retract it or ask the patient to retract it and look for chancres and carcinomas. Phimosis is the inability to retract the foreskin.

The inguinal area is examined for skin rashes (e.g., tinea cruris, *Candida*). Hernias present as inguinal or scrotal masses. A bulge that appears on straining is suggestive of a hernia. An incarcerated hernia cannot be reduced by pushing the contents back through the defect in the abdominal wall musculature. Other scrotal masses include varicoceles (dilated scrotal veins) and hydroceles (fluid collections are translucent on transillumination with a bright light). Testicular size and masses are noted. Testicular self-examination is important for early diagnosis of cancer. Testicular atrophy can accompany alcoholism. Testicular tenderness is noted in testicular torsion (an acute genitourinary emergency) or orchitis. Epididymal tenderness is present in epididymitis.

Female

The female pelvic examination is typically performed in the dorsal lithotomy (supine with legs in stirrups) position on a specialized examination table. The examination consists of an examination of the external genitalia, a speculum examination, and a bimanual examination of the pelvic organs. The speculum examination allows direct visualization of the vagina and cervix. Appropriate specimens are obtained to evaluate vaginitis or sexually transmitted diseases. The Papanicolaou (Pap) smear is taken to detect cervical cancer. The bimanual examination is so-named because both hands are used to examine the pelvic organs (one internally and the other externally, on the abdominal wall). The cervix is examined for cervical motion tenderness, suggesting pelvic inflammatory disease. The uterus and ovaries (adnexa) are examined for size, tenderness, and the presence of masses.

Rectal Examination

The rectal examination includes palpation of the prostate gland in men to screen for malignancy or enlargement. The prostate is examined for nodules (suggesting cancer) and tenderness (suggesting prostatitis). A normal prostate should feel rubbery, as when pushing the thumb tightly to the little finger. Firm areas identified on prostate examination should be referred for further evaluation.

The rectal examination in men and women should include visual inspection for lumps, ulcers, inflammation, rashes, or excoriations and palpation of the rectum in all directions to identify any masses. The tone of the anal sphincter, the presence of hemorrhoids (internal or external), fissures, or masses should be noted. If stool is present, it can be tested for occult blood (as a screen for malignancy or occult gastrointestinal bleeding). Normally the muscles of the anal sphincter close snugly around the finger. Altered anal sphincter tone may be a sign of neurologic dysfunction.

Peripheral Vascular System

To assess the peripheral vascular system, inspect the arms and legs, palpate pulses, and look for edema. See Figure 4.14 for location of peripheral pulses.

Exam of the Arms
- Size, symmetry, swelling, color.
- Radial and brachial pulses.

Exam of the Legs
- Size, symmetry, color.
- Femoral, popliteal, dorsal pedis, and posterior tibial pulses.
- Peripheral edema.

Several different grading systems are used to characterize peripheral pulses. One such system describes a gradation of pulse intensity from 0 to 4+, with 0 being the absence of a pulse, 3+ being normal, and

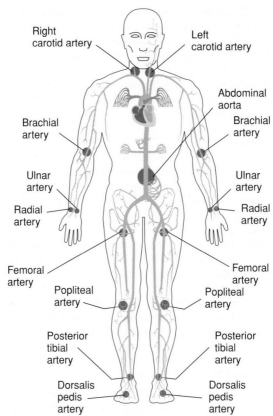

FIGURE 4.14 Locations of peripheral pulses. (Reprinted with permission from Longe RL, Calvert JC. In: Young LYY, ed. *Physical Assessment: A Guide for Evaluating Drug Therapy.* Vancouver, WA: Applied Therapeutics, Inc.; 1994.)

4+ denoting a bounding (strong and forceful) pulse. See example in Table 4.4.

Edema may be pitting or nonpitting. Pitting refers to a noticeable transient indentation in the tissue subsequent to firm pressure with the fingertips over a bony surface and reflects displacement of the excess interstitial fluid. Pitting is graded depending on severity from trace to

Table 4.4 SAMPLE RECORDING SYSTEM FOR PERIPHERAL PULSES

Pulse	Right	Left
Carotid	2/4	2/4
Brachial	2+	2+
Radial	3+	3+
Femoral	3+	3+
Popliteal	2+	2+
Dorsalis pedis (DP)	1+	0
Post tibial (PT)	1+	1+

4+. It is also important to note the location of the pitting edema (i.e., foot, ankle, midshin, knee, etc.).

Musculoskeletal System

The musculoskeletal system comprises the supporting structures of the body such as bones, joints, tendons, ligaments, and musculature.

Joint Examination

- Bony deformities, symmetry, alignment.
- Swelling or effusions.
- Temperature.
- Redness.
- Tenderness.
- Strength and range of motion.
- Surrounding tissue for nodules, skin changes, muscle atrophy, crepitus (an audible or palpable crunching during movements of ligaments or tendons over the bone).

Two common types of arthritis, osteoarthritis (OA) and rheumatoid arthritis (RA), have differing patterns of joint involvement. Osteoarthritis often affects the large weight-bearing joints—the knees, hips, and spine—causing swelling and bony proliferation. In the hands, osteoarthritis affects the proximal and distal interphalangeal (PIP and DIP) joints due to nodules known as Bouchard and Heberden nodes, respectively. Although RA can also affect weight-bearing joints, it classically causes symmetrical small joint arthritis, particularly of the hands, wrists, elbows, and feet. In contrast to OA, RA affects the metacarpophalangeal joints (MCP) and

PIP joints of the hands by causing joint inflammation, swelling, warmth, and pain and spares the DIP joints. A joint's range of motion can become limited by a number of diseases that affect the joint. Improvements in symptoms and examination findings can occur with disease-modifying agents for certain arthritic diseases.

The musculature or motor system is examined for bulk, strength, tone, tenderness, and the presence of abnormal spontaneous movements (e.g., fasciculations). Examination of the motor system is part of the neurologic examination and is discussed in that section.

Neurologic System

Mental Status

A detailed neurologic assessment is an important component of a geriatric physical examination. Impairment of cognitive and motor/sensory function in this population may severely affect quality of life issues and level of function.

Examine

- Appearance (dress, grooming, personal hygiene).
- Behavior (level of consciousness—alert, awake, obtunded, stupor, coma).
- Speech and language.
  - Quantity (talkative, silent, responsive to direct questioning, spontaneous comments).
  - Rate.
  - Loudness.
  - Articulation (clear, distinct, nasal quality).
  - Fluency (rate, flow, and melody of speech; content; and use of words).
- Mood and affect.
- Thoughts and perceptions.
  - Thought processes (logic, organization, relevance, coherence, repetition, confabulation).
  - Thought content (compulsions, obsessions, phobias, anxieties, delusions, feelings of unreality or depersonalization).
  - Perceptions (illusions, hallucinations).
  - Insight and judgment.
- Cognition: There are many tests available to screen for cognitive dysfunction or dementia such as the Mini Mental State Exam (MMSE)[2].
  - Orientation (time, place, person).
  - Attention (common tests include digit span, serial 7s, spelling backward).

▸ Remote memory (inquire about past historical events, birthdays, anniversaries, etc.).
▸ Recent memory (inquire about the events of the day that you can confirm).
▸ Information and vocabulary (e.g., name the last four presidents).
▸ Calculations (use simple addition and progress to multiplication).
▸ Abstract thinking (ask patient how an apple and an orange are alike).
▸ Constructional ability (ask the patient to draw a clock face complete with numbers and hands).

Cranial Nerves

The functions of the 12 cranial nerves (CN I to XII) are described in Table 4-5. A common mnemonic uses the first letter of each word in the following sentence: "*On Old Olympus' Towering Tops, A Finn And German Viewed Some Hops*" to identify the 12 cranial nerves (olfactory, optic, oculomotor, trochlear, trigeminal, abducens, facial, acoustic, glossopharyngeal, vagus, spinal accessory, and hypoglossal).

Motor System

When examining the motor system, pay attention to body position, involuntary movements, coordination, and the characteristics of the muscle (bulk, tone, strength). Use this sequence when examining the arms, legs, and trunk. If an abnormality is discovered, think about its origin (central or peripheral) and what nerves innervate the area.

- Body position (at rest and during movement).
- Involuntary movements (tremors, tics, fasciculations).
- Muscle bulk (compare size and contour).
- Muscle tone (resistance to passive stretching).
- Muscle strength (Table 4.6).
- Coordination (rapid alternating movements, point-to-point movements, gait, stance).

Sensory System

In evaluating a sensory abnormality, the clinician tests whether a deficit fits a dermatomal distribution, indicating dorsal root involvement (Figs. 4.15 and 4.16), or the distribution of a collection of spinal segments, constituting a peripheral nerve (peripheral neuropathy).

- Pain (use a sharp object for a pinprick to assess sharp versus dull).
- Temperature (hot versus cold; may omit if pain sensation is normal).
- Light touch (use soft piece of cotton).

Table 4.5 CRANIAL NERVES AND THEIR FUNCTIONS

Cranial Nerves	Function
Olfactory (I)	Sensory: smell reception and interpretation
Optic (II)	Sensory: visual acuity and visual fields
Oculomotor (III)	Motor: raise eyelids, most extraocular movements, changes of lens shape and papillary constriction
Trochlear (IV)	Motor: inward and downward eye movement
Trigeminal (V)	Motor: chewing, mastication, jaw opening and clenching Sensory: sensation to facial skin, ear, tongue, nasal and mouth mucosa, cornea, iris, lacrimal glands, conjunctiva, eyelids, forehead, and nose
Abducens (VI)	Motor: lateral eye movement
Facial (VII)	Motor: movement of facial expression muscles except jaw, close eyes, labial speech sounds (m, b, w, and round vowels) Sensory: taste, anterior two thirds of tongue, sensation to pharynx Parasympathetic: secretion of tears and saliva
Acoustic (VIII)	Sensory: hearing and balance of equilibrium
Glossopharyngeal (IX)	Motor: voluntary muscles for phonation or swallowing Sensory: sensation of nasopharynx, gag reflex, taste posterior one third of tongue Parasympathetic: secretion of salivary glands, carotid reflex
Vagus (X)	Motor: voluntary muscles of phonation (guttural speech sounds) and swallowing Sensory: sensation behind ear and part of external ear canal Parasympathetic: secretion of digestive enzymes, peristalsis, carotid reflex, involuntary action of heart, lungs, and digestive tract
Spinal accessory (XI)	Motor: turn head, shrug shoulders, some actions for phonation and swallowing
Hypoglossal (XII)	Motor: tongue movement for speech sound articulation (l, t, n) and swallowing

Table 4.6 MUSCLE STRENGTH GRADING

Grade	Muscle Strength
0	No muscle contraction
1	Flicker or trace of contraction
2	Movement possible, but not against gravity
3	Moves against gravity, but not against resistance
4	Can move against resistance
5	Normal strength

- Vibration (tuning fork of 128 Hz vibrating on pad of large toe, not the bone).
- Position (move digit upward or downward and have patient verbalize the direction of movement).
- Discriminative sensations (useful only if touch and position sense is intact; stereognosis: ability to identify an object by feeling it; patients eyes should be closed).

Reflexes

A reflex hammer is needed for evaluation of reflexes, which examines the spinal reflex arc. When an already partially stretched tendon is tapped briskly with a reflex hammer, stretch receptors in the tendon send an impulse to the spinal cord that elicits a contraction of the corresponding muscle. The spinal reflex arc is modified by control from the brain via descending corticospinal tracts. Typically, this often has an inhibitory influence. With damage to those higher centers, as in stroke or descending nerve tracts (i.e., the upper motor neurons), the spinal reflex arc is uninhibited and the reflexes are hyperactive. With damage to the peripheral nerve or particular dorsal roots (i.e., low motor neurons), the reflex arc is interrupted and the reflexes are diminished. Reflexes are graded on a scale from 0 to 4. A stick figure typically appears in the chart to designate the elicited reflexes (Fig. 4.17).

Reflex Response Exam

- Biceps reflex.
- Triceps reflex.
- Supinator or brachioradialis reflex.
- Knee reflex.
- Ankle reflex.

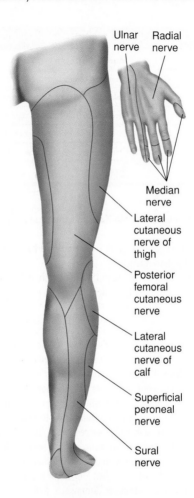

**AREAS INNERVATED BY
PERIPHERAL NERVES**

A

FIGURE 4.15 A: Areas innervated by peripheral nerves. (*continued*)

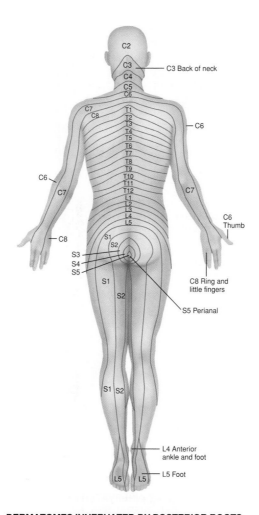

DERMATOMES INNERVATED BY POSTERIOR ROOTS

B

FIGURE 4.15 (*continued*) **B:** Dermatomes innervated by posterior roots. (Reprinted with permission from Bickley LS, Szilagyi PG. In: *Bates' Guide to Physical Examination and History Taking.* 9th ed. Philadelphia, PA: Lippincott Williams & Wilkins; 2007.)

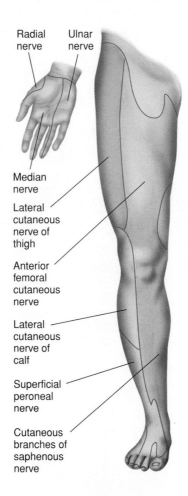

Radial nerve

Ulnar nerve

Median nerve

Lateral cutaneous nerve of thigh

Anterior femoral cutaneous nerve

Lateral cutaneous nerve of calf

Superficial peroneal nerve

Cutaneous branches of saphenous nerve

AREAS INNERVATED BY PERIPHERAL NERVES

A

FIGURE 4.16 A: Areas innervated by peripheral nerves. (*continued*)

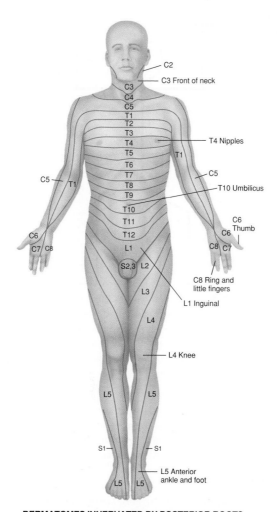

DERMATOMES INNERVATED BY POSTERIOR ROOTS

B

FIGURE 4.16 (*continued*) B: Dermatomes innervated by posterior roots. (Reprinted with permission from Bickley LS, Szilagyi PG. In: *Bates' Guide to Physical Examination and History Taking.* 9th ed. Philadelphia, PA: Lippincott Williams & Wilkins; 2007.)

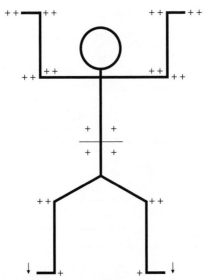

FIGURE 4.17 Example of deep tendons reflex (DTR) recording. Grading scale: 0 = no response; + = diminished; ++ = normal; +++ = hyperactive; ++++ = hyperactive, often with clonus. (Reprinted with permission from Longe RL, Calvert JC. In: Young LYY, ed. *Physical Assessment: A Guide for Evaluating Drug Therapy.* Vancouver, WA: Applied Therapeutics, Inc.; 1994.)

The plantar reflexes refer to the reflex motion of the great toe after a noxious stimuli is applied to the bottom of the foot. An upgoing toe, the Babinski sign, is suggestive of an upper motor neuron lesion (but can be normal in infants). A downgoing toe is normal.

References

1. Bickley LS, Szilagyi PG. *Bates' Guide to Physical Examination and History Taking.* 9th ed. Philadelphia, PA: Lippincott Williams & Wilkins; 2007.
2. Folstein MF, Folstein SE, McHugh PR. "Mini-mental state." A practical method for grading the cognitive state of patients for the clinician. *J Psychiatr Res.* 1975;12(3):189–198.

5 Interpretation of Clinical Laboratory Test Results

Kristina L. Butler

Clinical laboratory tests are valuable tools that may be used to gain additional information about the patient. Although not therapeutic on their own, these tests can be used to differentiate among possible diagnoses, confirm a diagnosis, assess current status, or evaluate response to therapy when history and physical exam alone cannot. Selection of laboratory tests are based on clinical judgment, with evidence-based medicine increasingly used to guide these decisions. This chapter contains many commonly encountered laboratory tests used in clinical medicine and is designed to provide the user with (a) brief descriptions of specific tests, (b) reference ranges in conventional and International System of Units (SI) units, and (c) descriptions of the clinical implications of values falling outside of the reference range. Examples of conditions that may increase or decrease the values obtained are also included, but these examples may not be all-inclusive.

If specific tests are not included or if more detailed information is desired, including an overview of the clinician's role in using laboratory tests, the reader is advised to consult the most recent edition of Frances T. Fischbach's *A Manual of Laboratory and Diagnostic Tests*, published by Lippincott Williams & Wilkins (Philadelphia, Pennsylvania); Mary Lee's *Basic Skills in Interpreting Laboratory Data*, published by American Society of Health-System Pharmacists (Bethesda, Maryland); R.A. Sacher and R.A. McPherson's *Widmann's Clinical Interpretation of Laboratory Tests*, published by F.A. Davis Company (Philadelphia, Pennsylvania); or John B. Henry's *Clinical Diagnosis and Management by Laboratory Methods*, published by W.B. Saunders (Philadelphia, Pennsylvania). Before using the information in this chapter, it is important to review the following general principles regarding laboratory tests.

Basic Concepts

For all laboratory tests, a *specimen* is needed for laboratory analysis. A specimen is a sample that may be obtained through *invasive* (needle, tube, scope, or other device used to penetrate the skin or enter the body) or *noninvasive* methods. See Table 5.1 for a list of common specimens. The substance measured by the laboratory assay is called the *analyte*. Some analytes exist in different forms (referred to as fractions, subtypes, isoenzymes, subforms, or isoforms), and therefore each will have a different *reference range* of values considered acceptable.

The reference range is a statistically derived numeric range obtained by testing a sample of individuals assumed to be healthy; usually established as the mean ± 2 standard deviations (SD). The upper and lower limits reflect points beyond which the probability of clinical significance begins to increase; they are not absolute (i.e., "normal" vs. "abnormal"), however, values that fall within the reference range are often referred to as "normal values." Reference ranges may vary between labs, depending on the analytic technique, reagent, and equipment.[1-5] Reference ranges may also vary between populations and may change as new data are published.

Laboratory tests may be *quantitative* or *qualitative*. The result of a quantitative test is reported as an exact number and assessed in context of a reference range. A *critical value* is a result that is far enough outside the reference range that it indicates impending morbidity. Laboratory test results are reported with various units, which can be confusing. In an

Table 5.1 COMMON LABORATORY SPECIMENS

Whole blood
Venous blood
Arterial blood
Plasma (watery acellular portion of blood)
Serum (liquid remaining after fibrin clot is removed from plasma)
Urine
Stool
Sputum
Sweat
Saliva
Gastric secretions
Vaginal fluid
Exhaled air
Cerebrospinal fluid
Tissues (including nails, hair)

attempt to standardize quantitative measurements worldwide, SI units were introduced in the 1960s; however most clinicians and the general public continue to use and understand conventional units. The result of a qualitative test is reported as positive or negative without comment on the degree of positivity or negativity; exact quantities may be measured but are reported qualitatively using predetermined reference ranges. The exception to this is a *semiquantitative* test, in which the result is reported as either negative or with varying degrees of positivity (e.g., 1+, 2+, 3+) without exact quantification.

Many factors can influence laboratory results (Table 5.2). Laboratory errors are uncommon, but may occur. Such errors should be suspected if one or more of the following occurs:

- Unusual trends develop.
- The magnitude of error is large.
- The result is not in agreement with confirmatory results.
- The result is inconsistent with clinical signs, symptoms, or other patient-specific information.

Abnormal values are not always clinically significant, and on occasion, values within the reference range can be considered abnormal in some diseases or conditions. Therefore, it is important to refer to published data or reference standards used by the laboratory performing the test and to consider potential interferences with the test in question.[1] The reference ranges in this chapter refer primarily to adults unless otherwise indicated and may vary between laboratories.

The clinical value of a laboratory test depends on its *sensitivity*, *specificity*, *accuracy*, *precision*, and the *incidence* of the disease/disorder in a given population. Accuracy and precision are measures of how well the test performs day-to-day in a laboratory, whereas sensitivity and specificity reflect the ability of the test to distinguish disease from absence of disease. The accuracy and precision of each test are pre-established and are frequently monitored by professional laboratory personnel. Sensitivity and specificity data are determined by research studies, are generally published in medical literature, and do not change with different populations. In contrast, the *predictive value* of a single test can vary with age, gender, and geographic location.[4] See Table 5.3 for definitions and formulas to further explain these concepts.

Laboratory tests can be categorized as *screening* or *diagnostic* tests. Screening tests detect disease early when interventions are likely to be effective and are generally fairly simple and highly sensitive tests,

Table 5.2 FACTORS THAT MAY INFLUENCE LABORATORY RESULTS

Patient-Specific Factors

Demographics	• Age • Gender • Ethnicity • Genetics (enzyme polymorphisms) • Occupation • Height • Weight • Body surface area
Food/nutrition	• Postprandial or fasting status • Type of food ingested/diet • Food-assay interactions • Nutritional status • Hydration status
Drugs	• Drug–drug interactions • Drug–disease interactions • Drug–assay interactions • Time of last dose (peak vs. trough) • Steady–state status • Nonadherence • Undisclosed drug, tobacco, or alcohol use
Clinical situation	• Disease acuity • Disease severity • Type of illness • Disease–assay interactions • Pregnancy • Stress • Organ function • Interfering diagnostic or therapeutic procedures
Posture	• Position/activity at time of specimen collection • Exercise/fitness level
Other	• Time of day (biologic rhythms) • Level of patient knowledge and understanding of testing process • Nonadherence with instructions and pretest preparation • Incorrect/incomplete patient preparation • Altitude

Laboratory-Specific Factors

Specimen Issues	• Specimen type (Table 5-1) • Incorrect order of draw • Wrong/absent preservative, wrong transport medium • Incomplete collection (especially timed samples), insufficient volume, insufficient number of samples • Hemolyzed blood sample • Old/deteriorating specimen • Air bubbles in tube

(continued)

Table 5.2   FACTORS THAT MAY INFLUENCE LABORATORY RESULTS *(continued)*

Laboratory-Specific Factors

Collector issues	• Delayed delivery • Improper collection, handling, storage, labeling, or preparation • Incorrect timing of sample (especially for peak/trough levels) • Discrepancy between test ordered and specimen collected
Testing issues	• Different/incorrect method of analysis • Free vs. bound analyte • Deteriorated reagents • Calibration errors • Technical/equipment error • Calculation errors • Misreading results • Computer entry/documentation errors

Source: Fischbach F. *A Manual of Laboratory Diagnostic Tests.* 6th ed. Philadelphia, PA: Lippincott Williams & Wilkins; 2004.

performed in individuals without signs or symptoms of common diseases. In comparison, diagnostic tests are performed in patients with signs, symptoms, or history of a specific disease or disorder, or an abnormal screening test. These tests tend to be more complex and highly specific, directed specifically to the individual patient. Related tests may be grouped into a set called a *profile* or a *panel* (Table 5.4); small differences may exist between panels and preferred panels, and their names may vary between laboratories/institutions. Abbreviations for specific laboratory tests and panels are common, and test results may be recorded in a patient's chart using various formats. With experience, clinicians are often able to identify particular laboratory tests by knowing the reference range.

Laboratory testing occurs in many environments, including hospitals, clinics, and the community. *Point-of-care* testing (POC or POCT) refers to tests done at the site of patient care, i.e., at the patient's bedside, clinic, pharmacy, or even home (usually referred to as *home-testing*). Point-of-care testing can provide rapid results with increased portability and convenience and may further engage patients in the management of their disease or condition. Other POC advantages include blood conservation, decreased specimen transport/storage/processing error, and overall cost

Table 5.3 LABORATORY TERMINOLOGY

Term	Definition	Formula
True-positive (TP)	Individuals with a given disease or condition who are detected by the test	
True-negative (TN)	Individuals without a given disease or condition who are not detected by the test	
False-positive (FP)	Individuals without a given disease or condition who test positive	
False-negative (FN)	Individuals with a given disease or condition who are not detected by the test	
Sensitivity	The ability of a test to correctly identify those individuals who have a given disease or condition; true-positive rate	$[TP \div (TP + FN)] \times 100\%$
Specificity	The ability of a test to correctly identify those individuals who do not have a given disease or condition; true-negative rate	$[TN \div (TN + FP)] \times 100\%$
Accuracy	The ability of a test to produce a result that approaches the absolute true value of the substance being measured	$[(TP + TN) \div (TP + TN + FP + FN)] \times 100\%$
Precision	The reliability of a test to produce similar results on repeated analysis of the same sample, with small amounts of random variation	
Incidence/prevalence	The rate of presence of a disease or condition within a (tested) population or community	$[(TP + FN) \div (TP + TN + FP + FN)] \times 100\%$
Predictive values	The ability of a screening test result to correctly identify the presence or absence of a given disease or condition in a population; predictive values may be positive (PPV) or negative (NPV)	
Positive predictive value (PPV)	The percentage of positive tests with true-positive results	$[TP \div (TP + FP)] \times 100\%$
Negative predictive value (NPV)	The percentage of negative tests with true-negative results	$[TN \div (TN + FN)] \times 100\%$

Sources: Fischbach F. A Manual of Laboratory Diagnostic Tests. 6th ed. Philadelphia, PA: Lippincott Williams & Wilkins; 2004; and Lee M. Basic Skills in Interpreting Laboratory Data. 3rd ed. Bethesda, MD: American Society of Health-System Pharmacists; 2004, with permission.

Table 5.4 COMMON LABORATORY PANELS

Panel (abbreviation)	Basic Metabolic Panel (BMP)	Comprehensive Metabolic Panel (CMP)	Electrolytes (Lytes)	Renal Function Panel	Hepatic Panel
Elements (abbreviation)	• Sodium (Na⁺) • Potassium (K⁺) • Chloride (Cl⁻) • Carbon dioxide (CO₂) • Blood urea nitrogen (BUN) • Creatinine (Cr or SCr) • Glucose • Calcium (Ca²⁺)	BMP plus • Albumin (Alb) • Total protein (TP, albumin/globulin [A/G] ratio) • Alkaline phosphatase (ALP, Alk phos) • Alanine aminotransferase (ALT, formerly known as SGPT) • Aspartate aminotransferase (AST, formerly known as SGOT) • Total bilirubin (T Bili, TBIL)	• Na⁺ • K⁺ • Cl⁻ • CO₂	BMP plus • Phosphorus • Lactic acid dehydrogenase (LDH) • Creatinine clearance (Cr-Cl) • TP, A/G ratio • Alb	• ALT • AST • ALP • T Bili • Direct bilirubin (D Bili, conjugated bilirubin) • Alb • TP, A/G ratio • Gamma glutamyl-transferase (GGT) • LDH

Panel (abbreviation) continued	Thyroid Function	Cardiac Markers	Lipid Profile	Enzymes	Hematology Panel (Hemogram)
Elements (abbreviation) continued	• Triiodothyronine (T₃) • T₃ uptake ratio (T₃ UR) • Total thyroxine (T₄) • Free T₄ • Thyroid-stimulating hormone (TSH)	BMP plus • Cardiac troponin (troponin) • Creatine kinase (CK) • Creatine kinase–myoglobin (CK-MB) • Homocysteine	• Total cholesterol (TC) • Triglycerides (TG) • High-density lipoprotein (HDL) • Low-density lipoprotein (LDL) May also include: • Very-low-density lipoprotein (VLDL) • Cholesterol/HDL ratio	• ALT • AST • Amylase • Lipase • GGT • LDH • CK	• Red blood cell (RBC) count • Hemoglobin (Hgb) • Hematocrit (Hct) • Platelet count • White blood cell (WBC) count • Mean corpuscular volume (MCV) • Mean corpuscular hemoglobin (MCH) • Mean corpuscular hemoglobin concentration (MCHC) • Red cell distribution width (RDW)

(continued)

Table 5.4 COMMON LABORATORY PANELS (continued)

Panel (abbreviation)	Complete Blood Count (CBC) with Differential (diff)	Iron Tests	Coagulation Panel	Arterial Blood Gases (ABG)	Urine Electrolytes
Elements (abbreviation)	Hemogram plus • WBC differential • Segmented neutrophils • Bands • Eosinophils • Basophils • Lymphocytes • Atypical lymphocytes • Monocytes	• Serum iron (Fe) • Total iron-binding capacity (TIBC) • Serum ferritin • Tranferrin	• Prothrombin time (PT)/International normalized ratio (INR) • Activated partial thromboplastin time (aPTT) • Fibrinogen • Hemogram with Platelet	• pH • PCO_2 • PO_2 • Base excess • Bicarbonate (HCO_3)	• Na^+ • K^+

savings. However, POC testing has the potential for misuse or misinterpretation of results, delays in seeking medical advice, loss of epidemiologic data, documentation errors, inappropriate material disposal, and quality assurance issues.[5]

Before obtaining the test specimen, a relevant history and assessment should be performed, with particular attention paid to any conditions that could affect the testing process or test results (e.g., allergies, phobias, pregnancy, diseases, cultural or language diversity, physical or mental impairments). Standard/universal precautions should be observed with every patient, and all patients should be monitored for complications following their specimen procurement, particularly if invasive tests are performed.[4]

Laboratory Tests

Hematologic Tests

A hemogram consists of a white blood cell count (WBC), red blood cell count (RBC), hemoglobin (Hgb or Hb), hematocrit (Hct), red blood cell indices, and a platelet count. A complete blood count (CBC) consists of a hemogram plus a differential WBC. The tests of a CBC provide information on both the quantity and quality of blood cells. Table 5.5 provides descriptions, reference ranges and clinical implications of CBC results in adults. The reference ranges of Hgb, Hct, WBC, and other hematologic tests vary for infants, children, and adolescents, but are often higher at birth and decrease over several years. However, values may be higher for adults than for older children and adolescents.

Iron is necessary for the production of Hgb, and iron tests measure the body's iron in its several components. Transferrin, serum iron (Fe), and total iron-binding capacity (TIBC) are used together in the differential diagnosis of anemia, assessing treatment of iron-deficiency anemia, and evaluating other blood disorders. Table 5.6 provides descriptions, reference ranges and clinical implications of iron study results in adults. Reference ranges for newborns and children can be found in other resources.

Hemostasis and coagulation tests are used to diagnosis, evaluate, and monitor patients with bleeding or clotting disorders or vascular injury or trauma. The common coagulation and hemostasis tests are presented in Table 5.7.

Table 5.5 HEMOGRAM REFERENCE RANGES FOR ADULTS

Test Name	Description	Reference Range Conventional Units	Reference Range SI Units	Increased With	Decreased With	Other Comments
Hematocrit (Hct)	Measures the amount of space RBCs take up in the blood, or RBC mass	Male: 37%–53% Female: 36%–46%	M: 0.37–0.53 F: 0.36–0.46	Erythrocytosis, dehydration, chronic obstructive pulmonary disease (COPD), polycythemia, shock	Anemia (various causes), hemolytic reactions, leukemia, cirrhosis, massive blood loss, hyperthyroidism	• Approximately 3 times Hgb • Usually parallels the RBC count when erythrocytes are of a normal size • Lacks clinical validity in sickle cell anemia, immediately after moderate blood loss or transfusion; may appear normal after acute hemorrhage • Decreased in iron-deficiency anemia because microcytic (small) cells pack into a smaller volume; however, RBC count may appear normal

| Hemoglobin (Hgb) | Measures amount of Hbg contained in RBCs; indication of oxygen capacity of blood | Male: 13–18 g/dL Female: 12–16 g/dL | M: 8.1–11.2 mmol/L F: 7.4–9.9 mmol/L | Dehydration, hemoconcentration (polycythemia, burns), excess production of RBCs in the bone marrow, hyperlipidemia, COPD, congestive heart failure (CHF), high altitudes | Anemia (various causes), cirrhosis, hemorrhage, hemolytic reactions, increased fluid intake, kidney disease, other chronic illnesses, aplastic anemia, leukemia, hyperthyroidism, pregnancy | • Consists of globin (4 protein subunits), a heme core, an iron atom, and a porphyrin ring
• When Hbg carries O_2, blood is scarlet (arterial); when it loses O_2, the blood becomes dark red (venous)
• One gram of Hgb carries 1.34 mL of O_2
• Used to assess anemia severity, response to treatment, or progression of associated disease(s)
• A decrease in the protein subtypes A_1, A_2, and F (fetal), and the appearance of type S Hgb is associated with sickle cell anemia
• Concentration fluctuates in patients with hemorrhages and burns because of fluid replacement and blood transfusions

(continued) |

Table 5.5 HEMOGRAM REFERENCE RANGES FOR ADULTS (continued)

Test Name	Description	Reference Range Conventional Units	Reference Range SI Units	Increased With	Decreased With	Other Comments
Red blood cell (RBC, erythrocyte count)	Quantification of RBCs; functional changes usually monitored by Hgb or Hct	Male: 4.4–5.9 × 10^6 cells/μL (or /mm^3) Female: 3.8–5.2 × 10^6 cells/μL (or /mm^3)	M: 4.4–5.9 × 10^{12} cells/L F: 3.8–5.2 × 10^{12} cells/L	Polycythemia vera, secondary polycythemia (hormone secreting tumors), diarrhea/dehydration, vigorous exercise, burns, high altitudes	Anemias, systemic lupus erythematosus (SLE)	• Decreased O_2 stimulates RBC production via erythropoietin • Usually released into the circulation as mature cells; if demand is high, immature cells (reticulocytes) will be released • RBCs have a life span ~120 days; older RBCs are removed from circulation by phagocytes in the spleen, hepatic, and bone marrow (reticuloendothelial system [RES])

RBC Indices

| Mean corpuscular volume (MCV) | = Hct/RBC Calculates the mean volume/size of RBCs | 78–100 μm^3 | 78–100 fL/cell | (Macrocytic) hepatic disease, alcoholism, folate/B_{12} deficiency, reticulocytosis, hyperglycemia, leukemia, drugs (antimetabolites, zidovudine, valproate, phenytoin, oral contraceptives, primidone, phenobarbital, methotrexate, pentamidine, sulfamethoxazole, triamterene, trimethoprim, colchicine, neomycin) | (Microcytic) iron-deficiency, pernicious anemia, thalassemia | • Expressed as normocytic (normal size), microcytic (small size, <75 fL), or macrocytic (large size, >105 fL)
 • Useful in the diagnosis of anemia.
 • Questionable value in sickle cell anemia, because the Hct is unreliable due to the abnormal RBC shape
 • A calculated value; therefore, possible to have a wide variation in macrocytes/microcytes and still have a normal MCV
 • Anemia of inflammatory disease may present with normal or low MCV
 (continued) |

Table 5.5 HEMOGRAM REFERENCE RANGES FOR ADULTS *(continued)*

Test Name	Description	Reference Range		Increased With	Decreased With	Other Comments
		Conventional Units	SI Units			
Mean corpuscular hemoglobin (MCH)	= Hgb/RBC. Calculates amount of Hgb inside RBCs	25–35 pg/cell	25–35 pg/cell	Folate/B₁₂ deficiency, hyperlipidemia	Iron deficiency	• Useful in the diagnosis of anemia • Affected by RBC size
Mean corpuscular hemoglobin concentration (MCHC)	= Hgb/Hct Amount of Hgb in terms of % volume of cell	31–37 g/dL	310–370 g/L	(Hyperchromia) hyperlipidemia, hereditary spherocytosis	(Hypochromia) iron deficiency, thalassemia, microcytic anemia, pyridoxine-responsive anemia, hypochromic anemia	• Expressed as normochromic (normal color), hypochromic (light color), or hyperchromic (dark color) • A better index of RBC Hgb than MCH, because MCHC is not affected by cell size
Reticulocyte (Retic) count	Quantification of immature, nonnucleated cells of the erythrocyte series in circulation	0.5%–2.5% of RBCs	0.005–0.025	Acute blood loss, sickle cell disease, hemolysis; indication that RBC production is accelerated	Untreated iron/vitamin B₁₂/folate deficiency; aplastic anemia, chronic infection, radiation therapy; indication that bone marrow RBC production is reduced	• If demand is high, reticulocytes will be released from the bone marrow into circulation prior to maturation to erythrocytes • If anemia present and reticulocyte count not increased, suggests insufficient production of erythrocytes by bone marrow

RBC distribution width (RDW)	Calculation of the variation in RBC size/volume (anisocytosis)	11.5%–15%	0.115–0.150	Iron/B_{12}/folate deficiency, hemolytic anemia, mixed anemias	• An increase in retics (~20%, maximum seen 7–14 days after treatment) reflects the effectiveness of anemias treatment • The greater the variation in RBC size, the larger the % • In some anemias (e.g., pernicious anemia), the anisocytosis (along with variation in shape, poikilocytosis) causes an increase in the RDW • Normal RDW is seen in thalassemia and in anemia of inflammatory disease
Platelet (PLT, thrombocytes) count	Quantification of platelets	$140–400 \times 10^3$ cells/μL (or /mm^3)	$140–400 \times 10^9$/L	(Thrombocythemia/ thrombocytosis) cancer, polycythemia vera, splenectomy, trauma, cirrhosis, myelogenous/ granulocytic leukemia, stress, iron-deficiency anemia, rapid blood regeneration, acute and chronic infection and inflammatory diseases, renal (Thrombocytopenia) idiopathic thrombocytopenia purpura (ITP), disseminated intravascular coagulation (DIC), pernicious, aplastic and hemolytic anemias, bone marrow lesions, toxemia or eclampsia in pregnancy,	• Necessary for clot formation. During adhesion/ aggregation, coagulation is triggered and thrombin is formed. Platelets then become interspersed with RBCs and WBCs to form a clot • Life span of ~7–12 days; 2/3 circulating and 1/3 in the spleen

(continued)

Table 5.5 HEMOGRAM REFERENCE RANGES FOR ADULTS (continued)

Test Name	Description	Reference Range — Conventional Units	Reference Range — SI Units	Increased With	Decreased With	Other Comments
				failure, recovery from bone marrow suppression	alcohol toxicity/abuse, CHF, inherited syndromes, hypersplenism, renal insufficiency, antiplatelet antibodies, thrombopoietin deficiency, drugs (amrinone, antineoplastic agents, gold salts, heparin, sulfonamides, quinidine, H_2 receptor antagonists, penicillins, penicillamine, valproic acid), radiation, human immunodeficiency virus (HIV) infection	• Spontaneous bleeding, prolonged bleeding time, petechiae, or ecchymosis may occur with values <20,000; the precise number necessary for hemostasis is not established • Aspirin and nonsteroidal anti-inflammatory drugs (NSAIDs) primarily affect platelet function rather than number
Mean Platelet Volume (MPV)	Measurement of the average size of platelets	6.4–11 μm^3	6.4–11 fL	ITP, septic thrombocytopenia, myeloproliferative disorders, myelogenous leukemia, massive hemorrhage, splenectomy, vasculitis, prosthetic heart valve, megaloblastic anemia	Aplastic anemia, Wiskott-Aldrich syndrome	• Platelet size is larger when the body is producing increased numbers of platelets; results can be used to make inferences about platelet production in bone marrow • Has been positively associated with measures of platelet activity; may be a useful indicator of the risk of vascular events

| White blood cell (WBC, leukocyte) count | Quantification of leukocytes (WBCs) | $4.4-11 \times 10^3$ cells/μL (or /mm^3) | $4.4-11 \times 10^9$ cells/L | (Leukocytosis) hemorrhage, trauma, drugs (mercury, epinephrine, corticosteroids), necrosis, toxins (eclampsia), leukemia; mild: food, exercise, emotion, menstruation, stress, seizures, cold baths | (Leukopenia) viral infections, hypersplenism, leukemia, drugs (antimetabolites, antibiotics, anticonvulsants, chemotherapy), pernicious/aplastic anemia | • Main functions are fighting infection, phagocytosis of foreign organisms, and production or transportation/distribution of antibodies. The two major types of WBCs are granulocytes (neutrophils, eosinophils, and basophils) and agranulocytes (lymphocytes and monocytes)
• Leukocytosis: WBC increase to 10.5–20 (slight); >30 (moderate); >50 (high); usually due to an increase of only one cell type (e.g., neutrophilia). Absence of anemia helps to distinguish infection from leukemia
• Leukopenia: WBC decrease to <4 |

(continued)

133

Table 5.5 HEMOGRAM REFERENCE RANGES FOR ADULTS (continued)

Test Name	Description	Reference Range Conventional Units	Reference Range SI Units	Increased With	Decreased With	Other Comments
Differential WBC count (diff)	Determines the specific patterns of WBCs in circulation					
Neutrophils (polymor- phonuclear segmented neutrophils, PMNs, polys, segs)	Most laboratories report neutrophils by combining segs and bands and reporting as an absolute number; also reported as % of WBCs. Absolute neutrophil count (ANC) = WBC × (% segs + % bands)	1.7–7.5×10^3 cells/μL (or /mm^3), 45%–74% ANC: 1.5–8×10^3 cells/μL (or /mm^3)	1.7–7.5×10^9/L, 0.45–0.75	(Neutrophilia) bacterial or parasitic infections, metabolic disturbances, hemorrhage, myeloproliferative disorders; mild/temporary: stress, excitement, exercise; notable increases compared to total WBC count may indicate a severe infection	(Neutropenia) decreased neutrophil production, increased cell disappearance, viral infection, blood diseases, hormonal disorders, toxic agents, massive infection	• Neutrophils fight bacterial infection (phagocytosis) and inflammatory disorders (rheumatoid arthritis [RA], asthma, and inflammatory bowel disease [IBD]) • A "shift to right" (an increase in segs, mature cells) occurs in hepatic disease, megaloblastic anemia due to B$_{12}$/folate deficiency, hemolysis, tissue breakdown, surgery, certain drugs (corticosteroids) • Degree of neutrophilia is proportionate to the amount of tissue involved in inflammation

Cell type	Reported as	Reference range	Reference range (SI)	Increased	Decreased	Notes
Bands	Reported as an absolute number or % of WBCs	0–0.4 × 10³ cells/μL (or /mm³), 0–5%	0–0.4 × 10⁹/L, 0–0.05	(Shift to left) infection, chemotherapeutic agents, a cell production disorder (leukemia), hemorrhage		• Bands are neutrophils in early stages of maturity
Eosinophils (EOS)	Reported as an absolute number or % of WBCs	0–0.5 × 10³ cells/μL (or /mm³), 0–8%	0–0.5 × 10⁹/L, 0–0.08	(Eosinophilia) neoplasm, Addison disease, allergic reactions, collagen vascular disease, parasitic infections, L-tryptophan (eosinophilic-myalgia syndrome)	(Eosinopenia) glucocorticoid excess (endogenous —bodily stress [infectious mononucleosis], Cushing disease—or exogenous)	• Eosinophils fight allergic disorders (ingest antigen-antibody complexes) and parasitic infections (phagocytosis) • EOS disappear early in pyogenic infections • Eosinophilia can be masked by steroid use
Basophils (mast cells)	Reported as an absolute number or % of WBCs	0–0.2 × 10³ cells/μL (or /mm³), 0–3%	0–0.2 × 10⁹/L, 0–0.03	(Basophilia) is granulocytic and basophilic leukemia, myeloid metaplasia, allergic reactions with high serum concentration of histamine	(Basopenia) acute infections, stress reactions, after prolonged steroid therapy	• Basophils fight blood dyscrasias and myeloproliferative disease; phagocytic cells that contain heparin, histamine, and serotonin
Monocytes (Monomorphonuclear monocytes)	Reported as an absolute number or % of WBCs	0.2–0.9 × 10³ cells/μL (or /mm³), 4%–11%	0.2–0.9 × 10⁹/L, 0.04–0.11	(Monocytosis) viral, bacterial and parasitic infections, collagen vascular and hematologic disorders	(Monocytopenia) secondary to stress, glucocorticoids, myelotoxic or immunosuppressive drugs	• The largest cells in the blood and serve as the body's second line of defense. Macrophages capable of phagocytosis and scavenger functions • Monocytes fight severe infections • Monocytes also produce interferon

(continued)

Table 5.5 HEMOGRAM REFERENCE RANGES FOR ADULTS (continued)

Test Name	Description	Reference Range		Increased With	Decreased With	Other Comments
		Conventional Units	SI Units			
Lymphocyte (monomorphonuclear lymphocytes)	Reported as an absolute number or % of WBCs	$1-3.5 \times 10^3$ cells/μL (or /mm^3), 16%–46%	$1-3.5 \times 10^9$/L, 0.16–0.46	(Lymphocytosis) viral diseases (mumps, mononucleosis, upper respiratory infections), bacterial diseases, hormonal disorders	(lymphopenia) Hodgkin disease, SLE, burns, trauma	• Lymphocytes are the second most common WBC; these small, mobile cells migrate during early and late stages of inflammation, elaborate immunoglobulins, and are important in cellular immune response. Located in the spleen, lymphatic tissue, and lymph nodes • Virocytes (stress lymphocytes, Downy type cells, atypical lymphocytes) are atypical cells than can also appear in viral, fungoid, and parasitic infections, after transfusions, and as a response to stress • Transformed lymphocytes are used as a measure of histocompatibility

Sources: http://www.labtestsonline.org. Accessed January 25, 2008; Kratz A, Lewandrowski KB. Case records of the Massachusetts General Hospital. Weekly clinicopathological exercises. Normal reference laboratory values. N Engl J Med. 1998;339:1063–1072; OHSU Test Directory of Lab and Pathology Services http://www.ohsu.edu/health/consult-and-refer/labtests/index.cfm. Accessed February 1, 2008; Fischbach F. A Manual of Laboratory Diagnostic Tests. 6th ed. Philadelphia, PA: Lippincott Williams & Wilkins; 2004; and Lee M. Basic Skills in Interpreting Laboratory Data. 3rd ed. Bethesda, MD: American Society of Health-System Pharmacists; 2004, with permission.

Table 5.6 IRON STUDIES AND RELATED HEMATOLOGIC TESTS

Test Name	Description	Reference Range		Increased With	Decreased With	Other Comments
		Conventional Units	SI Units			
Serum iron (Fe)	Measures the amount of iron bound to transferrin	30–175 μg/dl	5.4–31.3 μmol/L	Hemolytic anemia, pernicious anemia, thalassemia, acute hepatitis, acute porphyria, hemochromatosis, pyridoxine deficiency, excessive iron therapy, repeated transfusions, nephritis, lead poisoning, acute leukemia	Iron-deficiency anemia, remission of pernicious anemia, chronic blood loss, kwashiorkor, some systemic infections, idiopathic pulmonary hemosiderosis, hypothyroidism, paroxysmal nocturnal hemoglobinuria, pregnancy (third trimester), progesterone oral contraceptives, RA, SLE	• Many patients with iron-deficiency anemia have levels in the low-normal range (false-negative results). • Fe alone has limited utility for diagnosis or monitoring, as well as significant (<30%) diurnal and day-to-day variations *[continued]*

Table 5.6 IRON STUDIES AND RELATED HEMATOLOGIC TESTS (continued)

Test Name	Description	Reference Range		Increased With	Decreased With	Other Comments
		Conventional Units	SI Units			
Total iron-binding capacity (TIBC)	Indirect measure of serum transferrin	225–450 μg/dL	40.3–76.1 μmol/L	Iron-deficiency anemia, acute and chronic blood loss, acute hepatic damage, pregnancy, oral contraceptives	Hemochromatosis, anemias (of chronic diseases and infections), other non-iron-deficiency anemias, nephrosis, thalassemia, hypoproteinemia (malnutrition and burns), cirrhosis, hyperthyroidism	• Less sensitive to changes in iron stores than serum ferritin
Transferrin	Measures the transport protein that regulates iron absorption	250–425 mg/dL	2.5–4.25 g/L	Iron-deficiency anemia, estrogen therapy, pregnancy, hypoxia, oral contraceptives	Anemia of chronic disease, nephrosis, gastrointestinal (GI) losses, severe burns, chronic infections, malnutrition, genetic deficiency (atransferrinemia), kwashiorkor, severe hepatic disease, some inflammatory conditions, iron overdose	• High levels relate to the ability of the body to deal with infections

| Transferrin (iron) saturation | % = (100 × Fe) ÷ TIBC | ~30%
Male: 10%–50%
Female: 1%–50% | | Hemochromatosis, increased iron intake, thalassemia, hemosiderosis, acute hepatic disease | Iron-deficiency anemias, malignancy (standard and small intestine), anemia of infection and chronic disease, iron neoplasms | • Remaining unsaturated % reflects TIBC (though relationship is not linear) |
| Ferritin | Measure of iron stores; most reliable indicator of total-body iron status | Male: 20–322 ng/mL
Female: 10–291 ng/mL | M: 20–322 μg/L
F: 10–291 μg/L | Hemochromatosis, hemosiderosis, iron supplementation, alcoholic hepatic disease, end-stage renal disease, some malignancies, hyperthyroidism, non-iron-deficiency anemias, chronic inflammation | Iron-deficiency anemia | • More specific and sensitive than Fe or TIBC for diagnosing iron deficiency
• Decreases seen before anemia and other changes occur
• Levels should return to normal within a few days of the start of iron therapy; if remain low, consider nonadherence or continued iron loss
• Increases with age
• No value in alcoholic hepatic disease

(continued) |

Table 5.6 IRON STUDIES AND RELATED HEMATOLOGIC TESTS (continued)

Test Name	Description	Reference Range		Increased With	Decreased With	Other Comments
		Conventional Units	SI Units			
Glucose-6-phosphate dehydrogenase (G6PD) in erythrocytes	Identification of sex-linked disorder, with major variants in specific ethnic groups • Affects 13% of African American men and 3% of African American women (~20% carriers) • Decreased in ~50% of Iraqis, Kurds, Sephardic Jews, and Lebanese (less common in Greeks, Italians, Turks, and North Africans) • Decreased enzyme levels also seen in Southeast Asians	7–20.5 international U/g Hgb	0.11–0.34 nkat/g Hgb	G6PD deficiency, congenital nonspherocytic anemia, nonimmunologic hemolytic disease of the newborn (Asian and Mediterranean)	Untreated pernicious/megaloblastic anemia, thrombocytopenia purpura, hyperthyroidism, viral hepatitis, chronic blood loss, myocardial infarction (MI)	Deficiencies: • Class I: most severe; presents as chronic hemolysis in the absence of oxidative stress • Class II: G6PD <10% of normal; associated with severe episodic hemolysis • Class III: occasional hemolytic episodes with identifiable precipitating factors • Class IV: normal • Precipitating factors include aspirin, aminoquinoline antimalarials, salicylates, methylene blue, quinine, quinidine, large doses of ascorbic acid, nitrofurantoin, some sulfonamides and sulfones, fava beans, infections, and diabetic ketoacidosis; hemolysis generally occurs by day 3 of factor exposure • Degree of hemolysis depends on extent of deficiency and dose of precipitating agent

Vitamin B$_{12}$ (VB$_{12}$)	Antipernicious anemia factor	200–950 pg/mL 148–701 pmol/L	Leukemia, chronic renal failure, hepatic disease, cancer with hepatic metastasis, polycythemia vera, CHF, diabetes mellitus (DM), obesity, COPD, pregnancy, blood transfusion, high vitamin A and C doses, smoking	Pernicious/megaloblastic anemia, malabsorption syndromes (IBD, tapeworm, loss of gastric mucosa, Zollinger-Ellison syndrome (ZES), blind loop syndromes), vegetarian diet, folic acid deficiency, hypothyroidism	• Necessary for the production of RBCs • Increases with age • The Schilling test is used to determine whether vitamin B$_{12}$ deficiency is caused by malabsorption
Folic acid (folate)		1.9–20 ng/mL (serum) 140–628 ng/mL (RBC) 4.3–45.3 nmol/L (serum) 317–2,045 nmol/L (RBC)	blind loop syndrome, vegetarian diet, pernicious anemia, VB$_{12}$ deficiency	inadequate intake (Alcoholism, chronic disease, malnutrition, anorexia, lack of fresh vegetables), malabsorption (small bowel disease, high requirements (pregnancy), hypothyroidism), megaloblastic anemia, hepatic disease, celiac disease, vitamin B$_6$ deficiency, carcinomas, leukemia, Crohn disease, intestinal resection, drugs (anticonvulsants, methotrexate, antimalarials, alcohol, oral contraceptives, high-dose antacids)	• Needed for normal RBC and WBC function, and production of cellular genes

Sources: http://www.labtestsonline.org. Accessed January 25, 2008; Kratz A, Lewandrowski KB. Case records of the Massachusetts General Hospital. Weekly clinicopathological exercises. Normal reference laboratory values. *N Engl J Med.* 1998;339:1063–1072; OHSU Test Directory of Lab and Pathology Services http://www.ohsu.edu/health/consult-and-refer/labtests/index.cfm. Accessed February 1, 2008; Fischbach F. *A Manual of Laboratory Diagnostic Tests.* 6th ed. Philadelphia, PA: Lippincott Williams & Wilkins; 2004; and Lee M. *Basic Skills in Interpreting Laboratory Data.* 3rd ed. Bethesda, MD: American Society of Health-System Pharmacists; 2004; with permission.

Table 5.7 COAGULATION TESTS

Test Name	Description	Reference Range		Increased With	Decreased With	Other Comments
		Conventional Units	SI Units			
Bleeding time	Measures the primary phases of hemostasis; best test to screen for platelet function disorders	2–10 min		Platelet function disorders, thrombocytopenia, decreased or abnormal plasma factors (von Willebrand factor, fibrinogen), DIC, abnormalities in small blood vessel walls, vascular disease, leukemia, renal failure, hepatic failure, scurvy, excessive alcohol consumption, drugs (aspirin, dipyridamole, dextran, fibrinolytics)		• Extreme temperatures can alter test results • Edema or cyanosis of the extremity used will invalidate the test
Prothrombin time (Pro time, PT)	Directly measures for potential defects in the extrinsic thromboplastin system (factors I [fibrinogen], II [prothrombin], V, VII, and X)	10–15 s (can vary significantly by laboratory)		Extrinsic thromboplastin factor deficiencies, vitamin K deficiency, DIC, hemorrhagic disease of the newborn, premature newborns, hepatic disease, biliary obstruction, poor fat absorption, ZES, lupus or other endogenous circulating anticoagulants, salicylate intoxication, drugs (warfarin, heparin)	Increased vitamin K intake (green leafy vegetables)	• Not affected by platelet disorders (ITP), polycythemia vera, hemophilia A (factor VIII deficiency), Christmas disease (factor IX deficiency), von Willebrand disease, or tannin disease • Evaluation of bleeding is necessary if significantly prolonged • Prothrombin time ratio (PTR) = patient's PT ÷ control PT (lab's mean normal); therapeutic levels are 2.0–2.5

International normalized ratio (INR)	Standardizes PT results between laboratories; used for warfarin monitoring	0.8–1.2	Same as PT	Same as PT	• Conversion of PTR to INR requires knowledge of the sensitivity of the thromboplastin reagent used (expressed as an international sensitivity index [ISI]). INR = PTR[ISI] • Therapeutic range (during warfarin therapy) is usually 2–3.5 (depending on anticoagulation indication) • Evaluation of bleeding is necessary if significantly elevated
Activated partial thromboplastin time (aPTT)	Detects deficiencies in the intrinsic thromboplastin system (factors I, II, V, VIII, IX, X, XI, and XII); used for heparin monitoring	21–45 s (varies by laboratory)	von Willebrand disease, hemophilia, congenital deficiency of Fitzgerald/Fletcher factor, hepatic disease, DIC, drugs (heparin, streptokinase, urokinase, warfarin), vitamin K deficiency	Very early DIC, extensive cancer (except when hepatic involved), immediately after acute hemorrhage	• Therapeutic range (during heparin therapy) is usually 1.5–2.5 times normal (varies between laboratories) • Can be used to identify circulating anticoagulants (antibodies induced in hemophiliacs by plasma transfusions) *(continued)*

Table 5.7 COAGULATION TESTS (continued)

Test Name	Description	Reference Range		Increased With	Decreased With	Other Comments
		Conventional Units	SI Units			
Fibrinogen	Investigates abnormal PT, aPTT, and TT; screens for DIC and fibrin-fibrinogenolysis	200–450 mg/dL	2.0–4.5 g/L	Inflammatory diseases (RA), infections, acute MI (AMI), cerebral accidents/disease, cancer, nephrotic syndrome, pregnancy, eclampsia	DIC, hepatic disease, cancer, primary fibrinolysis, dysfibrinogenemia, hypofibrinogenemia, high FDP/FSP levels (fibrin degradation/split levels), elevated antithrombin III (AT III)	• High heparin levels interfere with test results • Critical values: ≤50 or ≥700 mg/dL
Fibrin degradation products (FDP, fibrin split products, FSP)	Identifies products (X, Y, D, and E) of fibrin when split by plasmin	Negative at 1:4 dilution or <2.5 µg/mL	<2.5 mg/L	DIC, primary fibrinolysis, venous thrombosis, thoracic and cardiac surgery, renal transplant, AMI, pulmonary embolism (PE), carcinoma, hepatic disease	Normal	• Used to diagnose DIC and other thromboembolic disorders • In DIC, FDPs usually begin to fall within 1 day; if very high at baseline, it may take ≥1 week to return to normal • Elevated urine levels suggest renal disease or rejection crisis following renal transplant • False elevations with exercise, stress, and traumatic venipuncture

Test	Description			Increased	Decreased	Comments
D-Dimer	Assesses for one FDP; consists of various size pieces of cross-linked fibrin	Negative or <0.5 µg/mL	<0.5 mg/L	DIC, arterial or venous thrombosis (deep vein thrombosis [DVT]), PE, renal or hepatic failure, late in pregnancy, preeclampsia, MI, malignancy, inflammation, severe infection, surgery, trauma	Normal	• False elevations with high titers of rheumatoid factor, tumor marker CA-125, estrogen therapy, and normal pregnancy
Thrombin time (TT)	A sensitive test for fibrinogen deficiency	Within 3 s of control value (control range 16–24 s, varies widely by laboratory and method used)		DIC, fibrinolysis, hypofibrinogenemia, multiple myeloma, high levels of FDPs, uremia, severe hepatic disease, drugs (heparin, low-molecular-weight heparins [LMWH])	Hct > 55%, hyperfibrinogenemia	• Tests the fibrinogen-to-fibrin conversion; affected by the concentration of fibrinogen and plasmin, and the presence of FDPs and antithrombotic agents • Elevated in ~60% of DIC cases; less sensitive and specific test for DIC than other tests • Most methods of measuring will give elevated results with heparin, urokinase, streptokinase, and asparaginase therapy • When assayed by the reptilase method, heparin does not elevate *(continued)*

145

Table 5.7 COAGULATION TESTS (continued)

Test Name	Description	Reference Range Conventional Units	Reference Range SI Units	Increased With	Decreased With	Other Comments
Antithrombin III (At III)	Heparin cofactor	Functional assay: 80%–130% normal pooled plasma (NPP) Immunologic assay: 17–39 mg/dL	0.8–1.3 170–390 mg/L	Acute hepatitis, vitamin K deficiency (warfarin), renal transplant, inflammation, menstruation, hyperglobulinemia	Congenital deficiency, DIC, DVT, PE, thrombophlebitis, hepatic transplant, partial hepatectomy, cirrhosis/chronic hepatic failure/disease, nephrotic syndrome, AMI, carcinoma, trauma, severe infection, pregnancy (last trimester), early postpartum period, midperiod of the menstrual cycle, heparin failure, protein-wasting disease	• Naturally occurring thrombin inhibitor; also inactivates the activated forms of factors II, IX, X, XI, and XII • Heparin's anticoagulant activity is due to accelerating AT III activity • Decreases may predispose patients to thrombus formation and failure of heparin anticoagulation • Test interferences include anabolic steroids, warfarin, heparin, asparaginase, estrogens, and oral contraceptives

Sources: http://www.labtestsonline.org. Accessed January 25, 2008; Kratz A, Lewandrowski KB. Case records of the Massachusetts General Hospital. Weekly clinicopathological exercises. Normal reference laboratory values. *N Engl J Med.* 1998;339:1063–1072; OHSU Test Directory of Lab and Pathology Services http://www.ohsu.edu/health/consult-and-refer/labtests/index.cfm. Accessed February 1, 2008; Fischbach F. *A Manual of Laboratory Diagnostic Tests.* 6th ed. Philadelphia, PA: Lippincott Williams & Wilkins; 2004; and Lee M. *Basic Skills in Interpreting Laboratory Data.* 3rd ed. Bethesda, MD: American Society of Health-System Pharmacists; 2004, with permission.

Chemistry Tests

Many chemical blood constituents are available to be tested, including electrolytes, enzymes, blood sugars, lipids, hormones, proteins, vitamins, minerals, and drug levels; other individual tests are available. It is common to need to test several of these to be able to establish patterns.

Electrolytes, Minerals, and Trace Elements

Determining serum electrolyte concentrations is one of most common laboratory tests and is routinely ordered as a basic metabolic panel (BMP). Some components included in metabolic panels are not electrolytes, minerals, or trace elements and will be addressed in the section most appropriate for that item. Table 5.8 presents descriptions, reference ranges (for adults), and clinical information for common electrolyte tests.

Arterial Blood Gases (ABGs)

Arterial blood gas concentrations are analyzed to assess the exchange of oxygen (O_2) and carbon dioxide (CO_2). An imbalance in these gases is also known as an acid-base imbalance. The specimen for ABGs must be an arterial blood sample and can be obtained by either an arterial puncture or from an indwelling arterial line. Table 5.9 describes the components of ABGs. Common indications for ABGs include the following:

Gas exchange abnormalities:
- Acute and chronic pulmonary disease.
- Acute respiratory failure.
- Cardiac disease.
- Pulmonary testing (at rest and with exercise).
- Monitoring O_2 therapy.
- Sleep disorder studies.

Acid-base disturbances:
- Metabolic acidosis.
- Metabolic alkalosis.

Laboratory Tests by Organ System

Although some laboratory tests provide information about a wide variety of body systems, others are used to diagnose, assess status, and monitor treatment of patients with organ system-specific diseases and conditions. Tests used for the cardiac system, endocrine system, gastrointestinal and hepatic system, and renal system will be presented.

Table 5.8 ELECTROLYTES

Test Name	Description	Reference Range Conventional Units	SI Units	Increased With	Decreased With	Other Comments
Sodium (Na^+)	Most abundant cation in extracellular fluid; maintains oncotic pressure and acid-base balance, aids in transmission of nerve impulses	135–145 mEq/L	135–145 mmol/L	(Hypernatremia) dehydration, aldosteronism, diabetes insipidus, osmotic diuretics, Conn syndrome, coma, Cushing disease, tracheobronchitis, drugs (anabolic steroids, corticosteroids, calcium, fluorides, iron)	(Hyponatremia) burns, diarrhea, vomiting, excessive intake of free water, Addison disease, nephritis, diabetic acidosis, cystic fibrosis, malabsorption, edema, hypothyroidism, syndrome of inappropriate antidiuretic hormone (SIADH), drugs (thiazide diuretics, chlorpropamide, carbamazepine, clofibrate, cyclophosphamide, heparin, laxatives, sulfates), some pulmonary disorders (tuberculosis, pneumonias), high triglycerides (false low), low	• Renal system, central nervous system (CNS), and endocrine system regulate Na^+ concentrations • Critical values: ≤120 or ≥160 • Clinical signs of hyponatremia: nausea, fatigue, cramps, psychosis, seizures, coma • Clinical signs of hypernatremia: cardiovascular and renal symptoms, heart failure • Total body water deficit = ~1 L for each 3 mmol/L of Na+ greater than normal

Potassium (K+)	Principle intracellular fluid cation; (with bicarbonate) serves as primary buffer	3.5–5.2 mEq/L	3.5–5.2 mmol/L	(Hyperkalemia) renal failure, dehydration, cell damage (trauma, burns, DIC, chemotherapy, surgery), acidosis, Addison disease, uncontrolled DM, RBC transfusion, pseudohyperaldosteronism, SLE, sickle cell disease, interstitial nephritis, renal transplant rejection, specimen hemolysis (false elevation)	protein (false low) (Hypokalemia) severe burns, vomiting, diarrhea, severe sweating, starvation, malnutrition, chronic alcoholism, draining wounds, primary aldosteronism, chronic stress, hepatic disease with ascites, renal tubular acidosis, respiratory alkalosis, Bartter syndrome, cystic fibrosis, drugs (diuretics, mineralocorticoids, antibiotics, cisplatin, ticarcillin, amphotericin), glucose tolerance testing or large ingestions of glucose (shifts glucose intercellularly), WBC >50,000/mm³ (falsely low)	• ~ 80%–90% excreted in the urine by the kidneys; aldosterone also regulates concentration • Critical values: ≤2.5 or ≥6.0 • ~10% (50 mmol) of total body K+ is extracellular; therefore, serum levels are a poor measure of total body K+, but do correlate with physiologic effects. Values do not vary with circulatory volume • Levels rise ~0.6 mEq/L for every 0.1 decrease in blood pH from normal (pH 7.4) • Specific electrocardiogram (ECG) changes are seen with changes in K+ levels • Hypokalemia clinical issues: enhanced effects of digitalis agents; need to also correct for hypomagnesemia; affects neuromuscular function • Hyperkalemia clinical issues: treat with insulin (and glucose); affects neuromuscular function • Each mmol/L decrease in the serum K+ represents a total body 200–400 mmol K+ deficit *(continued)*

149

Table 5.8 ELECTROLYTES (continued)

Test Name	Description	Reference Range Conventional Units	Reference Range SI Units	Increased With	Decreased With	Other Comments
Chloride (Cl⁻)	Major extracellular anion; involved in acid-base and water balance via influence on osmotic pressure	96–108 mEq/L	96–108 mmol/L	Dehydration, metabolic acidosis, hyperventilation, respiratory alkalosis, renal disorders (renal tubular acidosis), diabetes insipidus, Cushing syndrome, diarrhea, eclampsia, hypothalamic damage/head injury, primary hyperparathyroidism, salicylate intoxication	Vomiting, gastric suctioning, aggressive diuresis, burns, heat exhaustion, acute infection, diabetic acidosis, chronic respiratory acidosis, metabolic alkalosis, CHF, Addison disease, SIADH, overhydration, acute intermittent porphyria, salt-losing nephritis	• Cl⁻ concentration useful in diagnosis of acid-base disorders • Plasma concentration can be maintained near normal even in the presence of renal failure
Carbon dioxide (CO₂) content	Plasma CO₂ reflects bicarbonate (HCO₃) concentrations	22–32 mEq/L	22–32 mmol/L	Severe vomiting, emphysema, aldosteronism	Acute renal failure, diabetic acidosis, hyperventilation, salicylate toxicity	• Normal plasma CO₂ is ~95% bicarbonate (a base), which is regulated by the renal system; the remaining ~5% is dissolved CO₂ gas (an acid) and carbonic acid (H₂CO₃), which are regulated by the lungs • Critical values: ≤ 12 or ≥ 40

Calcium (Ca²⁺)	Measures total (protein-bound and free) serum calcium	8.5–10.5 mg/dL	2.1–2.6 mmol/L	(Hypercalcemia) hyperparathyroidism, neoplasms, parathyroid adenoma, Hodgkin disease, multiple myeloma, leukemia, bone metastasis, hyperplasia (associated with hypophosphatemia), renal failure, Addison disease, respiratory acidosis, immobilization, drugs (thiazide diuretics)	(Hypocalcemia) hyperphosphatemia, alkalosis, osteomalacia, hypomagnesemia, inadequate calcium replacement, sepsis, pancreatitis, renal failure, malnutrition, alcoholism, drugs (laxatives, furosemide, calcitonin, glucocorticoids, excessive thyroid hormone, exacerbated with bisphosphonates if inadequate calcium and vitamin D), pseudohypocalcemia (low protein/albumin may lead to low total serum Ca²⁺, but with less protein-bound, the level of free Ca²⁺ may be appropriate)

- Ca^{2+} plays an essential role in muscle contraction, cardiac function, transmission of nerve impulses, and blood clotting
- Critical values: ≤ 7.0 or ≥ 13.0
- Parathyroid hormone (PTH) is released when serum Ca^{2+} decreases. PTH increases renal conversion of vitamin D to the active form (stimulates intestinal Ca^{2+} absorption) and stimulates bone resorption (releases Ca^{2+} and PO_4 into the blood and enhances renal Ca^{2+} reabsorption)
- Because Ca^{2+} is 50% protein-bound, need to correct for abnormal binding (with low albumin) or measure free calcium
- Decreases in Alb of 1 g/dL will decrease the total serum Ca^{2+} by ~0.8 mg/dL (see Chapter 12, A Pharmacy Calculations Anthology)

(continued)

Table 5.8 ELECTROLYTES (continued)

Test Name	Description	Reference Range Conventional Units	Reference Range SI Units	Increased With	Decreased With	Other Comments
Ionized calcium (free calcium)	Measures only active (unbound/free) form of calcium	4.60–5.20 mg/dL	1.14–1.30 mmol/L	Same as calcium	Same as calcium	• Of the ~1%–2% of the body's total calcium that is in the blood, 50% is ionized/free (active form) and the remainder is bound to serum proteins, mainly albumin • When requesting ionized Ca^{2+} levels, blood pH should be measured concurrently
Phosphate (P, inorganic phosphorus, PO_4)	Measures serum phosphate	2.4–4.7 mg/dL	0.77–1.52 mmol/L	(Hyperphosphatemia) renal dysfunction, uremia, excessive phosphate intake, excessive vitamin D intake, hypoparathyroidism, hypocalcemia, bone tumors, respiratory acidosis, lactic acidosis, diabetic ketoacidosis (DKA), drugs (bisphosphonate therapy)	(Hypophosphatemia) hyperparathyroidism, hypercalcemia, rickets, vitamin D deficiency, diabetic coma, hyperinsulinism, continuous IV glucose administration in a person without DM, diuretic phase of severe burns, respiratory alkalosis, alcoholism, malnutrition, hypothyroidism, hypokalemia, drugs (antacids, overuse of diuretics)	• Phosphate (anion form) is required for generation of bony tissue, metabolism of glucose and lipids, maintenance of acid-base balance, and storage and transfer of energy within the body • Critical values: ≤0.9 mg/dL • ~85% of the body's total PO_4 is combined with Ca^{2+}; therefore, serum Ca^{2+} values must also be checked when evaluating phosphate levels

Uric acid	Measures uric acid levels	Male: 3.5–8.5 mg/dl Female: 2.3–6.6 mg/dl	M: 208–506 μmol/L F: 137–393 μmol/L	(Hyperuricemia) leukemia, lymphoma, shock, chemotherapy, metabolic acidosis, psoriasis, significant renal dysfunction, drugs (thiazide diuretics, low/moderate-dose salicylates, ethambutol, niacin, cyclosporine)	(Hypouricemia) Drugs (allopurinol, sulfinpyrazone, high-dose salicylates (>3 g/day) (Hypouricemia is not clinically significant)	• Formed from the breakdown of nucleic acids; serum levels are increased with excessive production/destruction of cells or an inability to excrete urate renally • Useful for monitoring gout therapy with allopurinol
Magnesium (Mg^{2+})	Measures serum magnesium levels	1.4–2.5 mg/dl	0.7–1.25 mmol/L	(Hypermagnesemia) renal dysfunction, diabetic acidosis, high-dose Mg^{2+} antacids with renal insufficiency, hypothyroidism, dehydration	(Hypomagnesemia) high PO_4 diets (suppress absorption), diarrhea, hemodialysis, malabsorption syndromes, lactation, acute pancreatitis, chronic alcoholism, drugs (thiazides, amphotericin B, cisplatin)	• Required for the utilization of adenosine triphosphate (ATP) as an energy source. Role in carbohydrate metabolism, protein synthesis, nucleic acid synthesis, and muscle contraction. Regulates neuromuscular irritability, the clotting mechanism, and Ca^{2+} absorption • Critical values: ≤0.9 or ≥5.0 mg/dl

(continued)

Table 5.8 ELECTROLYTES (continued)

Test Name	Description	Reference Range Conventional Units	Reference Range SI Units	Increased With	Decreased With	Other Comments
						• Hypomagnesemia can cause hypocalcemia and hypokalemia resulting in severe neuromuscular irritability and ventricular arrhythmias • Hypermagnesemia can act as a sedative and can depress cardiac and neuromuscular activity
Total serum protein (TSP, total protein [TP], albumin/globulin ratio, A/G ratio)	Commonly included in CMPs, hepatic and nutrition panels	6.0–8.0 g/dL	60–80 g/L	(Hyperproteinemia) hemoconcentration secondary to dehydration (both albumin and globulin increase), collagen diseases, SLE, acute hepatic disease, multiple myeloma	(Hypoproteinemia) increased loss of albumin in the urine, decreased formation in the liver, insufficient protein intake, severe burns	• Three major categories: (i) tissue or organ proteins, (ii) hemoglobin, and (iii) plasma/serum proteins (albumin and globulins), which reflect nutritional status and serve as buffers in the maintenance of acid-base balance

				• The A/G ratio decreases/is low if the globulin/TSP increases but the Alb concentration is unchanged, or if the globulin/TSP is unchanged but the Alb is low • See Table 5.12 for information on albumin
Zinc, Serum [Zn]	Measures serum zinc levels; often included in nutritional panels	Male: 75–291 μg/dL Female: 65–256 μg/dL	M: 11.5–44.5 μmol/L F: 9.95–39.2 μmol/L	(Uncommon) tissue injury, hemolysis, contaminated collection tubes	Abnormal losses (Crohn disease, pregnancy, fistulas, malabsorption), alcoholism, DM, proteinuria, renal disease, hepatic disease, porphyria, sickle cell disease, trauma, infection, stress, hypoalbuminemia, fasting obese patients, prolonged parenteral nutrition	• Cofactor of many enzymes (alkaline phosphatase, lactic dehydrogenase); ~80% of total in whole blood is in RBCs • Primary/normal losses are in pancreatic and intestinal secretions • Signs of deficiency include dermatitis, hair loss, diarrhea, depression, and hypogeusia • Levels affected by circadian variations, with peaks around 9 AM and 6 PM

Sources: http://www.labtestsonline.org. Accessed January 25, 2008; Kratz A, Lewandrowski KB. Case records of the Massachusetts General Hospital. Weekly clinicopathological exercises. Normal reference laboratory values. *N Engl J Med.* 1998;339:1063–1072; OHSU Test Directory of Lab and Pathology Services http://www.ohsu.edu/health/consult-and-refer/labtests/index.cfm. Accessed February 1, 2008; Fischbach F. *A Manual of Laboratory Diagnostic Tests.* 6th ed. Philadelphia, PA: Lippincott Williams & Wilkins; 2004; and Lee M. *Basic Skills in Interpreting Laboratory Data.* 3rd ed. Bethesda, MD: American Society of Health-System Pharmacists; 2004, with permission.

Table 5.9 ARTERIAL BLOOD GASES (ABGs)

Test Name	Description	Reference Range Conventional Units	Reference Range SI Units	Increased With	Decreased With	Other Comments
Oxygen saturation (SaO_2)	The amount of oxygen (O_2) carried by Hgb; expressed as a % of the capacity of O_2 to combine with Hgb	95%–99% O_2				• Used with pO_2 to evaluate the extent of oxygenation of Hgb and the adequacy of tissue oxygenation • RBCs are able to transport 65 times the amount of O_2 dissolved in plasma. This relationship is determined by pH, temperature, the concentration of 2,3 DPG (diphosphoglycerate), and the molecular species of Hgb
Partial pressure of oxygen (PaO_2, pO_2)	Measure of the partial pressure exerted by the amount of O_2 dissolved in the plasma	(Room air, age-dependent) >80 mm Hg	>10.6 kPa	Increased O_2 delivery by arterial means (nasal prongs, mechanical ventilation), hyperventilation by patient, polycythemia	COPD, restrictive airway disease (RAD, asthma), anemia, hypoventilation due to physical or neuromuscular impairment, compromised cardiac function	• Provides an estimate of the lung's ability to oxygenate blood • The partial pressure of O_2 dissolved in plasma determines the amount of O_2 bound to Hgb • Critical value: ≤50 mm Hg

Partial pressure of carbon dioxide (PaCO$_2$)	Measure of the pressure exerted by the CO$_2$ dissolved in the plasma	35–45 mm Hg	4.6–5.9 kPa	COPD, reduced function of the respiratory center, hypoventilation	Hypoxia, anxiety/nervousness, pulmonary embolism, hyperventilation	• Used to evaluate the effectiveness of alveolar ventilation and to determine the acid-base status of the blood • Critical values: ≤20 or ≥60–70 • In general, for each mEq decrease in HCO$_3$, the PaCO$_2$ will decrease 1.3 mm Hg
pH	Reflects the chemical balance of acids and bases within the body	7.35–7.45 pH units		Acidemia (due to increased formation of acids)	Alkalemia (due to acid loss)	• Hydrogen ion sources within the body include volatile acids and fixed acids (lactic acid, keto-acids) • When evaluating a pH value, pCO$_2$ and HCO$_3$ should also be obtained to estimate the respiratory or metabolic component contributing to the acid-base status • Critical values: ≤7.25 or ≥7.55–7.65
Anion gap (AG)	Calculated using available electrolyte	8–16 mEq/L (if K$^+$ included in calculation)		(+ High pH): extracellular volume contraction,	Hypoalbuminemia, multiple myeloma, hyponatremia	• Used clinically in the diagnosis of metabolic acidosis *[continued]*

157

Table 5.9 ARTERIAL BLOOD GASES (ABGs) *(continued)*

Test Name	Description	Reference Range		Increased With	Decreased With	Other Comments
		Conventional Units	SI Units			
	information to assist in quantifying unmeasured cations (including Ca^{2+} and Mg^{2+}) and anions (protein, PO_4^-, sulfate, and organic acids)	12–20 mEq/L (if K^+ not included in calculation)		administration of large-dose penicillins (+ low pH): MULEPAK (**m**ethanol ingestion, **u**remia, **l**actic acidosis, **e**thylene glycol ingestion, **p**araldehyde ingestion, **a**spirin intoxication, **k**etoacidosis)	caused by viscous serum, marked hypercalcemia, lithium toxicity Normal AG: metabolic acidosis from diarrhea, renal tubular acidosis, drugs (potassium-sparing diuretics, carbonic anhydrase inhibitors)	• Can be calculated using two different approaches: $AG = Na^+ - (Cl^- + HCO_3^-)$ $AG = (Na^+ + K^+) - (Cl^- + HCO_3^-)$ • See Chapter 12, A Pharmacy Calculations Anthology, and Chapter 9, Fluid and Electrolyte Therapy, for further discussions
Bicarbonate buffer system	Consists of carbonic acid (H_2CO_3) and bicarbonate (HCO_3)	22–26 mEq/L		Respiratory acidosis due to decreased ventilation	Respiratory alkalosis due to increased alveolar ventilation and removal of CO_2 and water, metabolic acidosis due to accumulation of body acids, loss of HCO_3 from the extracellular fluid	• The major buffer system in the extracellular body fluid • Calculated by: Total CO_2 content = $H_2CO_3 + HCO_3$

Sources: http://www.labtestsonline.org. Accessed January 25, 2008; Kratz A, Lewandrowski KB. Case records of the Massachusetts General Hospital. Weekly clinicopathological exercises. Normal reference laboratory values. *N Engl J Med.* 1998;339:1063–1072; OHSU Test Directory of Lab and Pathology Services http://www.ohsu.edu/health/consult-and-refer/labtests/index.cfm. Accessed February 1, 2008; Fischbach F. *A Manual of Laboratory Diagnostic Tests.* 6th ed. Philadelphia, PA: Lippincott Williams & Wilkins; 2004; and Lee M. *Basic Skills in Interpreting Laboratory Data.* 3rd ed. Bethesda, MD: American Society of Health-System Pharmacists; 2004, with permission.

Cardiac System Tests

While electrolytes and arterial blood gases can provide useful information when dealing with a cardiac patient, additional tests, such as cardiac enzymes and lipoprotein panels are often needed to evaluate cardiac issues more specifically (Table 5.10).

Endocrine System Tests

Diabetes mellitus (DM) and thyroid dysfunction are common endocrine disorders. Tests such as glycosylated hemoglobin and thyroid function tests, presented in Table 5.11, are commonly used to diagnose and monitor control of these conditions.

Gastrointestinal and Hepatic System Tests

Tests associated with gastrointestinal and hepatic disease include many enzymes, as well as some proteins, byproducts, and nutritional markers. Given the role of the liver in metabolism and clearance of many medications, liver function tests (LFTs)—more accurately described as hepatic enzyme tests—are routinely monitored and included in a comprehensive metabolic panel (CMP). Table 5.12 present the tests usually associated with this organ system.

Most liver injuries are hepatocellular or cholestatic in nature. Hepatocellular injury is often identified by disproportionately elevated serum transaminase levels ([alanine aminotransferase [ALT] and/or aspartate aminotransferase [AST]) compared with γ-glutamyl transferase (GGT) and alkaline phosphatase (alk phos, ALP, AP) levels. The opposite pattern typically signifies cholestatic injury.

Renal System Tests

In addition to electrolytes and hepatic enzyme tests, renal function tests are among the most common clinical laboratory tests used. Numerous factors, diseases, and conditions affect renal function and therefore, potentially impact the clearance of numerous substances and several regulatory functions. See Table 5.13 for laboratory tests pertinent to the renal system.

Other Blood Chemistry Tests

Table 5.14 includes other common blood tests, include those used for select immunologic and rheumatologic diseases or conditions.

Table 5.10 CARDIAC SYSTEM TESTS

Test Name	Description	Reference Range Conventional Units	Reference Range SI Units	Increased With	Decreased With	Other Comments
Creatine kinase (CK)	Measure of muscle enzyme (formerly known as creatine phosphokinase)	Male: 60–400 U/L Female: 40–175 U/L (higher in African Americans)	M: 1.00–6.67 µkat/L F: 0.67–2.91 µkat/L	MI (begins to rise 3–4 h after myocardial injury, peaking within 15–24 h and returning to normal within 3–4 days), cerebrovascular disease, muscular dystrophy, polymyositis, dermatomyositis, delirium tremens (DTs), chronic alcoholism, subarachnoid hemorrhage, CNS trauma		• High concentrations in heart and skeletal muscle • Used as a specific test for the diagnosis of MI and as a reliable measure of skeletal muscle diseases (muscular dystrophy, polymyositis) • Divided into three isoenzymes: BB (= CK1), MB (= CK2), and MM (= CK3) • Normal CK is virtually 100% MM
CK isoenzyme BB (= CK1)	Definitive indication of brain injury	0%		Biliary atresia, brain trauma, certain other brain injuries or tumors		• Brain tissue primarily composed of BB

CK isoenzyme MB (= CK2)	Definitive indication of myocardial injury	0–4% or ≤ 9 ng/mL	≤ 9 μg/L	MI, myocardial ischemia, muscular dystrophy	• In cardiac muscle • If negative throughout 48 h after onset of chest pain, MI usually ruled out
2CK isoenzyme MM (= CK3)	Indication of skeletal muscle injury	96%–100%		MI, muscle trauma, intramuscular (IM) injections, shock, after surgery	• In skeletal and cardiac muscle
Troponin I	High selectivity as a marker of cardiac damage	≤ 0.6 ng/mL	≤ 0.6 μg/L	> 1.5 ng/mL suggests current myocardial injury = MI (CK elevates within 6 h of myocardial injury; remains elevated for 7–10 days)	< 0.4 ng/mL indicates no myocardial injury within the previous several days 0.4–2.0 ng/mL is borderline and suggests possible MI; repeat testing recommended	• Globular proteins found in cardiac and skeletal muscle; key role in triggering muscle contraction in response to increased cytosolic calcium • Three cardiac troponins: troponin I (cTnI), T (cTnT), and C (cTnC). Subtype I is found specifically in the heart (C is not specific for the heart and T, while most commonly in heart tissue, can also be expressed in noncardiac tissue on injury) *(continued)*

Table 5.10 CARDIAC SYSTEM TESTS (continued)

Test Name	Description	Reference Range		Increased With	Decreased With	Other Comments
		Conventional Units	SI Units			
						• Levels of troponin I and T used to evaluate suspected MI (6 h–1 week after the incident)
Cholesterol (total cholesterol, TC)	Elevated cholesterol is a risk factor for cardiovascular disease	Desirable: ≤199 mg/dL Borderline: 200–239 mg/dL High Risk: ≥240 mg/dL	Desirable: ≤ 5.17 mmol/L Borderline: 5.17–6.18 mmol/L High Risk: ≥ 6.21 mmol/L	(Hypercholesterolemia) atherosclerosis, coronary artery disease (CAD), familial type II hypercholesterolemia, DM, hypothyroidism, metabolic syndrome, obstructive jaundice, pregnancy, drugs (anabolic steroids, beta-blockers, testosterone, epinephrine, oral contraceptives, vitamin D)	Malabsorption, hepatic disease, cancer, sepsis, hypolipoproteinemia, pernicious anemia, drugs (lipid-lowering agents such as statins, niacin, fibrates, cholesterol absorption inhibitors, bile acid sequestrants)	• Exists in tissues throughout the body; used to form steroid hormones, bile acids, and cell membranes • Levels of >200 mg/dL are considered to be high and require a TG evaluation

| Triglycerides (TGs), fasting | 10–150 mg/dL | 0.11–1.69 mmol/L | | Cirrhosis, anorexia nervosa, biliary obstruction, cerebral thrombosis, chronic renal failure, DM, Down syndrome, metabolic syndrome, hypertension (HTN), idiopathic hypercalcemia, hyperlipoproteinemia (types I, IIb, III, IV, and VI), glycogen storage diseases (types I, III, and VI), gout, ischemic heart disease, hypothyroidism, pregnancy, acute intermittent porphyria, respiratory distress syndrome, thalassemia major, viral hepatitis, Werner syndrome, high-carbohydrate diets, excessive alcohol consumption, | COPD, severe parenchymal hepatic disease, malnutrition, malabsorption, hyperthyroidism, hyperparathyroidism, hypolipoproteinemia, intestinal lymphangiectasia, drugs (some lipid-lowering agents such as statins, niacin, fibrates) | • Found in plasma lipids as chylomicrons and very-low-density lipoproteins (VLDLs)
 • Nutritional/fasting status most affects TGs (and therefore calculated LDL); patients should maintain usual diet for 3 days and must fast for 12 h before test. Alcohol should not be consumed 24 hours before test |

(continue

Table 5.10 CARDIAC SYSTEM TESTS (continued)

Test Name	Description	Reference Range Conventional Units	Reference Range SI Units	Increased With	Decreased With	Other Comments
				drugs (bile acid sequestrants, corticosteroids, estrogens, ethanol, oral contraceptives, spironolactone)		
High-density lipoprotein (HDL) cholesterol (HDLc)	Elevated HDLc is beneficial and protects against CHD	Desirable: >60 mg/dL Borderline: 35–60 mg/dL High risk: <35 mg/dL	Desirable: >1.55 mmol/L Borderline: 0.91–1.55 mmol/L High risk: <0.91 mmol/L	Chronic alcoholism, primary biliary cirrhosis, exposure to industrial toxins or polychlorinated hydrocarbons, exercise, moderate alcohol (especially red wine) intake, drugs (niacin, estrogens, oral contraceptives, phenytoin)	Cystic fibrosis, severe cirrhosis, DM, metabolic syndrome, Hodgkin disease, nephrotic syndrome, malaria, some acute infections, drugs (anabolic steroids, β-adrenergic blockers [mild])	• Products of liver and intestinal synthesis and TG catabolism • There is an inverse relationship between HDLc levels and CHD • Levels >60 mg/dL are protective and counted as a negative risk when calculating CHD risk (i.e., can subtract one risk factor)

| Low-density lipoprotein (LDL) cholesterol (LDLc) | Usually calculated with Friedewald equation; can be measured directly (may require specific order) | Desirable: <130 mg/dL
Borderline: 130–159 mg/dL
High: ≥160 mg/dL | Desirable: <3.36 mmol/L
Borderline: 3.36–4.11 mmol/L
High: ≥4.13 mmol/L | Familial and idiopathic hyperlipidemia coronary vascular disease, nonfasting status (especially if LDL value is calculated rather than measured directly), types IIa and IIb hyperlipoproteinemia, DM, metabolic syndrome, hypothyroidism, obstructive jaundice, nephrotic syndrome | Hypoproteinemia, abetalipoproteinemia, severe illness, drugs (estrogen, lipid-lowering agents such as statins, niacin, fibrates, cholesterol absorption inhibitors, bile acid sequestrants) | • Plays key role in transporting cholesterol to various tissues where it is needed for membrane synthesis and other functions
• Goal for patients with CHD or CHD risk equivalents (including DM): <100 mg/dL (2.59 mmol/L); for patients with DM and CHD (or multiple risk factors), optimal goal of <70 mg/dL (1.81 mmol/L) may be considered
• Friedewald equation: LDLc = TC − HDL − (TG/5) (only applicable if TG <400); various factors can affect accuracy of Friedewald calculation (may be less accurate if TG >200 or HDL <50, and affected by variable LDL size/type) |

(continued)

Table 5.10 CARDIAC SYSTEM TESTS (continued)

Test Name	Description	Reference Range Conventional Units	Reference Range SI Units	Increased With	Decreased With	Other Comments
Apolipo-protein A-1 (Apo A-1)	Main component of HDL	90–240 mg/dL	0.9–2.4 g/l	Familial hyper-α-lipoproteinemia	Tangier disease (hypo-α-lipoproteinemia), β-lipoproteinemia, Apo A-I Melano disease, Apo A-I-C-III deficiency, Apo C-II deficiency, hepatic disease, nephrotic syndrome/renal failure, poorly controlled DM, hypertriglyceridemia (familial), premature CHD, diet high in polyunsaturated fats, smoking	• <90 mg/dl indicates increased CAD risk • Patients must fast for 12 hours before test

Apolipoprotein B (Apo B)	Main component of LDL and VLDL	45–163 mg/dL	0.45–1.63 g/L	Hyperlipoproteinemia types IIa, IIb, and V, hepatic disease/obstruction, nephrotic syndrome/renal failure, Werner syndrome, Cushing syndrome, DM, hypothyroidism, premature CHD Fredrickson type IIa, porphyria, dysglobulinemia, drugs (statins, others)	Tangier disease (hypo-α-lipoproteinemia), hypo-β-lipoproteinemia, α-β-lipoproteinemia, Apo CII deficiency, type 1 hyperlipidemia, hypothyroidism, malnutrition/malabsorption, Reye syndrome, diet high in polyunsaturated fats, low-cholesterol diets	• >110 mg/dL indicates increased CAD risk • Patients must fast for 12 h before test • Important role in LDL catabolism, regulating cholesterol synthesis, and metabolism
Apo A-I/Apo B ratio	Correlates with increased risk for CAD	0.8–2.63				• Lower ratio = higher CAD risk
High-sensitivity C-reactive protein (hs-CRP)	Highly sensitive measure to detect lower levels of CRP	0.02–0.80 mg/dL	0.2–8 mg/L	MI, CAD risk		• Suggests risk for CAD • See Table 5.14 for general CRP

Sources: http://www.labtestsonline.org. Accessed January 25, 2008; Kratz A, Lewandrowski KB. Case records of the Massachusetts General Hospital. Weekly clinicopathological exercises. Normal reference laboratory values. *N Engl J Med.* 1998;339:1063–1072; OHSU Test Directory of Lab and Pathology Services http://www.ohsu.edu/health/consult-and-refer/labtests/index.cfm. Accessed February 1, 2008; Fischbach F. *A Manual of Laboratory Diagnostic Tests.* 6th ed. Philadelphia, PA: Lippincott Williams & Wilkins; 2004; Lee M. *Basic Skills in Interpreting Laboratory Data.* 3rd ed. Bethesda, MD: American Society of Health-System Pharmacists; 2004; and Grundy SM, Cleeman JI, Merz CN, et al. Implications of recent clinical trials for the National Cholesterol Education Program Adult Treatment Panel III guidelines. *Circulation.* 2004;110:227–239, with permission.

Table 5.11 ENDOCRINE SYSTEM TESTS

Test Name	Description	Reference Range Conventional Units	Reference Range SI Units	Increased With	Decreased With	Other Comments
Glucose (fasting blood glucose, [FBG], fasting blood sugar, [FBS])	Primarily a screening procedure to detect abnormalities in glucose utilization or production; included in BMP. Home and POC testing also available for day-to-day casual blood glucose (CBG) monitoring	70–100 mg/dl	3.89–5.55 mmol/L	(Hyperglycemia), impaired fasting glucose (IFG)/ prediabetes (FBS >100–125 mg/dl), DM (FBS >126 mg/dl), Cushing disease, chronic hepatic disease, potassium deficiency, chronic illness, pheochromocytoma, bacterial sepsis, acute distress (surgical procedures and anesthesia), parenteral glucose administration, pregnancy (gestational DM), drugs (alcohol, glucocorticoids, thiazide diuretics, estrogen, epinephrine, phenytoin)	(Hypoglycemia) insulin overdose, Addison disease, malnutrition, hepatic damage (alcoholism), alcohol use	• Abnormal values indicate the inability of the islet cells of the pancreas to produce insulin, the intestines to absorb glucose, cells to utilize glucose efficiently, and/or the liver to accumulate and break down glycogen • Critical values: ≤50 or ≥500

| Hemoglobin A1c (A₁c, HbA₁c, HgbA₁c, glycosylated hemoglobin) | Measures the blood glucose bound to Hgb; reflects the average blood sugar level in the 2–3 months preceding the test | 4.0%–6% of total Hgb

In patients with DM, American Diabetes Association goal: <7%; American Association of Clinical Endocrinologists goal: <6.5% | 0.04–0.06 fraction of total Hgb | DM with poor glucose control over the 2–3 months prior to the test, splenectomy, alcohol toxicity, lead toxicity, (falsely high) iron-deficiency anemia, sickle cell anemia, thalassemia | Pregnancy, chronic renal failure, (falsely low) hemolysis, hemolytic anemia, significant blood loss, sickle cell anemia, thalassemia | • Hgb A₁ has a life span of 120 days, undergoes glycosylation by a slow nonenzymatic process within the RBC, and is dependent on available glucose. The more glucose the RBC is exposed to, the higher the % of glycosylated Hgb
• Every 1% increase in A1c reflects a 35-mg/dl increase in blood glucose (A₁c 7% = mean plasma glucose 170 mg/dl)
• Used to monitor DM control; should not be used to diagnose DM
• Does not fully reflect temporary or new changes in glycemic control, hypoglycemia, or glycemic variability

(continued) |

Table 5.11 ENDOCRINE SYSTEM TESTS (*continued*)

Test Name	Description	Reference Range		Increased With	Decreased With	Other Comments
		Conventional Units	SI Units			
Fructosamine	Measurement of glycated protein; reflects the average blood sugar level in the 2–3 weeks preceding the test	170–285 µmol/L		DM with poor glucose control over the 2–3 weeks prior to the test	(Falsely low) decreased protein levels, increased protein loss, change in the type of protein produced by the body	• Serum proteins have a shorter life span than RBCs (~14–21 days) • May be useful in situations where the A1C cannot be reliably measured (rapid changes in DM treatment, gestational DM where tight control is essential, RBC loss or abnormalities) • Since fructosamine concentrations in well-controlled DM may overlap with patients without DM, fructosamine is not useful as a screen for DM • High levels of vitamin C, lipemia, hemolysis, and hyperthyroidism can interfere with test results

Insulin, free	Measures insulin levels	2–20 µU/mL	14.35–143.5 pmol/L	Insulinoma, type 2 DM (untreated), obesity, insulin administration, acromegaly, Cushing syndrome, pancreatic islet cell hyperplasia	Type 1 DM (severe), hypopituitarism	• Critical values: >35 µU/mL (243 pmol/L), fasting
Insulin C-peptide (C-peptide)	Monitors insulin production by the pancreatic beta cells and helps determine DM type and cause of hypoglycemia	0.5–2.7 ng/mL (varies by laboratory)	0.17–0.90 mmol/L	High levels of endogenous insulin production, insulin resistance (prediabetes, type 2 DM), insulinomas (insulin-producing tumors), pancreas or β-cell transplantation, hypokalemia, pregnancy, Cushing syndrome, renal failure (oral hypoglycemic drugs)	Insufficient insulin production by beta cells (type 1 DM), production suppressed by exogenous insulin, radical pancreatectomy, production suppressed with somatostatin suppression tests	• C-peptide can be used to help determine how much insulin the pancreas is still producing

(continued)

Table 5.11 ENDOCRINE SYSTEM TESTS (continued)

Test Name	Description	Reference Range		Increased With	Decreased With	Other Comments
		Conventional Units	SI Units			
Cortisol, plasma	Used primarily to diagnose Cushing or Addison disease	Morning: 6–24 μg/dL Evening: 3–12 μg/dL	Morning: 165–662 nmol/L Evening: 83–331 nmol/L	Hyperthyroidism, stress (circadian variation less apparent in this setting), obesity, Cushing syndrome, pregnancy, drugs (spironolactone, oral contraceptives); extreme increases in the morning and no variation later in the day suggest carcinoma	Hepatic disease, Addison disease, anterior pituitary hyposecretion, hypothyroidism	• Affects the metabolism of proteins, carbohydrates, and lipids and inhibits the effect of insulin; stimulates hepatic gluconeogenesis and decreases the rate of glucose use by the cells • In healthy patients with normal diurnal rhythms, cortisol secretion is higher in the morning (6–8 AM) and lower in the evening (4–6 PM)
Thyroid-stimulating hormone [TSH]	Measures TSH levels	0.5–5.0 μU/mL	0.5–5.0 mU/L	Primary hypothyroidism (T_4 should be low)	Hyperthyroidism *Normal TSH (with low T_3 and T_4): possible hypopituitarism	• Secreted from the anterior pituitary, stimulates thyroid hormone [triiodothyronine [T_3] and thyroxine [T_4] release from the thyroid gland. Secretion is under negative feedback control from T_3 and T_4

Thyroxine, total (T_4)	Measures the level of total circulating T_4	4–10.9 μg/dl Females taking estrogen: 6.5–12.5 μg/dl	51–140 nmol/L Females taking estrogen: 84–161 nmol/L	Hyperthyroidism, acute thyroiditis, pregnancy, early hepatitis, idiopathic thyroxine-binding globulin (TBG) elevation, estrogen use	Hypohyroidism, thyroiditis, nephrosis, cirrhosis, hypoproteinemia, malnutrition, idiopathic TBG decrease, drugs (anabolic steroids, salicylates, phenytoin, propranolol)	• Best screen for hypothyroidism (can differentiate primary hypothyroidism from pituitary/hypothalamic hypothyroidism) and hyperthyroidism; also used for monitoring thyroid replacement therapy • >95% of total T_4 is bound to TBG, prealbumin and albumin
Free thyroxine (free T_4)	Can be assessed in two ways: measured via equilibrium dialysis or indirectly calculated with the free thyroxine index (measure total T_4 and assess TBG binding capacity; see T_3UR)	Equilibrium dialysis: 0.8–2.7 ng/dl	0.010–0.035 nmol/L	Same as T_4	Same as T_4	• Only <5% of total T_4 is the free/unbound (biologically active) form. Assessment of free T_4 (along with total T_4 and TSH) is needed in thyroid disease workups

(continued)

Table 5.11 ENDOCRINE SYSTEM TESTS (*continued*)

Test Name	Description	Reference Range Conventional Units	Reference Range SI Units	Increased With	Decreased With	Other Comments
Triiodothyronine uptake ratio (T$_3$UR), thyroid hormone-binding ratio (THBI)	Indirect measurement of unsaturated TBG in the blood	25%–35%	0.25–0.35	Hyperthyroidism, nephrosis, severe hepatic disease, metastatic malignancy, pulmonary insufficiency; drugs (thyroxine [T$_4$] and desiccated thyroid therapy, heparin, androgens, anabolic steroids, phenytoin, large doses of salicylates)	Elevated levels of TBG, hypothyroidism, pregnancy, hyperestrogenic status; drugs (liothyronine [T$_3$] treatment)	• Main use of T$_3$UR is to help provide an indirect measure of free T$_4$, as described above

| Triiodothyro-nine (T_3) | Measures serum levels of T_3 | 45–181 ng/dL 0.69–2.78 nmol/L | Hyperthyroidism, T_3 thyrotoxicosis, acute thyroiditis, idiopathic TBG elevation, pregnancy, drugs (liothyronine >25 μg/day, levothyroxine >300 μg/day, estrogen, oral contraceptives) | Hypothyroidism (some clinically hypothyroid patients will have normal levels), starvation, idiopathic TBG depression, acute illness, drugs (anabolic steroids, androgens, high-dose salicylates, phenytoin) | • More metabolically active but shorter half-life than T_4. There is less T_3 than T_4 in the serum
• Diagnostic test for hyperthyroidism and T_3 thyrotoxicosis (elevated T_3 levels seen with normal T_4 levels)
• Little value in diagnosing hypothyroidism |

Sources: http://www.labtestsonline.org. Accessed January 25, 2008; Kratz A, Lewandrowski KB. Case records of the Massachusetts General Hospital. Weekly clinicopathological exercises. Normal reference laboratory values. *N Engl J Med.* 1998;339:1063–1072; OHSU Test Directory of Lab and Pathology Services http://www.ohsu.edu/health/consult-and-refer/labtests/index.cfm. Accessed February 1, 2008; Fischbach F. *A Manual of Laboratory Diagnostic Tests.* 6th ed. Philadelphia, PA: Lippincott Williams & Wilkins; 2004; Lee M. *Basic Skills in Interpreting Laboratory Data.* 3rd ed. Bethesda, MD: American Society of Health-System Pharmacists; 2004; American Diabetes Association. Diagnosis and classification of diabetes mellitus. *Diabetes Care.* 2008;31(Suppl 1):S55–S60; and American Association of Clinical Endocrinologists and the American College of Endocrinology. The American Association of Clinical Endocrinologists Medical Guidelines for the Management of Diabetes Mellitus: the AACE system of intensive diabetes self-management—2002 Update. *Endocr Pract.* 2002;8(Suppl 1):40–82, with permission.

Table 5.12 GASTROINTESTINAL AND HEPATIC ENZYME AND FUNCTION TESTS

Test Name	Description	Reference Range		Increased With	Decreased With	Other Comments
		Conventional Units	SI Units			
Amylase, serum	Measures enzyme concentrations in the serum	20–123 U/L	0.33–2.05 µkat/L	Acute pancreatitis, carcinoma (lung, esophagus, ovaries), acute exacerbation of chronic pancreatitis, partial gastrectomy, obstruction of pancreatic duct, perforated peptic ulcer, mumps, obstruction or inflammation of salivary duct or gland, acute cholecystitis, cerebral trauma, burns, traumatic shock, DKA, dissecting aortic aneurysm	Resolving acute pancreatitis, hepatitis, cirrhosis, toxemia of pregnancy	• An enzyme produced in the salivary glands, pancreas, liver, and fallopian tubes that converts starch to sugar

Lipase	Measures enzyme concentrations in the serum; reference values vary with methodology	10–140 U/L (varies widely by method of testing) 0.17–2.3 μkat/L	Pancreatitis, obstruction of the pancreatic duct, pancreatic carcinoma, acute cholecystitis, IBD, cirrhosis, severe renal disease	• Converts triglycerides to fatty acids and monoglyceride • The major source of lipase is the pancreas • With pancreatitis, elevation may not occur until 24–36 h after onset of illness; lipase may be high when amylase levels are normal; and lipase persists longer in the serum than amylase • Critical value: ≥500 U/L
Alanine aminotrans- ferase (ALT) (formerly serum glutamic pyruvic transaminase [SGPT])	Measures enzyme concentrations in the serum	10–50 U/L 0.17–0.83 μkat/L	Hepatocellular disease, active cirrhosis, obstructive jaundice/biliary obstruction, hepatitis, drugs (many)	• High enzyme concentrations present in the liver; also found in the heart, muscle, and kidney • More liver-specific than AST; used in the diagnosis of hepatic disease and to monitor the course of treat- ment for hepatitis, postne- crotic cirrhosis, and hepa- totoxic effects of drugs • An increase more than three times upper limit of normal [ULN] is generally considered clinically significant *(continued)*

Table 5.12 GASTROINTESTINAL AND HEPATIC ENZYME AND FUNCTION TESTS (continued)

Test Name	Description	Reference Range Conventional Units	Reference Range SI Units	Increased With	Decreased With	Other Comments
Aspartate aminotransferase (AST) (formerly serum glutamic oxaloacetic transaminase [SGOT])	Measures enzyme concentrations in the serum	5–40 U/L	0.08–0.67 μkat/L	MI, hepatic disease, acute pancreatitis, trauma, acute hemolytic anemia, acute renal disease, severe burns, drugs (many)	Acidotic patients with DM	• Enzyme of high metabolic activity found in heart, liver, skeletal muscle, kidney, brain, spleen, pancreas, and lung. Any injury or death of these cells or disease that causes change in these highly metabolic tissues will release the enzyme into circulation
Alkaline phosphatase (Alk Phos, ALP, AP)	Measures enzyme concentrations in the serum	30–130 U/L	0.5–2.17 μkat/L	Obstructive jaundice, hepatic lesions, cirrhosis, Paget disease, metastatic bone disease, osteomalacia, hyperparathyroidism, total parenteral nutrition, hyperphosphatemia, following IV administration of albumin (moderate)	Hypophosphatemia, malnutrition, hypothyroidism	• Enzyme mainly from bone, liver, and placenta, with different isoenzymes from different tissues. High concentrations are found in biliary canaliculi; also found in the kidney and intestines • In hepatic disease, levels rise when excretion is impaired due to biliary tract obstruction • Bone AP is a marker of bone formation

Test	Clinical significance	Reference values	Causes of abnormality	Comments
γ-Glutamyl transferase (GGT)	Beneficial in detecting acute or chronic alcohol consumption, obstructive jaundice, cholangitis, and cholecystitis	Male: ≤94 U/L Female: ≤70 U/L M: ≤1.5 μkat/L F: <1.12 μkat/L	Cholecystitis, cholelithiasis, cirrhosis, biliary obstruction, drugs (barbiturates, hepatotoxic drugs [especially those that induce the cytochrome P450 system])	• In most clinical instances, routine AP does not distinguish the isoenzymes. It is possible to measure these separately (for research purposes or patients who may have both hepatic and bone disease) to distinguish the source • Present mainly in the liver, kidney, spleen, and prostate (men have higher levels); liver is considered the source of normal serum activity, even though the kidney has the highest enzyme levels • Believed to function in the transport of amino acids and peptides • If AP and GGT are elevated, then increased AP is likely to be hepatic in origin • GGT is very sensitive but not specific; elevations of just GGT (not AST, ALT) do not necessarily indicate hepatic damage

(continued)

Table 5.12 GASTROINTESTINAL AND HEPATIC ENZYME AND FUNCTION TESTS (continued)

Test Name	Description	Reference Range		Increased With	Decreased With	Other Comments
		Conventional Units	SI Units			
Bilirubin (Bili, T. Bili)	Important in evaluating hepatic function, hemolytic anemias, and hyperbilirubin-emia (in newborns)	Total: <1.4 mg/dL Conjugated/ Direct: <0.4 mg/dL	Total: <23.9 μmol/L Conjugated/ Direct: <7 μmol/L	Unconjugated bilirubin: hemolytic anemia, trauma with evidence of a large hematoma, pulmonary infarcts; conjugated bilirubin: pancreatic cancer, cholelithiasis; both forms: hepatic metastasis, hepatitis, cirrhosis, cholestasis secondary to drugs; accompanied by jaundice: hepatocellular injury,		• Hgb breaks down into bilirubin (orange-yellow pigment); primarily removed by the liver and excreted into the bile, with a small amount found in the serum • Two forms of bilirubin: indirect/unconjugated (protein-bound), and direct/conjugated (circulates freely in the serum) • Increased conjugated bilirubin is usually associated with increased

			destruction of RBCs; increased unconjugated bilirubin is more likely due to dysfunction or blockage of the liver
			disease of parenchymal cells, bile duct obstruction, red cell hemolysis; hemolyzed blood samples (falsely elevated)
Lactate dehydrogenase (LD) (formerly LDH)	Levels are nonspecific but aid in confirmation of MI or pulmonary infarction in combination with other findings; may also be helpful in diagnosing muscular dystrophy and pernicious anemia	90–210 U/L (values vary considerably) 1.5–3.5 μkat/L	Acute leukemia, skeletal muscle necrosis, skin disorders, shock, megaloblastic anemia, lymphomas, acute MI (LD_1:LD_2 ratio usually "flips" to >1; levels increase within 12–24 h of MI and usually peak 3–4 days after), pulmonary infarction (increased within 24 h after onset of pain), drugs (various) Reflect a good response to cancer therapy	• Intracellular glycolytic enzyme, widely distributed in the tissues, particularly in the liver, kidney, heart, lungs, and skeletal muscle • Catalyzes the interconversion of lactate and pyruvate • More specific information can be determined if specific isoenzymes are requested

(continued)

181

Table 5.12 GASTROINTESTINAL AND HEPATIC ENZYME AND FUNCTION TESTS (continued)

Test Name	Description	Reference Range — Conventional Units	Reference Range — SI Units	Increased With	Decreased With	Other Comments
Albumin (Alb)	Measure of nutritional status	3.5–5.0 g/dL	35–50 g/L	(Uncommon) IV infusions, dehydration	Inadequate iron intake, severe hepatic disease, malabsorption, severe burns, starvation states, nephrotic syndrome, DM, SLE, may increase free drug (and effect) for agents that are highly protein bound (phenytoin, aspirin, valproate)	• Formed in the liver and helps maintain normal water distribution (colloidal osmotic pressure); aids in the transport of blood constituents (ions, bilirubin, hormones, enzymes, drugs) • Long half-life (21 days); slow to respond to changes in nutritional status
Prealbumin (PAB, transthyretin)	Preferred measure of nutritional status	17–42 mg/dL	170–420 mg/L		0–5 mg/dL = severe protein depletion; 5–10 mg/dL = moderate protein depletion; 10–15 mg/dL = mild protein depletion	• Shorter half-life (2 days) than albumin; responds quickly to changes in nutritional intake and restoration

| Ammonia (NH₃) | Evaluates metabolism as well as the progress of severe hepatic disease and response to treatment | ≤48 μmol/L | ≤48 μmol/L | Hepatic disease, hepatic coma, pericarditis, severe CHF, acute bronchitis, emphysema, urinary tract obstruction, azotemia, Reye syndrome, exercise | | • Formed by bacterial metabolism of proteins in the intestine; levels vary with protein intake Normally removed from the blood by the liver, converted to urea and excreted by the kidney
• Critical value: ≥150 |
| Hemoccult (guaiac or benzidine method) | Used to measure the presence of blood in stools, nasogastric output, and other bodily secretions | Negative | | Bleeding in gastrointestinal tract, (false positives: large doses of iron, iodides, phenazopyridine, or red meat within 3 days of the test) | (False negative: high doses of ascorbic acid) | • Blood in stools requires further investigation |

Sources: http://www.labtestsonline.org. Accessed January 25, 2008; Kratz A, Lewandrowski KB. Case records of the Massachusetts General Hospital. Weekly clinicopathological exercises. Normal reference laboratory values. N Engl J Med. 1998;339:1063–1072; OHSU Test Directory of Lab and Pathology Services http://www.ohsu.edu/health/consult-and-refer/labtests/index.cfm. Accessed February 1, 2008; Fischbach F. A Manual of Laboratory Diagnostic Tests. 6th ed. Philadelphia, PA: Lippincott Williams & Wilkins; 2004; and Lee M. Basic Skills in Interpreting Laboratory Data. 3rd ed. Bethesda, MD: American Society of Health-System Pharmacists; 2004, with permission.

Table 5.13 RENAL SYSTEM TESTS

Test Name	Description	Reference Range		Increased With	Decreased With	Other Comments
		Conventional Units	SI Units			
Blood urea nitrogen (BUN)	Provides an index of glomerular filtration	7–25 mg/dL	2.5–8.9 mmol/L	(Azotemia) inadequate excretion secondary to renal disease or urinary obstruction, decreased renal function (shock, dehydration, infection, DM, advanced age), major GI bleeding with subsequent catabolism of blood to nitrogen, increased protein intake, nephrotoxic drugs (aminoglycosides, amphotericin B)	End-stage hepatic failure, overhydration (dilutional), impaired absorption disorders (inability to absorb nitrogen or digest protein)	• Urea is a nonprotein, nitrogenous end product of protein catabolism, formed in the liver, carried by the blood to the kidneys, and excreted in urine • BUN can be affected by tissue necrosis, protein catabolism, and hydration status • Not as sensitive an indicator of renal function as creatinine or creatinine clearance • BUN/Cr ratio of >20 indicates prerenal azotemia; <20 when BUN is elevated is associated with intrinsic renal disease and azotemia

| Creatinine (Cr, serum creatinine, SCr) | Provides an index of glomerular filtration rate (GFR) | 0.6–1.3 mg/dL 62–115 µmol/L | Impaired renal function (nephritis, urinary tract obstruction, muscle disease, severe dehydration); drugs (many); may be normal despite impaired renal function in elderly and malnourished patients due to decreased muscle mass | Muscular dystrophy, atrophy (spinal cord injury), malnutrition, decreased muscle mass of aging | • Cr is a by-product of muscle creatine/phosphocreatine metabolism and is excreted renally. Since Cr is freely filtered by renal glomeruli and is not appreciably reabsorbed in the tubules under normal conditions, SCr and CrCl reflect GFR
• Several drugs can interfere with the measurement of SCr independent of their effects on renal function (ascorbic acid, cimetidine, levodopa, methyldopa)
• Serum half-life is ~1 day; therefore, it can take several days for new steady-state SCr to reflect changes in renal function
• Changes in SCr are not a linear representation of renal function; 2 and 3 mg/dL SCr correspond to ~50% and ~30% of normal renal function, respectively

(continued) |

Table 5.13 RENAL SYSTEM TESTS (*continued*)

Test Name	Description	Reference Range Conventional Units	Reference Range SI Units	Increased With	Decreased With	Other Comments
Creatinine clearance (CrCl)	Reflection of GFR	90–140 mL/min/1.73 m² body surface area (BSA)		High cardiac output, pregnancy, burns, carbon monoxide poisoning	Impaired renal function, renal disease/infection, shock, dehydration, hemorrhage, COPD, CHF Stages of chronic kidney disease (CKD): stage 1 = GFR >90; stage 2 = GFR 60–89; stage 3 = GFR 30–59; stage 4 = GFR 15–29; stage 5 = kidney failure with GFR <15 or dialysis	• Calculated creatinine clearance (CrCl) is a better reflection of renal function and takes into account the age and weight of the patient; measured CrCl is better still, but requires measurement of Cr in a timed urine collection and SCr. • Overestimates GFR in severe renal impairment; SCr is more accurate in this situation
Creatinine, urine	Used when measuring CrCl from a timed sample and albumin-to-creatinine ratio (urine microalbumin)	11–26 mg/kg/d	97–230 μmol/kg/d	Same as SCr, acromegaly, gigantism, DM, hypothyroidism, high-protein diet	Same as SCr, hyperthyroidism, anemia, polymyositis, inflammatory muscle disease, leukemia, advanced renal disease or renal stenosis	• To calculate CrCl, values for SCr and the total amount of creatinine excreted in urine over a fixed time (usually 24 h) are required [see Chapter 12, A Pharmacy Calculations Anthology] • If the value is lower than expected (see reference values), then it is likely that the urine collection was not complete and will not allow accurate assessment of CrCl

| Microalbumin/albumin, urine | Assesses small amounts of protein in urine | <30 µg/mg creatinine (random) | Microalbuminuria: 30–299 µg/mg creatinine; macro (clinical)-albuminuria: >300 µg/mg creatinine
Diabetic nephropathy, end-stage renal disease (ESRD), marker for increased cardiovascular disease (CVD) risk | • Preferred method: albumin-to-creatinine ratio in a random spot collection; 24-h or timed collections are more burdensome and add little to prediction or accuracy
• Measuring urine albumin only (immunoassay or dipstick specific for micro-albumin), without simultaneously measuring urine Cr, is not recommended (false negatives and positives due to variations in urine concentration with hydration and other factors)
• Albumin excretion can be variable, so 2/3 of specimens collected within 3–6 mo should be abnormal before considering new diagnosis
• Numerous factors (recent exercise, infection, fever, CHF, pronounced hyperglycemia or HTN) may elevate urinary albumin excretion over baseline values |

(continued)

Table 5.13 RENAL SYSTEM TESTS (continued)

Test Name	Description	Reference Range Conventional Units	Reference Range SI Units	Increased With	Decreased With	Other Comments
Urine sodium (Na$^+$)	Assesses fluid balance, aldosterone effects, and renal concentrating ability	40–220 mEq/24 h	40–220 mmol/24 h	Diuretic use, Addison disease, SIADH, renal tubular acidosis, renal tubular necrosis (>30 mmol/L with oliguria)	Dehydration, CHF, hepatic, disease, nephrotic syndrome	• Wide range of reference values reflects variations in diet, posture, stress, and endocrine effects
Urine potassium (K$^+$)	Used in workup of aldosteronism, renal tubular acidosis, and alkalosis	25–125 mEq/24 h	25–125 mmol/24 h	Chronic renal failure, DM, renal tubular acidosis, dehydration, primary aldosteronism, Cushing disease	Acute renal failure, malabsorption/diarrhea syndromes	• Concentration is dependent on diet • Urine pH is decreased in patients who have decreased potassium levels (hydrogen secreted in exchange for potassium) because less potassium is available for exchange

Test	Purpose	Reference Range	Comments
Na^+/K^+ ratio, urine	Evaluates renal function, fluid and electrolyte balance, acid-base balance, and extent of aldosterone effects on electrolyte composition of the urine	0.9–3.88	• Diurnal variation occurs • Timed collection is required for an accurate measurement; a single collection may be used to assess responses to spironolactone therapy (>1 with effective therapy)
Urine chloride (Cl^-)	Used in workup of acid-base status to determine whether metabolic alkalosis is chloride responsive	110–250 mEq/24 h 110–250 mmol/24 h	• Normal values are dependent on diet and perspiration • Only has meaning if Na^+/K^+ intake and output are also known • Can serve as a guide in monitoring individuals eating salt-restricted diets

Sources: http://www.labtestsonline.org. Accessed January 25, 2008; Kratz A, Lewandrowski KB. Case records of the Massachusetts General Hospital. Weekly clinicopathological exercises. Normal reference laboratory values. N Engl J Med. 1998;339:1063–1072; OHSU Test Directory of Lab and Pathology Services http://www.ohsu.edu/health/consult-and-refer/labtests/index.cfm. Accessed February 1, 2008; Fischbach F. A Manual of Laboratory Diagnostic Tests. 6th ed. Philadelphia, PA: Lippincott Williams & Wilkins; 2004; and Lee M. Basic Skills in Interpreting Laboratory Data. 3rd ed. Bethesda, MD: American Society of Health-System Pharmacists; 2004; and American Diabetes Association. Diagnosis and classification of diabetes mellitus. Diabetes Care. 2008;31(Suppl 1):S55–S60, with permission.

Table 5.14 MISCELLANEOUS BLOOD TESTS

Test Name	Description	Reference Range Conventional Units	Reference Range SI Units	Increased With	Decreased With	Other Comments
Erythrocyte sedimentation rate (ESR, sed rate)	Nonspecific test that is used for monitoring infections and inflammatory diseases	Males: 1–20 mm/h Females: 1–30 mm/h		Increased plasma fibrinogen, globulin, or cholesterol, infections (tuberculosis [TB]), inflammatory diseases (RA), tissue destruction (acute MI, neoplasms), multiple myeloma, advanced age, female sex, macrocytic anemia, normocytic anemia, pregnancy	CHF, microcytic anemia, sickle cell anemia, polycythemia vera, carcinomas, hepatic disease, corticosteroids	• Increases with age • Useful for following certain diseases (MI, rheumatic fever, RA, TB)
C-reactive protein (CRP)	Marker of inflammatory processes	<0.12 mg/dL	<12 mg/L	Severe trauma, infections (rheumatic fever), inflammation (RA), surgery, cancer		• Sensitive acute-phase reactant • Used to assess activity of inflammatory disease, detect infections after surgery, detect transplant rejection, and monitor inflammatory processes

Test	(Clinical use)	Reference values	(Conditions)	Comments
Beta₂-microglobulin (B₂M)	Monitoring may allow diagnosis of renal graft rejection before changes in SCr are seen, allowing for earlier treatment	Urine: <120 μg/24 h Serum: 1.2–2.5 mg/L	Inflammatory reactions, active chronic lymphocytic leukemia, glomerular disease (serum), tubular dysfunction (urine), aminoglycoside toxicity	Glomerular disease (urine), tubular dysfunction (serum), treatment of acute renal graft rejection (serum B₂M decreases faster than SCr)	• Serum B₂M values depend on GFR, whereas urinary B₂M values vary with the functional activity of proximal renal tubular cells • Useful for evaluating kidney allograft rejection in transplant patients; will often change in advance of SCr
Prostate-specific antigen (PSA)	Used for screening and early detection of prostate cancer	0–4.0 ng/mL	0–40 μg/L	Prostate cancer (80% of patients), benign prostatic hypertrophy [benign prostatic hyperplasia [BPH], <8 ng/mL)	• In both normal prostatic epithelial and carcinoma cells • Most prognostically reliable marker for monitoring recurrence or prostatic carcinoma; however, does not have sensitivity or specificity to be an ideal tumor marker

Sources: http://www.labtestsonline.org. Accessed January 25, 2008; Kratz A, Lewandrowski KB. Case records of the Massachusetts General Hospital. Weekly clinicopathological exercises. Normal reference laboratory values. *N Engl J Med.* 1998;339:1063–1072; OHSU Test Directory of Lab and Pathology Services http://www.ohsu.edu/health/consult-and-refer/labtests/index.cfm. Accessed February 1, 2008; Fischbach F. *A Manual of Laboratory Diagnostic Tests.* 6th ed. Philadelphia, PA: Lippincott Williams & Wilkins; 2004; and Lee M. *Basic Skills in Interpreting Laboratory Data.* 3rd ed. Bethesda, MD: American Society of Health-System Pharmacists; 2004, with permission.

Table 5.15 URINALYSIS

Test Name	Description	Reference Range Conventional Units	Reference Range SI Units	Increased With	Decreased With	Other Comments
Specific gravity	Evaluates patients with renal disease	1.001–1.030		Glucosuria, iodinated contrast media, massive proteinuria (>2 g/24 h)		• >1.025 in the morning indicates good concentrating ability • 1.010–1.012 means the urine is isotonic with plasma (285–295 mOsm)
Appearance		Straw-colored, yellow				
pH		5.0–7.5		(Alkalinized) urea splitting organisms (Proteus sp., Klebsiella sp., Escherichia coli), renal tubular acidosis caused by amphotericin		
Protein	A 24-h urine specimen is collected to quantitate the urinary protein	0–trace (Tr)		Renal disease, DM, prolonged standing (trace amounts), alkaline urine (false positive with dipstick method)		• The urinary protein may be normal, indicating increased glomerular permeability or a renal tubular disorder; or abnormal because of multiple myeloma and Bence-Jones proteins

Glucose	More commonly found in routine UA; no longer routinely used for DM monitoring	Negative	DM	• The correlation of urine glucose with serum glucose can be helpful in monitoring and adjusting hypoglycemic medications (rarely used for this anymore)
Ketones		Negative	Starvation, poorly controlled DM, alcoholism	
Blood		Negative		
Sediment analysis		Cell count for RBC, WBC (see Table 5.16)		• No particular type of urine cast is pathognomonic for a specific renal disorder. However, the presence of RBC or WBC casts may signal a clinically significant issue (Table 5.2)
Gram stain		Negative		

Sources: http://www.labtestsonline.org. Accessed January 25, 2008; Kratz A, Lewandrowski KB. Case records of the Massachusetts General Hospital. Weekly clinicopathological exercises. Normal reference laboratory values. N Engl J Med. 1998;339:1063–1072; OHSU Test Directory of Lab and Pathology Services http://www.ohsu.edu/health/consult-and-refer/labtests/index.cfm. Accessed February 1, 2008; Fischbach F. A Manual of Laboratory Diagnostic Tests. 6th ed. Philadelphia, PA: Lippincott Williams & Wilkins; 2004; and Lee M. Basic Skills in Interpreting Laboratory Data. 3rd ed. Bethesda, MD: American Society of Health-System Pharmacists; 2004, with permission.

Table 5.16 CELL TYPES IN THE URINE SEDIMENT

Cell Type	Reference Range	Clinical Considerations
RBC	0–2 per high-power field (hpf)	• Cystitis is the most frequent cause of hematuria, although slight hematuria may occur with exertion, trauma, or febrile illness • Yeast cells may be confused with RBCs; to distinguish between the two, adding acetic acid will cause RBCs, but not yeast cells, to lyse
Epithelial	0–2/hpf	• Epithelial cells increase with tubular damage or heavy proteinuria • Should be squamous epithelial cells only
Bacteria	0	• Presence of bacteria on Gram stain of unspun specimen correlates well with culture growth of 10^5 organisms (= urinary tract infection) • A culture and sensitivity (C&S) is useful to confirm the presence of bacteria
WBC	0–5/hpf	• Polymorphonuclear leukocytes are the most common form of WBCs observed; if seen, and two routine cultures are negative, the culture should be tested for tubercle bacilli
Casts	0–occasional per low-power field	• Red cell casts usually signify active glomerular disease • Fatty and waxy casts may be seen with inflammatory or degenerative renal disease • Leukocyte casts are usually associated by pyelonephritis • Hyaline or granular casts may also be present normally, $\leq$0–1 per hpf

Sources: http://www.labtestsonline.org. Accessed January 25, 2008; Kratz A, Lewandrowski KB. Case records of the Massachusetts General Hospital. Weekly clinicopathological exercises. Normal reference laboratory values. *N Engl J Med.* 1998;339:1063–1072; OHSU Test Directory of Lab and Pathology Services http://www.ohsu.edu/health/consult-and-refer/labtests/index.cfm. Accessed February 1, 2008; Fischbach F. *A Manual of Laboratory Diagnostic Tests.* 6th ed. Philadelphia, PA: Lippincott Williams & Wilkins; 2004; and Lee M. *Basic Skills in Interpreting Laboratory Data.* 3rd ed. Bethesda, MD: American Society of Health-System Pharmacists; 2004, with permission.

Tests for infectious diseases, including hepatitis and human immunodeficiency virus (HIV), are numerous and are beyond the scope of a general review such as this. Standard practices in the therapies, goals, and tests used for this disease are ever-evolving; therefore specific infectious disease references should be consulted when diagnosing, assessing, or monitoring these patients.

Urinalysis (UA)

A urinalysis provides many pieces of information (Tables 5.15 and 5.16) and can be used to evaluate patients with renal disease, diabetes, infections, and other conditions.

Acknowledgment

The previous authors, Mary B. Elliot, Richard C. Christopherson, and Karen E. Vick Smith, are acknowledged for their work on this chapter in the first two editions.

References

1. www.labtestsonline.org. Accessed January 25, 2008.
2. Kratz A, Lewandrowski KB. Case records of the Massachusetts General Hospital. Weekly clinicopathological exercises. Normal reference laboratory values. *N Engl J Med.* 1998;339:1063–1072.
3. OHSU Test Directory of Lab and Pathology Services http://www.ohsu.edu/health/consult-and-refer/labtests/index.cfm. Accessed February 1, 2008.
4. Fischbach F. *A Manual of Laboratory Diagnostic Tests.* 6th ed. Philadelphia, PA: Lippincott Williams & Wilkins; 2004.
5. Lee M. *Basic Skills in Interpreting Laboratory Data.* 3rd ed. Bethesda, MD: American Society of Health-System Pharmacists; 2004.
6. Grundy SM, Cleeman JI, Merz CN, et al. Implications of recent clinical trials for the National Cholesterol Education Program Adult Treatment Panel III guidelines. *Circulation.* 2004;110:227–239.
7. American Diabetes Association. Diagnosis and classification of diabetes mellitus. *Diabetes Care.* 2008;31(Suppl 1):S55–S60.
8. American Association of Clinical Endocrinologists and the American College of Endocrinology. The American Association of Clinical Endocrinologists Medical Guidelines for the Management of Diabetes Mellitus: the AACE system of intensive diabetes self-management—2002 Update. *Endocr Pract.* 2002;8(Suppl 1):40–82.

Other Suggested Readings and Resources

Beer MH, Porter RS, Jones TV, eds. *The Merck Manual of Diagnosis and Therapy.* 18th ed. Whitehouse Station, NJ: Merck & Co., Inc.; 2006.

Burtis CA, Ashwood ER, Bruns DE, eds. *Tietz Fundamentals of Clinical Chemistry*. 6th ed. Philadelphia, PA: WB Saunders; 2007.

Burtis CA, Ashwood ER, Bruns DE, eds. *Tietz Textbook of Clinical Chemistry and Molecular Diagnostics*. 4th ed. Philadelphia, PA: WB Saunders; 2005.

Henry JB, Davey FR, Herman CJ, et al., eds. *Clinical Diagnosis and Management by Laboratory Methods*. 20th ed. Philadelphia, PA: WB Saunders; 2001.

Howanitz JH, Howanitz PJ, eds. *Laboratory Medicine: Test Selection and Interpretation*. Philadelphia, PA: WB Saunders; 1991.

National Committee for Clinical Laboratory Standards. *How to Define and Determine Reference Intervals in the Clinical Laboratory: Approved Guideline*. 2nd ed. Wayne, PA: NCCLS; 2000.

Pagana KD, Pagana TJ, eds. *Mosby's Manual of Diagnostic and Laboratory Tests*. 3rd ed. St. Louis, MO: Mosby; 2005.

Ravel R. Clinical Laboratory Medicine—Clinical Application of Laboratory Data. 6th ed. St. Louis, MO: Mosby; 1994.

Sacher RA, McPherson RA. *Widmann's Clinical Interpretation of Laboratory Tests*. 11th ed. Philadelphia, PA: FA Davis Co; 2000.

Tierney LM, McPhee SJ, Papadakis MA, eds. *Current Medical Diagnosis and Treatment*. 47th ed. New York, NY: McGraw-Hill; 2008.

Wu AHB, ed. *Tietz Clinical Guide to Laboratory Tests*. 4th ed. Philadelphia, PA: WB Saunders; 2006.

6 Diagnostic Procedures

Roberta A. Aulie, Robert M. Breslow,
Katherine E. Rotzenberg, and Kathleen A. Skibinski

General Procedures

Biopsy[1,2]

Description

A biopsy is performed by means of an aspiration or cutting needle, fine needle, scalpel, or punch. Biopsies may be closed (i.e., not requiring a surgical incision) or open (i.e., requiring a surgical incision). The technique and equipment used are dependent on the location and type of tissue to be sampled. Common biopsy sites include the bone marrow, breast, bone, cervix, endometrial tissue, kidney, liver, lung, lymph node, muscle, myocardium, nerve, pleura, prostate, skin, small bowel, and thyroid. A local or general anesthetic may be administered before the procedure. Diagnostic modalities such as radiographs, computed tomography (CT), and ultrasound (US) are used to guide the needle to the appropriate site.

Purpose

The purpose of a biopsy is to gather a small piece of tissue for microscopic analysis (either histologic or cytologic) to determine if the tissue is cancerous or noncancerous, to determine if infection is present, or to determine if other diagnostic findings are due to inflammation, scarring, or organ rejection. Biopsy usually follows other diagnostic procedures, such as CT or magnetic resonance imaging (MRI), that can identify changes but cannot diagnose the cause of those changes.

Findings

Normal and abnormal findings are dependent on the histology or cytology of the specific tissue undergoing biopsy.

Pharmacy Implications

- Patients may require sedation with a parenteral benzodiazepine such as midazolam or diazepam. Patients should be monitored for oversedation and respiratory depression.
- If a local anesthetic such as lidocaine or bupivacaine is to be used, the patient should be asked about a history of allergic reactions.
- In those patients requiring general anesthesia, an anticholinergic such as parenteral atropine or glycopyrrolate, a sedative such as diazepam or midazolam, or an analgesic such as morphine or meperidine may be required 15 to 30 minutes before anesthesia.
- It is recommended that antiplatelet agents should be discontinued before open and needle biopsies. Aspirin should be discontinued 7 to 10 days before the procedure. Nonsteroidal anti-inflammatory drugs (NSAIDs) (e.g., ibuprofen, naproxen) that reversibly inhibit the enzyme cyclooxygenase should be discontinued 2 to 4 days before the procedure. Based on early evidence, it appears that COX-2 inhibitors may not require discontinuation before biopsy.

Computed Tomography (CT)[3–7]

Description

Computed tomography (CT or CAT), is a painless, noninvasive method for obtaining a three-dimensional picture of body structures using cross-sectional (transverse) slice x-ray views. A complete scan consists of many pictures.

When performing a CT scan, an x-ray source or beam, together with a gamma ray detector, rotates around the patient in a 360-degree arc. The x-ray beam is very narrow, allowing little internal scatter of radiation. The detector simultaneously measures the intensity of radiation. A computer calculates the amount of radiation absorbed by each volume of tissue and assigns a gray scale number to it. The computer analyzes the numbers and reconstructs a cross-sectional picture that can be displayed on a screen or produced as a hard copy for a permanent record and later interpretation.

Contrast media such as diatrizoate, iohexol, iopamidol, iothalamate, metrizoate, or metrizamide may be injected intravenously to enhance the images of brain, abdominal structures, and vasculature. Several doses of oral contrast media (diatrizoate) as a 2% solution (4 mL/200 mL H_2O) is administered before abdominal CT scans to provide contrast enhancement of certain abdominal structures.

Purpose

CT scans can confirm the diagnosis of suspected malignancies, assist in determining the staging and extent of neoplastic disease, and determine the effectiveness of therapy. CT scans of the brain and skull (cranial CT) may be performed to define the nature of head trauma, hydrocephalus, increased intracranial pressure, cerebrovascular lesions, degenerative brain diseases, and infections. CT scans of the body (body CT) that examine the neck, thorax, abdomen, and extremities may provide information on the cause of jaundice, inflammatory processes, pleural or chest wall abnormalities, and suspected abnormal collections of blood or fluid. A spinal CT is performed to evaluate disorders of the spine and spinal cord.

Findings

Normal and abnormal findings are dependent on the organs being evaluated.

Pharmacy Implications

- Because patients must lie completely still for an extended period, uncooperative patients are sedated with benzodiazepines (e.g., midazolam, diazepam, or lorazepam) or a sedative such as chloral hydrate. The typical sedative doses for these agents are as follows:
  - *Midazolam.* Children: 0.05–0.1 mg/kg via an intravenous (IV) route or 0.1 mg/kg via an intramuscular (IM) route; adults: 0.05–0.1 mg/kg IV or 0.07–0.08 mg/kg IM.
  - *Diazepam.* Adults: 0.1–0.3 mg/kg IV.
  - *Lorazepam.* Adults: 0.04 mg/kg IV or 0.5 mg/kg IM up to 4 mg.
  - *Chloral hydrate.* Children: 50–70 mg/kg up to 2.5 gm.
- IV iodine contrast media should be used cautiously in patients with known or suspected hypersensitivity to iodine. Ionized contrast media are more likely to produce hypersensitivity reactions. Nonionized products rarely produce reactions and are used in patients with previously documented histories of iodine hypersensitivity.

Gallium Scan[4,6–8]

Description

Radioactive gallium citrate (Ga^{67}) is administered intravenously 24–48 hours before the scan. The gallium scan is performed over the entire body by the use of a gamma scintillation camera or a rectilinear scanner. The scanning device measures the radiation emissions of Ga^{67} and shows the distribution or uptake patterns of Ga^{67} throughout the body. These emissions are converted into images that can be displayed in a video format or can be photographed for later use and interpretation. The degree of radioactivity Ga^{67} possesses is minimal and not harmful. A complete scan takes approximately 30 to 60 minutes.

Purpose

Gallium scans are used to detect or evaluate primary or metastatic neoplasms; inflammatory lesions of bacterial, autoimmune, or other origin; malignant lymphoma or recurrent tumors after chemotherapy or radiation therapy; and lung cancer. In addition, these scans aid in the diagnosis of focal defects in the liver.

Findings
Normal

Ga^{67} uptake is seen in the liver, spleen, bones, and large bowel.

Abnormal

Ga^{67} uptake is seen in abscesses, inflamed tissues, and some tumors.

Pharmacy Implications

Ga^{67} is excreted into the feces. This could interfere with the detection of inflammatory or neoplastic diseases of the colon. Therefore, a cleansing enema should be administered before the scan. Patients do not need to restrict food or fluid intake before the scan.

Magnetic Resonance Imaging (MRI)[4,9-14]

Description

With conventional MRI, the patient is placed inside a large circular magnet. The magnetic field causes the protons inside the body's atoms to spin in the same direction. A radio frequency signal is then beamed into the magnetic field, which causes the protons to move out of alignment. When the radio signal is terminated, the protons move back into the position produced by the magnetic field, releasing energy as this occurs. A receiver coil measures the energy released and the time it takes for the protons to return to the aligned position. This provides information about the type and condition of the tissue from which the energy emanates. A computer then processes all the information and constructs a two- or three-dimensional picture of the tissues examined, which appears on a television screen. A permanent copy of this image is produced on film or magnetic tape.

Open MRI uses the same technology as conventional MRI but does not have a closed tube into which the patient is placed to perform the imaging.

This open technology is advantageous for the patient who experiences claustrophobia in narrow closed spaces.

MRI combines the advantage of anatomic imaging with excellent soft tissue characterization. Although MRI does not use ionizing radiation and does not require a contrast agent to identify vascular structures, a specialized contrast material such as gadolinium is now being used in certain circumstances to enhance MRI images.

Purpose

MRI is especially useful for diagnosis of brain and nervous system disorders, cardiovascular disease, and cancer. MRI provides very precise and detailed images of internal organs.

Findings

Normal and abnormal findings are dependent on the anatomy being evaluated.

Pharmacy Implications

- Successful imaging requires patients to lie very still. Uncooperative patients, patients who are claustrophobic, and children should be sedated (see CT scan recommendations). No contrast media are required.
- MRI is contraindicated in patients with cardiac pacemakers, surgically inserted metal hardware such as aneurysm clips, intrauterine devices, and recently inserted metal prostheses.

Ultrasonography[4,15]

Description

Ultrasound (US) is a noninvasive, nontoxic (without dyes) diagnostic procedure that examines internal structures by using high-frequency sound waves. As sound travels through the body tissues, it is modified (weakened as it goes through tissues) and travels at different speeds depending on the density and elasticity of the tissues. This is referred to as the acoustic impedance of the tissue.

In ultrasonography, a transducer produces short pulses of sound. When the sound wave produced by the transducer encounters an interface (the border between two adjacent structures), some of the waves are reflected (echoed) back to the transducer and an electric current is produced. The current is amplified, and the resultant image is displayed on a cathode ray tube (CRT).

US produces a good image when there are small differences in tissue density of the adjacent structures. However, when there are large differences, as between bone and soft tissue or air-filled spaces and soft tissue, the image is unintelligible because most of the sound waves are reflected back.

Traditionally, US could not be used to evaluate bone or air-filled spaces. A new generation of equipment used to screen for osteoporosis uses US principles to assess bone density. Because US can measure sound frequency shifts due to motion, US can be used to evaluate blood flow, free fluid, and amniotic fluid.

Purpose
- Examine internal soft tissue organs and structures including the eye, thyroid, breast, heart, liver, spleen, gallbladder, bile ducts, pancreas, uterus, ovary, bladder, and kidneys.
- Detect and evaluate masses, abscesses, stones, motion, fluid, and other reasons for obstruction.
- Determine size, shape, and position of the organ under study.
- Differentiate solid, cystic, and complex masses.

Several enhancement techniques are now used to provide better contrast and visualization of various body structures and to provide more recognizable images with greater detail.

Findings
Normal
Absence of masses, obstructions, and abscesses. Normal shape, size, and position of organs.

Abnormal
Presence of masses, obstructions, or abscesses. Abnormal size, shape, or location of organs.

Pharmacy Implications
None.

 ## Allergy/Immunology

Candida, Histoplasmin, and Mumps Skin Test [4,16,17]
Description
Skin testing is a method of detecting an individual's sensitivity to certain allergens (antigens) or microorganisms responsible for disease. Skin

testing may also be used to assess the integrity of a person's cell-mediated immune system. Three types of skin tests are generally used: scratch, patch, and intradermal tests. Reaction to a skin test demonstrates a hypersensitivity to the tested antigen. This indicates immunity to a disease or product or can indicate the presence of the active or inactive disease being studied.

An antigen is made from serum in which the organism responsible for the respective infection is present. The antigen is injected (0.1 mL) intradermally as a bleb on the volar (flexor) surface of the forearm by use of a tuberculin syringe and a small (25- to 27-gauge) needle. Tests are usually evaluated at 48 to 72 hours.

Purpose

Although each test can be used by itself to determine whether a patient has had the respective infection, the primary purpose of these recall antigens (those to which a patient has had, or may have had, previous exposure or sensitization) is to evaluate the competence of the cell-mediated immune system by attempting to provoke an immune response These skin tests are referred to as controls because they are used to determine whether a negative response to a skin test (e.g., tuberculin) is the result of negative exposure to the antigen or to incompetent cell- mediated immunity.

Findings
Normal

A positive reaction indicates previous exposure and resistance to the antigen. A positive test is observed when an induration ≥ 10 mm in diameter appears after injection of the antigen.

Abnormal

A negative reaction indicates that the patient has not been exposed to the antigen or is suggestive (more likely) of a compromised immune system (anergy). No erythema and a lesion <10 mm in diameter indicates a negative test.

Pharmacy Implications

Skin tests are refrigerated before use. Concurrent or recent use of corticosteroids can produce a false-negative result due to suppression of the cell-mediated (delayed hypersensitivity) immune response. Antihistamines and H_2-blockers interfere with the cutaneous histamine response of the immunoglobulin E (IgE)-mediated immediate hypersensitivity reaction and can produce false-negative results.

Tuberculin Skin Test (PPD)[4,7,16]

Description

Tuberculin is a protein fraction (purified protein derivative) of the soluble growth product of *Mycobacterium tuberculosis* or *Mycobacterium bovis*. The antigen is administered intradermally (0.1 mL), creating a bleb at the intradermal injection site (usually the volar or dorsal aspect of the forearm). The antigen is available in three concentrations described as tuberculin units (TU): 1 TU, 5 TU, and 250 TU. The test is evaluated within 48 to 72 hours.

Purpose

The tuberculin antigen is administered to determine if the patient has active or dormant tuberculosis. However, the test cannot differentiate active from dormant infections.

Findings

Normal

Absence of redness or induration. This is referred to as a negative skin test.

Abnormal

Induration of the skin, erythema, edema, and central necrosis. The larger the wheal diameter in millimeters around the injection site, the more positive is the result (negative, <5 mm; doubtful or probable, 5–9 mm; positive, ≥ 10 mm). A positive skin test indicates prior exposure to the tubercle bacilli (TB) or previous bacille Calmette-Guérin (BCG) vaccination.

Pharmacy Implications

PPD (purified protein derivative of tuberculin) is refrigerated and must be drawn up just before use. The 5-TU concentration is used most frequently; however, the 1-TU concentration is sometimes used as initial screening in patients with suspected tuberculosis to lessen the severity of the reaction. The 250-TU concentration, although rarely used, can be used when tuberculosis is suspected and a state of anergy may be present.

Concurrent or recent use of corticosteroids and other immunosuppressive agents can produce false-negative results due to suppression of the cell-mediated (delayed hypersensitivity) immune system. Antihistamines and H_2-blockers interfere with the cutaneous histamine response of the IgE-mediated immediate hypersensitivity reaction and can produce false-negative results. Lymphoid disease can produce a false-positive result. Viral and certain bacterial infections can cause false-negative results due to suppression of the delayed hypersensitivity reaction. Prior administration of BCG vaccine and recent vaccination with attenuated live virus vaccines can result in a false-positive reaction.

Cardiology

Cardiac Catheterization[11,12]

Description

Cardiac catheterization is performed by inserting a catheter (a thin, flexible tube) through a small incision made in an artery or vein in the neck, arm, or groin after administration of a local anesthetic at the intended insertion site to minimize patient discomfort. The catheter is then threaded into the right or left side of the heart with the assistance of fluoroscopy to help guide the placement of the catheter. Patients are mildly sedated before the test but remain awake throughout the procedure. Cardiac catheterization is usually performed in conjunction with coronary angiography, which uses an IV contrast material to visualize the coronary arteries. Fluoroscopy provides immediate visualization of the coronary circulation.

Purpose

Cardiac catheterization is performed to evaluate cardiac valvular disease, heart function, and congenital heart anomalies as well as to determine the need for cardiac surgery. When combined with angiography, the coronary arteries can be evaluated for obstruction (occlusion) to assess patient risk for myocardial infarction (MI). Catheterization can also be used to perform angioplasty and place stents to open up and prevent reocclusion of coronary arteries.

Findings
Normal

Heart size, motion, thickness, blood supply, and blood pressure within normal limits.

Abnormal

Presence of coronary artery disease, valvular heart disease, ventricular aneurysms, or enlargement of the heart.

Pharmacy Implications

- Patients receiving daily digoxin should receive their dose on the day of the procedure.
- It is likely that patients will receive diazepam or lorazepam 30 minutes before the procedure.

- Patients should be evaluated for a history of sensitivity to local anesthetics or IV contrast material.

Echocardiography[4,7,11,12,15,18,19]

Description

Echocardiography is a specialized two-dimensional ultrasonographic technique by which a transducer is placed on the chest where there is no bone or lung tissue. High-frequency sound waves are directed at the heart. The heart reflects these waves (echoes) back to the transducer. These sound waves are then converted to electrical impulses and relayed to an echocardiography machine, which creates a diagram on an oscilloscope.

Conventional (transthoracic echocardiography) is performed by placing the transducer on the exterior chest wall. The problem encountered with this technique is a degraded heart image due to bony structures (sternum and ribs) and an extensive lung interface. Transesophageal echocardiography was developed to overcome these barriers to image quality. This technique involves the placement of an echo transducer on the tip of a gastroscope. Following administration of a local anesthetic spray to the back of the throat, a gastroscope is advanced orally into the esophagus, permitting placement of the transducer in closer proximity to the heart. This approach serves to eliminate chest cage and lung interference seen with the conventional technique. Because the transducer can be placed closer to the heart, transesophageal echocardiography can use higher-frequency transducers that significantly improve the resolution of the images. Two-dimensional conventional or transesophageal echo can be complemented with the addition of three-dimensional Doppler echocardiography, which is used to gather hemodynamic information because of its ability to measure the velocity of the red blood cells.

Purpose

- Diagnose or rule out valvular abnormalities or pericardial effusion.
- Measure the size of heart chambers.
- Evaluate chambers and valves of the heart.
- Detect atrial tumors and cardiac thrombi.
- Evaluate cardiac function or wall motion after MI.
- Evaluate blood flow through the heart chambers and valves.

Findings
Normal

No mechanical or gross anatomic abnormalities. Normal cardiac function. Normal blood flow patterns and blood velocity through the heart chambers and valves.

Abnormal

Abnormal motion, pattern, and structure of the four cardiac valves, left ventricular dysfunction, valve abnormalities, wall thickening, tumors or thrombi in the heart, abnormal size of the heart or chamber, or pericardial effusion. Abnormal blood flow.

Pharmacy Implications
Conventional Echocardiography
None.

Transesophageal Echocardiography
- Patients should be questioned about allergies to topical anesthetic spray.
- Patient will require parenteral sedation (e.g., midazolam) and analgesia (e.g., morphine).

Electrocardiography (ECG)[4,7,11,12,16,20]
Description
ECG is a graphic recording of the electrical impulses of the heart that tracks the cardiac cycle from depolarization through repolarization. The electrical current generated by myocardial depolarization is naturally conducted to the surface of the body, where it is detected by electrodes placed on the patient's limbs and chest. The waves produced by this electrical activity are amplified for greater visibility before being printed on a moving graph paper strip. To capture the multidirectional electrical activity, 12 ECG leads are used simultaneously to achieve a comprehensive view of the electrical activity of the heart. Leads I, II, III, AVF, AVL, and AVR are attached to the limbs and provide an electrical view of the frontal plane of the heart; leads V1, V2, V3, V4, V5, and V6 are attached to the chest and produce a horizontal view of the heart's electrical activity. The tracing produced by the ECG shows the voltage of the waves, the time duration of waves, and the interval between them.

Purpose
ECG is used in the diagnosis of coronary artery disease, MI, pericardial effusion, pericarditis, rhythm disturbances as a result of ischemia or electrolyte abnormalities, and disorders of impulse formation and conduction. It is also helpful for evaluation of the effect of drugs on the heart.

Findings
Normal
See Table 6.1.

Table 6.1 DESCRIPTION OF ECG WAVE AND NORMAL FINDINGS

Wave/Interval	Explanation	Normal Finding
P wave	Impulse from SA node to atria (atrial depolarization)	Normal size, shape, and deflection
PR interval	P wave to QRS complex	0.1–0.2 s
QRS complex	Depolarization of the ventricle	<0.12 s
ST segment	Interval between depolarization and repolarization	No elevation or depression
T wave	Recovery phase after contraction (ventricular polarization)	No inversion

SA, sinoatrial.

Abnormal

Abnormal heart rate, rhythm, axis, or position of the heart; myocardial hypertrophy; or MI. Conclusions can be reached about heart function after comparing the waves and intervals of the particular tracing against a normal tracing. However, this information cannot be used to depict the actual mechanical state of the heart or the integrity of the heart valves.

Pharmacy Implications

Cardioactive drugs (e.g., digoxin, quinidine, beta-blockers) have various specific effects on the ECG tracing.

Electrophysiology Study (EPS)[16,18,21]

Description

Solid electrode catheters are most commonly inserted into the venous system and advanced into the right atrium, across the septal leaflet of the tricuspid valve and into the right ventricle in a fashion similar to cardiac catheterization. Discrete conduction intervals are measured by recording electrical conduction during the slow withdrawal of a bipolar or tripolar electrode catheter from the right ventricle through the His bundle to the sinoatrial (SA) node. As part of the study, ECG leads are attached to the patient's chest. After baseline values have been determined, pacing (electrical stimulation of the heart) is used to induce arrhythmias. When an ectopic site takes over as pacemaker, EPS can help pinpoint its origin. If a sustained arrhythmia is induced, an attempt will usually be made to capture the heart by pacing to terminate the arrhythmia. If the patient's cardiovascular system cannot compensate for the arrhythmia, the patient may require cardioversion to convert the dysrhythmia into a normal sinus rhythm (NSR).

Purpose

- To aid in the diagnosis of disorders of the heart's conduction system. EPS can also provide insight into the etiology and mechanism of ventricular arrhythmias and other disturbances within the atrioventricular (AV) conduction system.
- To aid in the selection of an antiarrhythmic drug and/or evaluation of the effectiveness of antiarrhythmic drug therapy.
- To assess the need for an implanted pacemaker in some patients.
- To perform a workup for patients with syncope and sick sinus syndrome.

Findings
Normal

Normal conduction intervals, refractory periods, recovery times, and absence of arrhythmias. Normal conduction intervals in adults are as follows: H-V interval, 35 to 55 ms; A-H interval, 45 to 150 ms; P-A interval, 20 to 40 ms.

Abnormal

Prolonged conduction intervals (Table 6.2), abnormal refractory periods, abnormal recovery times, and induced arrhythmias.

Table 6.2 CONDUCTION INTERVALS AND POTENTIAL CAUSES

Interval Prolonged	Possible Cause
H-V	Acute or chronic disease
A-H	Atrial pacing, chronic conduction system disease, carotid sinus pressure, recent MI, and drugs
P-A	Acquired, surgically induced, congenital atrial disease, and atrial pacing

H-V, time from the onset of bundle of His deflection to ventricular activation; A-H, time from atrial activation to onset of His deflection; P-A, time from onset of the p wave on the ECG to atrial deflection; MI, myocardial infarction.

Pharmacy Implications

- Patients are not permitted to have food or fluids for at least 6 hours before the study.
- EPS is contraindicated in patients with severe coagulopathy, recent thrombophlebitis, and acute pulmonary embolism.

Exercise Electrocardiography (Stress Test)[4,7,11,12,18,22,23]

Description

Electrical cardiac principles are the same as for the ECG; however, the exercise stress test requires more preparation and patient participation. The electrode sites are shaved if necessary, and the skin is cleansed to remove the superficial epidermal skin layer and excess skin oil. The chest electrodes are placed according to the lead system selected to provide the desired tracing. Electrodes are held in place by adhesive or a rubber belt. The lead wire cable is draped over the patient's shoulder, with the lead wires connected to the previously placed electrodes. A baseline rhythm strip is run and checked for dysrhythmias. Blood pressure is checked, and a stethoscope is used to listen for the presence of S_3 and S_4 gallops or chest rales. The patient then steps onto a treadmill moving at a slow speed. A monitor is continuously observed for any changes in cardiac electrical activity, and a rhythm strip is checked at preset intervals for any abnormalities as the treadmill speed is increased. Blood pressure is monitored at predetermined intervals, and changes in systolic blood pressure are recorded. The speed and incline of the treadmill are increased every 2 to 3 minutes. The test is terminated when the maximum (target) heart rate is reached or if unstable changes occur pertaining to the ECG, blood pressure, heart rate, or patient status (i.e., exhaustion or angina). Once the exercise stops, the patient lies down and an ECG tracing is recorded every minute for 5 minutes or until ischemic changes have returned to normal or until the heart rate has returned to normal.

Purpose

- Test cardiac reaction to increased demands for oxygen.
- Help diagnose the source of chest pain or other cardiac pain.
- Help determine the functional capacity of the heart after cardiac surgery or MI.
- Screen for coronary artery disease.
- Establish the limits of an exercise program.

- Identify dysrhythmias.
- Evaluate the effectiveness of antiarrhythmic or antianginal drug therapy.

Findings
Normal
A normal ECG tracing with expected wave forms and intervals (see ECG).

Abnormal
The most prominent abnormal findings are a flat or down-sloping ST-segment depression and an up-sloping but depressed ST segment.

Pharmacy Implications
- Use of beta-adrenergic blockers may make the stress test difficult to interpret because the heart will be prevented from reaching the maximal target rate. Digoxin may limit the value of the stress test due to its affect on ST waves. The physician may elect to perform stress echocardiography or nuclear imaging instead for patients on these medications.

Holter Monitoring[3,7]
Description
Holter monitoring, also known as ambulatory electrocardiography, continuously records heart rate and rhythm for a period of time (24–72 hours). Although a Holter monitor is primarily used by ambulatory patients, it also can be used by patients restricted to bed. Three to five electrodes are placed on the chest, and heart rate and rhythm are recorded on magnetic tape. The tape is then analyzed for evidence of cardiac arrhythmias that would normally not have been present during a routine ECG test.

Purpose
- Diagnose supraventricular and ventricular cardiac arrhythmias.
- Evaluate therapy (drugs and pacemakers) for cardiac arrhythmias.
- Identify asymptomatic patients at high risk for sudden cardiac death.
- Evaluate syncopal episodes in which arrhythmias are not evident.
- Detect myocardial ischemia.

Findings
Holter monitoring can demonstrate the relationship between symptoms such as syncope, palpitations, or shortness of breath and a cardiac arrhythmia. Unfortunately, symptom(s) and the Holter monitor abnormality must occur during the same testing period.

Pharmacy Implications

Patients keep a diary of all activities and symptoms during the period tested. All medications are recorded at the exact time taken.

MRI of the Heart[24,25]

Description

MRI of the heart, also referred to as noninvasive cardiac evaluation, creates a three-dimensional image of the heart and lungs. The images may be used to estimate left ventricular end-diastolic and end-systolic volumes. These measurements can help calculate stroke volume, ejection fraction, and cardiac output. Typical exam time is approximately 1 hour.

Purpose

- Determine cardiopulmonary transit times.
- Aid in determination of extent of damage to the myocardium (infarct size and location).
- Predict if cardio revascularization is beneficial.
- Provide qualitative assessment of left ventricular wall motion and mitral valve function.
- Quantify cardiac parameters (cardiac index, stroke volume, left ventricular ejection fraction, etc.).
- Assist in diagnosis and management of heart failure.

Findings

Normal

No infarct present. All cardiac parameters are within normal limits. No unusual left ventricular wall motion. Mitral valve functioning properly (no regurgitation).

Abnormal

Presence of infarcted tissue or any wall motion abnormalities. Decreased cardiac parameters (ejection fraction <40%). Cardiomegaly. Prolonged cardiopulmonary transit times.

Pharmacy Implications

- Many medications affect cardiac parameters (cardiac index, stroke volume, heart rate, etc.).
- Atrial fibrillation may interfere with the accuracy of study results.
- Contrast media may be used to enhance results (allergies and contraindications need to be assessed).

Multiple Gated Acquisition Scan (MUGA)[4,21,26,27]

Description

Most commonly, erythrocytes labeled with a radioactive isotope (technetium 99-m pertechnetate) are injected into the patient's venous circulation. As the isotope-labeled erythrocytes pass through the ventricle of the heart, a scintillation camera, triggered by and synchronized with the patient's ECG signals, records 14 to 64 points of a single cardiac cycle. This produces sequential images that can be viewed as a motion picture film. A MUGA scan allows evaluation of ventricular performance including wall motion, ejection fraction (EF), and other indices of cardiac function. The MUGA scan can also be performed after exercise. When compared to the results at rest, changes in ejection fraction and cardiac output (CO) can be assessed. The test is also known as cardiac blood pool scanning, because the blood, not the heart itself, is imaged.

Purpose

- Evaluate left ventricular function to assess prognosis in patients after acute MI.
- Evaluate the efficacy of coronary artery disease therapies.
- Differentiate ventricular hypokinesis from left ventricular aneurysms.
- Detect intracardiac shunting in patients with congenital heart disease or septal rupture after MI.
- Detect right ventricular failure.
- Provide useful information in patients with aortic regurgitation.

Findings
Normal

The left ventricle contracts symmetrically and the isotope appears evenly distributed in the scans. EF (amount of blood in the left ventricle propelled forward with each contraction) is 50% to 65%.

Abnormal

Asymmetric blood distribution in the myocardium, the presence of coronary artery disease as seen by segmental abnormalities of ventricular motion, the presence of cardiomyopathies as seen by globally reduced EFs, right-to-left shunting as seen by early arrival of activity in the left ventricle or aorta, and the presence of aneurysms in the left ventricle.

Pharmacy Implications

None.

Myocardial Biopsy[7,11,12,28]

Description

Myocardial biopsy is performed similarly to or as part of cardiac catheterization (see Cardiac Catheterization). When myocardial biopsy is performed alone, the jugular vein in the neck is the most common point of insertion for the IV catheter. The catheter is carefully threaded into the right side of the heart through the superior vena cava by using fluoroscopy. A local anesthetic may be used to minimize patient discomfort. Once in the right ventricle of the heart, a cutting instrument is used to remove heart muscle for analysis.

Purpose

Diagnose cardiac disease (e.g., cardiomyopathy, myocarditis, cardiac amyloid) and assess suspected rejection of a transplanted heart.

Findings
Normal

Normal pathology and histology.

Abnormal

- Signs of rejection in a transplanted heart. These are graded 0 through 4 based on the degree of interstitial lymphocytic infiltration.
- Presence of amyloid protein.
- Bacterial, viral, or parasitic causes of myocarditis.

Pharmacy Implications

- Antiplatelet agents are discontinued before the procedure. Aspirin should be stopped 7 to 10 days before, and other NSAIDs should be stopped 2 to 4 days before the procedure.
- As with cardiac catheterization, patients are assessed for sensitivity to local anesthetics.

Swan-Ganz Catheterization[7]

Description

Swan-Ganz catheterization can be performed by using the internal jugular vein, subclavian vein, femoral vein, or brachial vein as the point of insertion. The procedure should be performed in a setting in which vital signs and heart rhythm can be monitored closely. The procedure may be performed with or without the use of fluoroscopy. The skin at the insertion site is prepared with an antiseptic such as betadine. If the internal jugular or subclavian veins are used, the patient is often placed in a Trendelenburg position to increase central venous distension. Sedation may be necessary if the patient is unable to cooperate. A local anesthetic, such as lidocaine, is injected into the subcutaneous layer and deeper tissues to provide patient comfort. A thin-gauge needle (21 gauge, 1.5 in.) is usually attached to a 5-mL syringe and used to locate the vessel of interest. Once the vessel has been located, a large-gauge needle (16 or 18 gauge) is attached to a syringe and placed into the vessel, following the course of the "finder needle." When blood is aspirated easily into the syringe, the syringe is disconnected from the needle and a flexible guidewire is threaded through the needle into the vein. The guidewire must be controlled carefully to prevent serious complications and death if lost in the patient. Once the needle is removed, a dilator is advanced over the guidewire and through the skin, to facilitate passage of a venous introducer. The introducer should be flushed with heparinized saline before insertion to avoid air emboli. Once the tract along the guidewire is dilated, the dilator should be slipped off the guidewire (maintaining guidewire position in the vein). The introducer and dilator can then be put together as a unit (dilator within introducer) and slid over the guidewire into the vein, again taking care to control the tip of the guidewire outside the patient's body. After the placement of the introducer and guidewire assembly, the guidewire and dilator should be removed from the patient. This leaves only the venous introducer sheath within the patient. At this point, if the introducer has a side-port lumen, venous blood should be aspirated and the introducer then flushed. If blood cannot be aspirated via a side-port lumen, the introducer is incorrectly placed and must be reinserted. No blood should come from the center of the introducer since this piece is usually accompanied by a one-way ball valve that does not allow blood leakage. The introducer is secured to the patient's skin with sutures. When the venous introducer has been placed, the Swan-Ganz catheter can then be inserted. The catheter can then be guided via the introducer, through the central venous system, through the right atrium, right ventricle, pulmonary artery, and into the wedge position. The catheter usually passes smoothly through the circulation, with the aid of the inflated balloon at its tip. The catheter should never be withdrawn with the balloon inflated. Catheter position can be ascertained by pressure wave forms, although fluoroscopy can be quite helpful in guiding the catheter into the wedge position. A chest radiograph is usually obtained after catheter insertion to verify position and to rule out the possibility of pneumothorax if the subclavian or internal jugular approach was used.

Purpose

- Monitor acute MI with hemodynamic instability.
- Evaluate severe hypotension of unknown cause.
- Monitor selected cases of septic shock.
- Confirm the diagnosis of noncardiogenic pulmonary edema (normal wedge pressure).
- Aid in fluid and ventilator management of patients with adult respiratory distress syndrome.
- Confirm the diagnosis of cardiac tamponade, monitor hemodynamics during pericardiocentesis, and follow response to therapy.
- Evaluate suspected papillary muscle rupture.
- Diagnose possible ventricular septal defect or atrial septal defect following MI.
- Monitor congestive heart failure responding poorly to diuretics, especially when intravascular volume status is uncertain.
- Provide intraoperative monitoring of patients undergoing open heart surgery, particularly coronary artery bypass procedures involving multiple vessels; patients undergoing abdominal aortic aneurysm repair may also benefit from pulmonary artery (PA) catheterization perioperatively.
- Monitor drug overdose, especially when the risk of acute lung damage is high (e.g., heroin, aspirin).
- Monitor exacerbations of chronic obstructive lung disease requiring intubation; hemodynamic monitoring may detect occult or superimposed causes of respiratory failure not suspected clinically (e.g., left ventricular dysfunction).
- Evaluate and monitor end-stage liver failure with deteriorating renal function.
- Diagnose pulmonary hypertension.

Findings

See Table 6.3.

Pharmacy Implications

- Patients should be evaluated for hypersensitivity to local anesthetics.
- Sedation may be induced by a benzodiazepine such as midazolam or a parenteral analgesic such as morphine.
- Aspirin and NSAIDs should be discontinued in advance of the procedure. However, use of these agents is not an absolute contraindication to performing the procedure.
- The effects of heparin or warfarin should be reversed before catheterization.

Table 6.3 NORMAL FINDINGS FOR SWAN-GANZ CATHETERIZATION

Parameter of Interest	Normal Resting Hemodynamic Value
Right atrium	Mean: 0–8 mm Hg; A wave: 2–10 mm Hg; V wave: 2–10 mm Hg
Right ventricle	Systolic: 15–30 mm Hg; End diastolic: 0–8 mm Hg
Pulmonary artery	Systolic: 15–30 mm Hg; end diastolic: 3–12 mm Hg
Wedge	A wave: 3–15 mm Hg; wave: 3–12 mm Hg; mean: V 5–12 mm Hg
AVO_2 difference (mL/L)	30–50
Cardiac output (L/min)	4.0–6.5 (varies with patient size)
Cardiac index (L/min/m²)	2.6–4.6
Pulmonary vascular resistance (dynes/s/cm²)	20–130
Systemic vascular resistance (dynes/s/cm²)	700–1600

Thallium Stress Test/Scan[7,29,30]

Description

This nuclear medicine study can be performed while the patient is at rest or while exercising on a treadmill. The procedure incorporates the radionuclide thallium[201], which has biologic properties similar to potassium. These similarities account for its intracellular uptake when administered intravenously. Blood flow then distributes the radionuclide to the myocardium and other organs. A gamma camera is used to measure the radioactivity throughout the myocardium. Healthy myocardium rapidly takes up the thallium, whereas areas of infarcted myocardium show little or no radioactivity.

The stress test is performed using a multistage treadmill test and ECG monitoring with thallium[201] being administered at the time of peak exercise. The patient exercises for an additional 30 to 60 minutes with imaging performed immediately after. Three hours later, the myocardium is reimaged, and myocardial perfusion is further assessed following redistribution of the thallium. For those patients unable to exercise, adenosine, dipyridamole, or dobutamine is administered intravenously along with the thallium to simulate the change in cardiac blood flow that would normally occur with exercise.

Purpose
- Evaluate regional myocardial perfusion.
- Detect evidence of recent or remote MI.
- Identify viable myocardium in a previously infarcted portion of the myocardium.

Findings
Normal
Homogeneous distribution of thallium throughout the myocardium.

Abnormal
A thallium defect demonstrates a region of decreased myocardial blood flow. Infarcted areas can be demonstrated on the images immediately after injection and at the time of delayed imaging. Ischemic areas are detected on the early images as defects but disappear with delayed imaging due to thallium redistribution.

Pharmacy Implications
- Patients should not eat for several hours before the test to prevent increased distribution of the thallium to the gut. Caffeine and theophylline products should be withheld for 36 to 48 hours before dipyridamole and for 12 hours before adenosine.
- Beta-adrenergic blockers should be withheld for 24 to 48 hours before the test if exercise is to be performed to prevent a blunted response to exercise. Calcium channel blockers (diltiazem and verapamil) can also blunt maximal heart rate and should be withheld for 24 to 48 hours before the examination.
- Angiotensin-converting enzyme inhibitors should be withheld for 24 to 48 hours and nitrates for 6 hours before dobutamine.
- Chest pain, headache, nausea, and dizziness occur frequently with dipyridamole. Chest pain, headache, and flushing are common with adenosine. Chest pain, palpitations, arrhythmia, and flushing are common with dobutamine.
- IV aminophylline can be administered (75–250 mg) to counteract the systemic adverse effects of IV dipyridamole.

- The dobutamine dose is 10 μg/kg per minute titrated up to 40 μg/kg per minute.
- The adenosine dose is 50–140 μg/kg per minute given over 6 minutes (21–60 mg).
- A typical dipyridamole dose for a 70-kg adult is 40 mg given over 4 minutes.

Endocrinology

Adrenocorticotropic Hormone Stimulation Test (Cosyntropin)[4,31-33]

Description
Cosyntropin (a synthetic derivative of adrenocorticotropic hormone [ACTH]), 250 μg IM or IV (preferred route), is administered following baseline blood sampling to measure the patient's cortisol level. Additional blood samples are drawn at 30 and 60 minutes after the cosyntropin has been administered, and serum cortisol concentrations are determined from these samples by radioimmunoassay.

Purpose
The ACTH stimulation test is a useful screening test to aid in the differentiation of primary and secondary adrenal failure and is used to diagnose adrenal insufficiency.

Findings
Normal
Serum cortisol will rise at least 10 μg/dL above the baseline determination. Generally, a doubling of the baseline level is a normal response. Baseline determinations are affected by the time of day due to diurnal variation.

Abnormal
Baseline cortisol level will be low and will display an inadequate response by rising <10 μg/dL over the baseline. This does not fully differentiate primary (adrenal) failure from secondary (pituitary) failure. Further testing is necessary.

Pharmacy Implications
- The patient may fast overnight, but this is not always done.
- If cosyntropin is to be given intravenously, the injection time should not exceed 2 minutes.

- Estrogens, spironolactone, cortisone and its analogues, lithium, amphetamines, vasopressin, insulin, and metyrapone can interfere with the test.
- Dexamethasone does not affect the test due to its noninterference with the assay technique.
- Smoking, obesity, and alcohol can produce increased cortisol levels.

Dexamethasone Suppression Test (DST)[4,11,12,31–33]

Description

The low-dose dexamethasone suppression test involves the administration of 1 mg of dexamethasone at midnight. At 8:00 AM the following morning, a blood sample is drawn to measure the plasma cortisol level. Variants of this low-dose study include dexamethasone 500 μg every 6 hours for 2 days or 2 mg every 6 hours for 2 days. In both cases, the plasma cortisol level is measured on the second day. The radioimmunoassay (RIA) method of measuring the plasma cortisol concentration is generally preferred. For use in evaluating depression, 1 mg of dexamethasone is administered at 11:00 PM and cortisol levels are measured at 4:00 PM and 11:00 PM the following day.

Purpose

- The DST is a screening test for the presence of Cushing syndrome. It is most useful for ruling out Cushing syndrome as the diagnosis. The overnight test does not easily differentiate among pituitary, adrenal, or ectopic causes. The 2-day test provides more information and may be more diagnostic with respect to etiology. Nevertheless, it is performed less frequently due to the time required.
- The DST also aids in the diagnosis of major endogenous depression.

Findings
Normal
Plasma cortisol <5 μg/dL.

Abnormal
- Failure to suppress (cortisol >5 μg/dL) suggests that the pituitary-adrenal axis is not suppressible and Cushing disease may be present.
- Failure to suppress appears in only approximately 50% of patients with major depression. Consequently, the usefulness of the DST as a screening test for depression is limited.

- Patients with significant psychiatric disorders, thyrotoxicosis, obesity, or acromegaly; pregnant patients; and alcoholic patients often have elevated plasma cortisol levels. This may confound the screening test. Diurnal rhythm (time of day) can also influence the result.

Pharmacy Implications
- The patient must fast overnight.
- ACTH, cortisone, estrogens, hydrocortisone, oral contraceptives, ethanol, lithium, or methadone taken 2 weeks before testing increases plasma test results. Phenytoin and androgenic steroids may decrease plasma cortisol levels.

Oral Glucose Tolerance Test (OGTT)[4,11,12,42–46]

Description
A blood sample to determine the fasting (baseline) blood glucose for the patient is drawn first. Then, the patient drinks a highly concentrated glucose solution (75 g/300 mL for nonpregnant adults and 100 g/400 mL for pregnant women). Subsequently, a timed series of blood glucose tests is performed at 30, 60, 90, and 120 minutes for nonpregnant adults and 1, 2, and 3 hours for pregnant women to determine the rate of removal of glucose from the bloodstream. This test is not performed if the fasting blood sugar is >126 mg/dL in nonpregnant adults, because virtually all such patients will have blood glucose determinations that meet or exceed the diagnostic criteria for diabetes mellitus.

Purpose
Diagnose or rule out overt diabetes, glucose intolerance, Cushing syndrome, and acromegaly. The OGTT is more sensitive and specific than fasting plasma glucose for diagnosing diabetes; however fasting plasma glucose is the preferred test for this condition as it is less costly, more reproducible, more convenient, and easier to administer.

Findings
Normal—Adult (Nonpregnant)
Fasting blood glucose: 70 to 110 mg/dL
After 75 g of oral glucose:

30 minutes	<200 mg/dL
60 minutes	<200 mg/dL
90 minutes	<200 mg/dL
120 minutes	<14 to 110 mg/dL
180 minutes	70 to 110 mg/dL

Abnormal—Adult

- *Diabetes mellitus.*
  - › Fasting plasma glucose $\geq$126, or
  - › Two-hour OGTT blood glucose level $\geq$200 mg/dL.
  - › Reading must be confirmed on a subsequent day unless there is unequivocal evidence of hyperglycemia.
- *Impaired glucose tolerance.* Two-hour OGTT blood glucose level $\geq$140 and <200 mg/dL.
- *Impaired fasting glucose.* Fasting plasma glucose of $\geq$100 mg/dL and <126 mg/dL.
- *Gestational diabetes.* Some institutions screen pregnant women before administering the diagnostic 100-g glucose load, whereas those with a high prevalence of gestational diabetes only administer the diagnostic test without screening.
- Screen: 50-g glucose load (nonfasting).
  - 1 hour $\geq$130 or 140, proceed to diagnostic step
- Diagnostic: 100-g glucose load (fasting); diagnosis is made if the reading is equal to or greater than the values below on two occasions:

Fasting	95 mg/dL
1 hour	180 mg/dL
2 hours	155 mg/dL
3 hours	140 mg/dL

- Patients should be rescreened for diabetes 6 to 12 weeks postpartum.

Pharmacy Implications

- The patient should be instructed to fast overnight ($\geq$8 hours).
- Seventy-five grams of glucose (Glucola) are given to nonpregnant adults and 100 g are given to pregnant women on the morning of the test.
- Insulin or oral hypoglycemic agents should not be taken until the test is completed.
- The following drugs should be discontinued $\geq$3 days before the test: hormones (including oral contraceptives), salicylates, diuretics, hypoglycemic agents. Other drugs and substances may also influence test results; clinical judgment should be used. These may include (not exhaustive) alcohol, alpha-blockers, amphetamines, androgens, beta-blockers, caffeine, calcitonin, cannabis, cimetidine, clofibrate, diazoxide, diethylstilbetrol, felodipine, guanethidine, haloperidol, imipramine, interferon-α, iron, isoniazid, lisinopril, lithium, MAO (monoamine

oxidase) inhibitors, mefenemic acid, niacin, nicotine, nifedipine, phenothiazines, phenytoin, steroids, thyroid hormone, verapamil.

Thyroid Uptake/Scan[7]

Description
Uptake
Radioactive iodine (I^{131} or I^{123}) is ingested by the patient in either solid oral dosage form or as an oral liquid. Six hours and 24 hours after ingestion, a gamma probe placed over the thyroid measures the amount of radioactivity in the thyroid gland. This result is compared against the dose of radioactive iodine administered to the patient, and a percent uptake is calculated.

Scan
Technetium-99m pertechnetate is administered intravenously and is concentrated in the thyroid gland like iodine. A gamma camera is used to scan the thyroid gland approximately 30 minutes after injection. The information gathered by the scanner is sent to a computer, which creates a two-dimensional image of the thyroid gland and thyroid nodules on x-ray film or as a computer printout. Alternatively, the patient can ingest I^{131} or I^{123} as in the thyroid uptake test. Six and 24 hours later, the thyroid gland is scanned and two-dimensional images produced.

Purpose
Uptake
To evaluate thyroid function when blood tests of thyroid function are abnormal. The test is able to detect and quantify the extent of thyroid disease and can be useful in distinguishing between primary and secondary thyroid disease.

Scan
To evaluate the location, size, anatomy, and function of the thyroid gland.

Findings
Normal
Percent uptake of radioactive iodine is in the normal range at 6 and 24 hours. The thyroid gland is of normal size, shape, location, and color. There is a homogeneous and symmetric distribution of radioactive material throughout the thyroid gland.

Abnormal

The percent of radioactive iodine uptake is less than or greater than the range for normal. This will indicate either hypothyroid or hyperthyroid disease. Scanning can reveal a thyroid tumor, goiter, thyroid nodules, thyroiditis, or ectopic thyroid tissue. The color of the thyroid gland will appear lighter or darker than the normally expected color.

Pharmacy Implications

- Barbiturates, estrogen, lithium, and phenothiazines can increase iodine uptake.
- ACTH, antihistamines, corticosteroids, Lugol solution, nitrates, potassium iodide solution, thyroid drugs, antithyroid drugs, tolbutamide, iodinated contrast agents, and cough syrups containing iodine compounds suppress radioactive iodine uptake.
- Patients should discontinue thyroid and antithyroid drugs 1 to 2 weeks before uptake or scanning studies.

Thyrotropin-Releasing Hormone Test (Protirelin)[41,42]

Description

The test is performed by administering IV protirelin (thyrotropin-stimulating hormone [TRH]), 500 μg, over 15 to 30 seconds following pretest blood sampling to determine the patient's baseline thyroid-stimulating hormone (TSH). Plasma TSH levels are drawn 30 and 60 minutes after TRH is administered.

Purpose

- Diagnose suspected hyperthyroidism in individuals whose routine thyroid function tests are not fully diagnostic.
- Assess the integrity of the pituitary thyrotropes to aid in differentiating hypothyroidism due to intrinsic pituitary disease from hypothalamic dysfunction.
- Aid in the diagnosis of mild hypothyroidism.

Findings
Normal

TSH rise >5 mU/L above the baseline TSH excludes the diagnosis of hyperthyroidism.

Abnormal

- *Hyperthyroidism.* No TSH rise or <5 μU rise.
- *Primary hypothyroidism.* Initially high baseline levels of TSH (exaggerated response).
- *Secondary hypothyroidism.* Little or no response when pituitary failure is present.
- *Hypothalamic hypothyroidism.* TSH will rise at 45 or 60 minutes after TSH.

Pharmacy Implications

- Results can be affected by patients receiving thyroid supplementation.
- A 14-hour overnight fast is recommended.

Gastroenterology

Abdominal Radiograph (KUB)[4,7,43,44]

Description

The patient lies on his or her back, and a radiograph is taken of the kidneys, ureters, and bladder (KUB). A KUB radiograph is also called a "scout film." No contrast media are used for this study. When performed in the erect position, gas fluid levels within the small and large intestine and free air in the peritoneum can be better visualized. Patients who cannot stand can be placed on their side (lateral decubitus position). A posterior-anterior (PA) view of the chest is sometimes done along with the KUB to evaluate pulmonary pathology as a possible cause of abdominal pain.

Purpose

- Diagnose intra-abdominal abnormalities such as nephrolithiasis, intestinal obstruction, tissue masses, abnormal accumulation of gas, free air in the abdomen, or enlargement or perforation of the tissues.
- Evaluate size, shape, and position of the liver, spleen, and kidneys.

Findings
Normal

No masses, smooth peritoneal space, and normal size and position of organs. Right kidney is slightly lower than the left.

Abnormal

Foreign bodies, abnormal fluid, ascites, abnormal kidney location or shape, urinary calculi, calcification of blood vessels, cysts, or tumors.

Pharmacy Implications

- Normally, there is no patient preparation.
- The presence of feces or gas can obscure the film, which may necessitate the administration of a laxative (milk of magnesia) at bedtime the night before the examination or 75 mL of senna fruit concentrate at 4:00 PM on the day before the film. However, this is not frequently done.
- The presence of barium obscures the clarity of the film. The KUB should be scheduled before examinations requiring the administration of oral contrast media.

Barium Enema[11,12,45,46]

Description

Barium contrast is instilled through the rectum by inserting a rectal tube up to the ileocecal valve. The rectal tube remains in place while the films are taken. The rectal tube may be equipped with a small balloon at the tip, which can be inflated to prevent leakage of the barium. Examination of the large intestine is performed using x-ray views and fluoroscopy. These show position, filling, and movement of the colon. The barium contrast opacifies the bowel mucosa and outlines folds of the large intestine.

Abdominal CT scan or US are now considered first-line procedures for the initial evaluation of suspected abdominal masses.

Purpose

- Diagnose colorectal masses and inflammatory bowel diseases such as ulcerative colitis.
- Detect the presence of polyps or diverticula.
- Evaluate the structure of the large intestine.
- Diagnose intestinal stricture or obstruction.

Findings
Normal

Normal position, contour, filling, rate of passage of barium, movement, and patency of colon.

Abnormal

Presence of tumors, diverticula, obstructions, inflammation, or other abnormal findings.

Pharmacy Implications

A typical procedure protocol includes the following:

Typical Procedure Variant 1

- Ingesting a liquid diet 2 days before procedure.
- Drinking 32 oz of water the day before the examination (from noon to 11:00 PM).
- Drinking 300 mL magnesium citrate at 5:00 PM the day before the procedure. If severe renal disease is present, the patient should drink 1 bottle (75 mL) senna fruit concentrate.

Typical Procedure Variant 2

- Taking 4 5-mg bisacodyl tablets at 7:00 PM the day before the procedure. Tablets should be swallowed whole and should not be taken within 1 hour of antacids or milk.

Typical Procedure Variant 3

- Taking metoclopramide, 10 mg, by mouth or intravenously (IV) at 3 to 4 PM the day before the procedure.
- Ingesting GI lavage solution until the evacuated fluid is clear. When using GI lavage solution, the patient should be evaluated for pre-existing fluid overload conditions or fluid restrictions.
- Ingesting no food or drink after midnight the night before the procedure.
- Performing a 2,000-mL cleansing enema before the procedure.
- Taking 30 mL milk of magnesia orally as a cathartic after the procedure. In a patient with compromised renal status, 30 mL sorbitol 70% should be given orally after the procedure.

Use of magnesium citrate or magnesium hydroxide cathartics should be avoided in patients with renal failure.

Barium Enema with Air Contrast[4,45,46]

Description

This test is often referred to as double-contrast barium enema or pneumocolon. It involves the same principles as a standard barium enema but includes the instillation of air into the bowel in addition to the contrast medium. This method improves detection of subtle changes in the colon but is not as thorough an examination as a colonoscopy.

Purpose

See Gastroenterology, Barium Enema.

Findings

See Gastroenterology, Barium Enema.

Pharmacy Implications

See Gastroenterology, Barium Enema.

Enteroclysis[11,12,47–49]

Description

Enteroclysis is a radiographic examination of the small bowel performed by delivering barium directly into the jejunum by way of an orogastric or nasogastric tube (12- or 14-gauge French catheter), followed by a radiolucent methylcellulose solution. Enterolysis provides an improved and more detailed view of the entire small bowel compared with the standard small bowel series. It is the procedure of choice in evaluating suspected small bowel malabsorption.

Purpose

Evaluate malabsorption, inflammatory bowel disease, and the presence of a small bowel obstruction. It should be performed only after other diagnostic procedures have been attempted or performed.

Findings
Normal

The presence of normal-appearing bowel mucosa, small bowel wall thickness, and normal fluid transit time. The absence of lesions, obstructions, or fistulas.

Abnormal

Inflamed mucosa, motility disorder, presence of masses, obstruction, narrowed lumen, fistulas, and small bowel bleeding.

Pharmacy Implications

- See Gastroenterology, Barium Enema.
- Metoclopramide, 10 mg IV, may be administered 20 to 30 minutes before the procedure to aid in intubation of the small bowel.
- Apprehensive patients may benefit from administration of a low-dose anxiolytic such as diazepam or lorazepam to aid in intubation.

Barium Swallow (Upper GI with Small Bowel Follow-Through [UGI/SBFT])[4,47,48]

Description

A fluoroscopic radiographic examination of the pharynx, esophagus, stomach, duodenum, and upper jejunum comprises the upper GI portion of the examination. An oral contrast medium (barium) is swallowed, permitting visualization of the lumen in these areas. To evaluate the remainder of the jejunum and the ileum (small bowel follow-through), a series of hourly films may be required to track the contrast medium through the small bowel. This portion of the examination is complete when the ileocecal valve has filled with the contrast material.

Purpose

Detect or diagnose congenital abnormalities of the bowel, esophageal stricture, esophageal cancer, tumors, pyloric stenosis, varices, diverticula, ulcers, polyps, hiatal hernia, gastritis, regional enteritis, malabsorption, gastroesophageal reflux, obstruction, and motility disorders.

Findings
Normal

Normal size, contour, motility, and peristalsis.

Abnormal

Deformed contour from intrinsic tumor, filling defects, or stenosis with dilation. Ulcers and other irregularities also may be seen.

Pharmacy Implications

- Barium sulfate or diatrizoate (Gastrografin) must be given during procedure.
- No oral ingestion (including medications, antacids) after 10:00 PM the day before the examination.
- Administration of 30 mL of milk of magnesia after the procedure as a cathartic. In a patient with compromised renal status, 30 mL sorbitol 70% should be given after the procedure.

Cholangiography (Percutaneous Transhepatic)[7,11,12,50–52]

Description

With the patient lying supine, a local anesthetic is administered in the right upper quadrant of the abdomen. A 20- to 22-gauge, 6-inch-long flexible needle is used to puncture the skin and is passed into the intra-hepatic biliary tree with the help of fluoroscopy. Contrast material is then administered via this needle into the biliary tree. A fluoroscopic examination is performed, and individual radiographs are taken.

Purpose
- Aid in the diagnosis of obstructive jaundice (differentiate intrahepatic and extrahepatic causes of cholestasis).
- Outline the detail of the intrahepatic and extrahepatic ducts and the biliary tree.
- Identify the presence of stones, tumors, lesions, strictures, and biliary duct fistula.

Findings
Normal
Normal-sized ducts and duct anatomy (duct is smooth). Absence of stones or lesions.

Abnormal
Extrahepatic obstructive jaundice is associated with dilated ducts with an accompanying biliary system obstruction caused by stones, biliary carci-noma, sclerosing cholangitis, stricture, cholangiocarcinoma, gallbladder carcinoma, or pancreatic carcinoma impinging on the common bile duct.

Intrahepatic cholestasis is associated with normal-sized ducts and no obstruction.

Pharmacy Implications
- The patient should take nothing by mouth (NPO) 4 hours before the procedure.
- Contrast dye may produce a hypersensitivity reaction.
- The patient may receive a parenteral benzodiazepine anxiolytic before the procedure.
- Prophylactic antibiotics may be administered (e.g., ampicillin, an aminoglycoside, cefoxitin or cefotetan, cefoperazone or ceftriaxone) before and after the procedure to prevent infection from Enterobac-teriaceae, enterococci, and bacteroides.
- Aspirin should be discontinued 7 to 10 days before the procedure and NSAIDs 2 to 4 days before the procedure.
- Patients should be evaluated for non–drug-related impaired coagu-lopathy.

- If the international normalized ratio (INR) is abnormal, oral or parenteral (preferably subcutaneous [SC] or IM) vitamin K may be given daily before the procedure. Alternatively or in addition, fresh frozen plasma (FFP) as a source of vitamin K and clotting factors can be administered to correct coagulopathy.

Cholangiography (T-Tube)[4,7]

Description

An iodine contrast dye is injected into a T tube (a self-retaining drainage tube attached to the common bile duct during gallbladder surgery), and a fluoroscopic examination is made. The T tube is then unclamped, and the contrast material drains out. This test is often referred to as postoperative cholangiography.

Purpose

Evaluate the patency of the common bile duct following gallbladder surgery and evaluate the presence of an extrahepatic obstruction.

Findings

Normal

Patent common bile duct with no obstructions.

Abnormal

Extrahepatic obstruction noted.

Pharmacy Implications

Contrast dye may produce a hypersensitivity reaction.

CT of the Abdomen

See General Procedures, Computed Tomography (CT).

Endoscopy[4,11,12,47]

Endoscopy is the visual examination of various internal body structures using a fiber-optic instrument. The fiber-optic instrument is composed of a flexible tube and a lighted mirror lens system. The diameter of the endoscope will vary depending on the orifice into which the endoscope is inserted. Endoscopy can be used for diagnostic purposes, because the device allows direct visualization. Endoscopy can be used to perform therapeutic procedures and tissue biopsies.

Colonoscopy[7,11,12]

Description

Colonoscopy is examination of the colon and terminal ileum by use of a flexible fiber-optic endoscope. Following cleansing of the bowel the evening before or morning of the procedure, the patient is placed on his or her left side with knees drawn up toward the abdomen. The colonoscope is inserted through the anus and advanced to the terminal small bowel. To aid in direct observation of the bowel, air is inserted through the scope. Suction is used to keep the bowel clear of secretions. Better views of the bowel occur during withdrawal of the scope, permitting a more careful examination of the bowel during this phase of the procedure. Colonoscopy is considered more sensitive for early detection of select abnormalities than colon x-ray procedures.

Purpose

- Further evaluate an abnormal barium enema result.
- Help determine the cause of lower GI bleeding.
- Screen (serve as surveillance) for the presence of cancer.
- Evaluate patients with colonic cancer or inflammatory bowel disease.
- Determine the cause of unexplained diarrhea.
- Perform polypectomy.
- Arrest the bleeding from lesions.
- Decompress a dilated colon, reduce an intestinal volvulus, or dilate strictures.
- Remove foreign objects from the large bowel.
- Perform tissue biopsies to aid in the diagnosis of suspected disease.

Findings

Normal

Absence of inflammation, normal mucosa, and normal anatomy.

Abnormal

Presence of polyps or tumors, areas of inflammation, signs of bleeding, presence of foreign objects, and abnormal anatomy.

Pharmacy Implications

- Preparation for colonoscopy with lavage is thought to be more effective than standard cathartics (either evening before or morning of colonoscopy) and includes:
  - Metoclopramide, 10 mg (IM, IV, or by mouth [PO]) 30 minutes before GI lavage solution.

- › GI lavage solution (polyethylene glycol-electrolyte solution), 1.2 to 1.8 L/hour until bowel evacuations are clear (usually 4 L). Lavage is stopped if the patient develops vomiting or severe abdominal pain. If the patient is unable to tolerate the solution by mouth, a nasogastric tube may need to be placed.
- ■ Alternate preparation for a typical procedure protocol includes the following:
  - › A clear liquid diet 2 days before the procedure.
  - › On the evening before the procedure: administration of magnesium citrate, 300 mL PO at 5:00 PM (senna concentrate 75 mL is used instead of magnesium citrate in patients with renal disease); administration of a bisacodyl tablet, 10 mg PO at 7:00 PM; encouragement of clear fluids; and NPO after midnight.
  - › On the morning of procedure: administration of a 1,500 mL saline enema. Repeat the enema one time. Administration of meperidine IM on call or 30 minutes before the procedure.

Endoscopic Retrograde Cholangiopancreatography (ERCP)[4,7,11,12,54,55]

Description

Following administration of a local anesthetic spray to the pharynx with the patient lying in the left lateral decubitus position, a special side-viewing flexible duodenoscope is passed orally into the duodenum and advanced to the papilla of Vater (the point of junction where the pancreatic duct and the common bile duct enter the duodenum). A catheter (cannula) is then placed into the papilla, and a radiographic contrast medium is injected. Radiographs are taken of the ducts. Areas visualized include the common bile duct, intrahepatic ducts, gallbladder, and pancreatic ducts. This direct diagnostic method is thought to be the most reliable approach to evaluating pancreatic and biliary tract disease. Other techniques such as ultrasonography and CT do not provide as detailed a view of the ductal anatomy and specific pathology.

Purpose

- ■ Aid in the diagnosis and treatment of certain biliary tree and pancreatic diseases by helping to differentiate surgical from nonsurgical disease.
- ■ Evaluate the anatomy of the pancreas and ductal system prior to possible therapeutic intervention in patients with suspected obstructive jaundice, disease of the biliary system, pancreatic cancer, and recurrent pancreatitis.

- Place biliary stents (devices used to keep the biliary or pancreatic duct open).
- Perform sphincterotomy, remove common duct gallstones, and perform other minor surgical procedures related to the pancreatic and common bile duct.

Findings
Normal
Normal ductal anatomy (pancreatic duct and common bile duct) and the absence of lesions, stones, and other causes of obstruction.

Abnormal
Ductal dilation and/or strictures as well as presence of stones or tumors.

Pharmacy Implications
- Patients should be NPO for ≥ 8 hours before the procedure.
- IM atropine is administered 30 minutes before the procedure to decrease secretions and to prevent a vagal response due to stimulation from the endoscope.
- IM meperidine is administered 30 minutes before the procedure to reduce pain perception. Meperidine is thought to have less of an effect on the sphincter of Oddi compared with other narcotic analgesics. The clinical significance of this finding is unclear. Morphine or hydromorphone can be administered as alternatives.
- IV benzodiazepines (diazepam, midazolam, or lorazepam) are sometimes used to alleviate anxiety and provide an amnesic effect.
- Aspirin should be discontinued 5 days before the procedure and NSAIDs 2 days before, especially if biopsy or sphincterotomy are planned.
- Glucagon in 0.2-mL doses may be given to decrease motility and improve visualization.
- Contrast dye may produce a hypersensitivity reaction.

Esophagogastroduodenoscopy (Upper Endoscopy)[4,11,12,56]

Description
Esophagogastroduodenoscopy is direct visual examination of the esophagus (esophagoscopy), stomach (gastroscopy), and duodenum (duodenoscopy) using an endoscope. Following the application of a local anesthetic spray to the throat to prevent gagging, the endoscope is placed through the mouth and throat and passed along the esophagus into the stomach and duodenum. Air is placed into the esophagus and stomach for better visualization.

Purpose
- Determine the cause of upper GI bleeding.
- Determine the presence of inflammation, ulcerations, tumors, and esophageal strictures.
- Visualize directly abnormalities seen on an upper GI series.
- Evaluate ulcer healing following pharmacotherapy.
- Investigate gastric emptying and swallowing abnormalities.
- Perform polypectomy, sclerotherapy of esophageal varices, esophageal and gastric dilation, and tissue biopsies.
- Remove foreign objects.
- Coagulate bleeding sites.
- Place feeding tubes and percutaneous gastrostomy tubes.

Findings
Normal
Absence of inflammation, lesions, and bleeding. Mucosa and anatomy appear normal.

Abnormal
Inflammation (reddened mucosa) of the examined structures, identified area of bleeding (hemorrhage), hiatal hernia, lesions (benign or malignant), visible ulcers, and esophageal narrowing.

Pharmacy Implications
- NPO for at least 6 hours before the examination.
- No antacids after 10:00 PM on the day before the examination, or before the examination if being performed on an emergency basis.
- IM atropine is administered 30 minutes before the procedure to decrease secretions and prevent reflex bradycardia secondary to vagal stimulation from insertion of the scope. Caution is required when giving IM injections to a patient who has a low platelet count, has a bleeding disorder, or is receiving anticoagulant therapy.
- Parenteral narcotics and benzodiazepines (e.g., midazolam) may be administered just before the examination to produce sedation, reduce anxiety, and decrease the perception of discomfort. The patient must be alert enough to assist in swallowing.
- Local anesthetics may be used to anesthetize the throat. If used, the patient should not eat or drink for 1 to 2 hours after the procedure to reduce the risk of aspiration when swallowing. Initially, clear liquids are administered and the patient is closely observed for swallowing difficulties.

Proctoscopy[4,57]

Description

Proctoscopy, also known as anoscopy, is direct instrumental examination of a 12-inch area of the rectum and anal canal using a proctoscope. A proctoscope is a rigid metal or plastic tube with a lighted mirror and lens at the end.

Purpose

- Confirm or rule out ulcerative, pseudomembranous, or granulomatous colitis.
- Examine the rectosigmoid area for the presence of tumors, polyps, hemorrhoids, foreign bodies, suspected anal or rectal fissures, perianal abscesses, and fistulae.
- Aid in the diagnosis of irritable bowel syndrome and Crohn disease.
- Evaluate rectal bleeding.
- Perform a biopsy.

Findings
Normal

No tumors or inflammation. Rectal mucosa is smooth and pink. The rectum has normal anatomy.

Abnormal

Edematous, red, or denuded mucosa. Presence of grainy minute masses. The tissue is easily broken or pulverized. Visible ulcers or pseudomembranes. Spontaneous bleeding on examination.

Pharmacy Implications

- Laxatives and an enema (tap water or phosphate) are given the evening before the procedure.
- One or two phosphate enemas or a suppository (bisacodyl) may be given 1 hour before the procedure.
- Barium administered within the previous week could interfere with the examination.
- The patient should take nothing by mouth 2 hours before the examination.

Sigmoidoscopy (Flexible)[4,7,11,12,58]

Description

Sigmoidoscopy is direct visual examination of the distal 60 cm (24 in.) of the rectum and sigmoid colon using a flexible fiber-optic scope. The patient is placed in the left lateral decubitus position. After lubricating the sigmoidoscope, it is inserted into the rectum and advanced to the sigmoid colon. Air is introduced into the bowel to aid in visualization. This diagnostic procedure may be preferable to rigid proctoscopic examination. However, anoscopy is thought to be superior to sigmoidoscopy for visualization of the rectum and anal canal.

Purpose

- Visualize and biopsy abnormalities in the rectosigmoid area.
- Evaluate lesions seen on radiographs.
- Evaluate patients who have undergone bowel resection and the cause of bloody diarrhea or rectal bleeding.
- Diagnose and monitor inflammatory bowel disease and the effectiveness of therapy.
- Reduce a sigmoid volvulus.
- Screen for colon cancers and monitor patients with a history of colon cancer.

Findings
Normal

Absence of inflammation, bleeding, and lesions. Normal anatomy.

Abnormal

Reddened or bleeding mucosa, presence of neoplastic disease.

Pharmacy Implications

- No preparation for patients who present with a primary complaint of diarrhea, who are suspected of having inflammatory bowel disease, or have a history of acute bright red rectal bleeding.
- Usual preparation includes withholding breakfast on the morning of the procedure and the rectal administration of two phosphate enemas (130 mL each) given 30 minutes before the procedure.

Hepatobiliary Scintigraphy (HIDA, PAPIDA, or DISIDA Scan)[4,59]

Description

A radionuclide tracer, (^{99m}Tc) IDA (technetium-labeled iminodiacetic acid derivatives), is injected intravenously, undergoes uptake by the liver, and is excreted into the biliary tree. Using a scintillation camera, serial images are taken (an image every 5 minutes for 1 hour) that show the radioactivity in the liver, bile ducts, gallbladder, and duodenum.

Purpose

- Diagnose cholecystitis, biliary tract stones, tumors, cancer, obstruction, leaks, and anatomic anomalies of the biliary tree.
- Evaluate the biliary ducts for patency after surgical intervention.
- Evaluate liver function and determine liver rejection after transplantation.

Findings
Normal

The gallbladder, bile ducts, liver, and a portion of the small bowel are visualized within 1 hour of radionuclide administration showing normal size, shape, and function of the biliary system.

Abnormal

Radioactivity in the liver, but little or none in the gallbladder and duodenum, indicates biliary obstruction. Decreased or absent radioactivity in the gallbladder, bile ducts, and duodenum or delayed uptake by the liver indicates hepatocellular disease.

Pharmacy Implications

Administration of cholecystokinin or sincalide intravenously may be used to improve the procedure by stimulating contraction of the gallbladder to hasten movement of the tracer into the bile ducts. The dose of sincalide is 0.02 μg/kg administered over a 30- to 60-second interval. A second dose of 0.04 μg/kg may be administered if the first dose does not produce satisfactory results.

Laparoscopy

See Gynecology, Laparoscopy.

Liver Biopsy[4,7,53,60]

Description

This procedure is performed at bedside and uses a percutaneous needle aspiration of a core of tissue from the liver via a Menghini needle (a long, large-bore needle), the Jamshidi, or the Tru-Cut needle. The needle is inserted through an intercostal space anterior to the midaxillary line just below the point of maximal dullness on expiration. The biopsy may be guided by using US or CT. The biopsied tissue is then sent for histologic analysis.

Purpose

- Diagnose the cause of hepatocellular disease such as cirrhosis or hepatitis.

- Confirm alcoholic liver disease.
- Assess the cause of persistently elevated liver function tests such as AST, ALT, bilirubin, and alkaline phosphatase.
- Assess the cause of cholestasis of unknown origin after other testing has been inconclusive.
- Assess the course of and response to therapy of various hepatic cellular diseases.
- Assist in diagnosing and staging lymphomas and other malignancies.
- Assist in the diagnosis of metabolic disease, multisystem disease, and granulomatous infections.
- Assess the effect of hepatotoxic drugs (e.g., methotrexate).
- Evaluate suspected rejection of a transplanted liver.

Findings
Normal
Presence of normal pathology and histology.

Abnormal
Presence of tumors or cysts, hepatic cellular changes consistent with cirrhosis or hepatitis, signs of organ rejection, and signs of drug toxicity.

Pharmacy Implications
- It is recommended that antiplatelet agents be stopped before open and needle biopsies. Aspirin should be discontinued 7 to 10 days before the procedure. NSAIDs (e.g., ibuprofen, naproxen) that reversibly inhibit the enzyme cyclooxygenase should be discontinued 2 to 4 days before the procedure.
- Preprocedure medications such as parenteral analgesics (e.g., meperidine, morphine) and parenteral sedatives/anxiolytics (e.g., lorazepam, diazepam, midazolam) may be administered.
- A local anesthetic (e.g., lidocaine) may be necessary. The patient's history should be checked for allergic reactions.

MRI of the Abdomen
See General Procedures, Magnetic Resonance Imaging (MRI).

Paracentesis[4,7,61]
Description
Paracentesis is the puncture of any cavity for the aspiration of fluid; however, the withdrawal of fluid from the abdomen (abdominal paracentesis) is the most commonly encountered. First, the patient is asked to empty

his or her bladder. Second, the area between the umbilicus and the pubis is prepared with iodine and anesthetized with a local anesthetic such as lidocaine. Third, a long 22-gauge needle is inserted through the abdominal wall into the peritoneum 1 to 2 in. below the umbilicus. For diagnostic purposes, 50 to 100 mL of fluid are aspirated and sent to the laboratory for analysis. When performed for therapeutic purposes, fluid volumes of 1.5 to 5 L may be removed.

Purpose

- Aid in the diagnosis of a suspected infection (peritonitis) or malignancy.
- Assess the electrolyte and protein makeup of the fluid.
- Remove ascitic fluid therapeutically from the abdomen of patients with cirrhosis or abdominal malignancy.
- Determine if abdominal bleeding is present.

Findings
Normal
Peritoneal fluid: see Table 6.4.

Abnormal

Cloudy or turbid appearance, elevated protein content, elevated glucose, presence of RBCs or bloody fluid, WBCs >300/mL, and cytology positive for malignant cells.

Pharmacy Implications
The patient should be assessed for allergies to local anesthetics and iodine.

Table 6.4 NORMAL PARACENTESIS FINDINGS

Appearance	Clear and yellowish
Volume	<50 mL
Protein content	0.3–4.1 g/dL
Glucose	70–100 mg/dL
RBCs	None
WBCs	<300/mL
Bacteria and fungi	None
Cytology	No malignant cells

Small Bowel Series[11,12]

See Gastroenterology, Barium Swallow (Upper GI With Small Bowel Follow-Through [UGI/SBFT]).

Small Bowel Biopsy[4,7,53,62]

Description

Small bowel biopsy is usually performed using a suction apparatus called the Rubin tube. It is passed orally into the small bowel, and a piece of jejunal tissue is harvested or duodenal fluid is aspirated. Alternatively, a Carey capsule directed by gravity may be used to perform the biopsy. The specimen obtained with this device is more broad and less deep than the samples obtained with the Rubin tube. Fluoroscopy is used to check the position of the tube. However, biopsy samples are obtained in a blind fashion. Histologic, microbiologic, and fluid analysis are performed on the samples. A similar procedure can be undertaken with upper endoscopy permitting direct visualization of the small bowel. However, the endoscope can only reach the duodenum, thus limiting its usefulness when sampling of the ileum or jejunum must be performed.

Purpose

- Determine the cause of malabsorption or diarrhea.
- Assess response to drug or nondrug therapies.
- Verify a suspected malignancy.
- Diagnose and assess inflammatory bowel disease.
- Collect pancreatic fluid and bile fluid for analysis to assess gallbladder disease.
- Diagnose bacterial overgrowth or giardiasis.

Findings
Normal

Presence of normal pathology, histology, and fluid composition.

Abnormal

Presence of histologic changes characteristic of inflammatory bowel disease or malignancy, the presence of *Giardia* sp. or bacterial overgrowth, or the presence of cholesterol crystals and WBCs in bile fluid.

Pharmacy Implications

- The patient should take nothing by mouth for ≥ 6 to 8 hours before the procedure.

- The patient's throat is sprayed with a local anesthetic (e.g., benzocaine, Cetacaine, or lidocaine) to reduce the likelihood of gagging when the tube is passed.
- Preprocedure medications such as parenteral analgesics (e.g., meperidine) and parenteral sedatives/anxiolytics (e.g., lorazepam, diazepam, or midazolam) may be administered. However, the patient needs to be cooperative and somewhat alert to be able to swallow the tube.
- Metoclopramide, 10 mg PO or IV, may be used to help advance the tube or capsule into the small bowel.
- Antiplatelet agents such as aspirin and other NSAIDs should be discontinued ≥ 5 days in advance of the biopsy. Anticoagulants such as warfarin may be a contraindication to this test.
- An elevated prothrombin time (PT) or activated partial thromboplastin time (aPTT) for a non–drug-related reason is a contraindication to performance of this procedure unless coagulopathy can be corrected in advance of the procedure.

Ultrasonography of the Abdomen

See General Procedures, Ultrasonography.

Gynecology

Breast Biopsy (Needle and Open)[4,11,12,63]
Description
Needle
A needle is introduced into the breast mass where fluid (if present) is aspirated. Tissue obtained from the biopsy is sent for cytologic study. Diagnostically, this procedure is limited by the small tissue sample obtained from a needle biopsy; it may not be representative of the entire breast mass. There is also an increased risk of seeding the needle tract with potentially malignant cells, thus causing further spread of the disease. Therefore, a needle biopsy is generally reserved for a fluid-filled cyst or an advanced malignant lesion.

Open
In an open biopsy of the breast, an incision is made to expose the breast mass. If the mass is small enough (<2 cm) and looks benign, the mass is excised. If the mass is larger or looks malignant, a representative amount of tissue is incised from the mass. This complete or partial excision of the

mass is called lumpectomy. The tissue is sent for receptor assay analysis and frozen section. Frozen section involves quick freezing of the tissue sample so it can be cut into microscopic sections and examined by the pathologist to determine if the tissue is malignant and if the tissue margins indicate adequate excision. This entire process takes 10 to 15 minutes and provides valuable information on whether more malignant tissue needs to be excised or if the wound can be closed.

Purpose

Needle and open breast biopsies are performed to determine if breast tumors are benign or malignant. Receptor assays are done on malignant tissues to determine if the tumor is estrogen-receptor (ER) and/or progesterone-receptor (PR) positive or negative. ER(+) and PR(+) tumors will respond best to hormonal chemotherapy such as tamoxifen, anastrazole, exemestane, letrozole, raloxifene, toremifene, or fulvestrant.

Findings
Normal

Results from a breast biopsy will reveal adequate amounts of cellular and noncellular connective tissue with proper development of tissue.

Abnormal

Presence of a benign tumor (such as adenofibroma) or presence of a malignant tumor (such as adenocarcinoma, inflammatory carcinoma, or sarcoma). Plasma cell mastitis or the presence of intraductal papilloma.

Pharmacy Implications

- Local anesthetics are administered before needle and some open breast biopsies. Some open biopsies require the use of a general anesthetic, in which case the patient is not to eat or drink after midnight the night before the procedure.
- A penicillinase-resistant antibiotic (e.g., dicloxacillin, cephradine, cefazolin, ampicillin/sulbactam) is sometimes used after an open breast biopsy as prophylaxis against penicillinase-producing staphylococcal infections.

Colposcopy[4,11,12]

Description

Colposcopy is a visual examination of the cervix and vagina by using a colposcope, an instrument containing a magnifying lens and a light. A speculum is used to open the birth canal. The cervix is swabbed with acetic acid to remove the surface layer of mucus and to highlight abnormal tissue if present. The colposcope is placed at the opening of the vagina, and the entire area is examined. Biopsies of abnormal tissue may be performed.

Purpose
- Observe the cervix and vagina directly.
- Perform a tissue biopsy of the cervix and vagina.
- Confirm intraepithelial neoplasia or invasive carcinoma.
- Evaluate other vaginal or cervical lesions.
- Monitor antineoplastic therapy.

Findings
Normal
Vaginal and cervical mucosa and epithelium of normal color and appearance.

Abnormal
Presence of color tissue changes or lesions.

Pharmacy Implications
The patient may be instructed to take an over-the-counter NSAID (such as ibuprofen, 400–600 mg, or naproxen, 125–250 mg) the night before the procedure to minimize the cramping that can occur with the colposcopy and biopsy.

Hysterosalpingography[4,7]
Description
Hysterosalpingography, also known as a uterogram, is a radiographic examination performed to visualize the outline of the uterine cavity and the fallopian tubes by means of a contrast medium injected through a cannula inserted into the cervix. The uterus and fallopian tubes are viewed under fluoroscopy, and radiographs are taken.

Purpose
Evaluate tubal patency as part of an infertility workup or to evaluate the fallopian tubes following tubal ligation or reconstruction.

Findings
Normal
Normal anatomy with no tubal or uterine abnormalities.

Abnormal

Tubal adhesions or occlusions. Uterine abnormalities including foreign bodies, fibroid tumors, congenital malformations, or fistulas.

Pharmacy Implications

A sedative may be administered before the procedure.

Laparoscopy[4,8]

Description

Laparoscopy is the direct visual examination of the peritoneal cavity (omentum, liver peritoneum, gallbladder, portions of the spleen, diaphragm, and serosal surfaces of the small bowel and colon) with an endoscope (laparoscope) through the anterior abdominal wall. In women, the ovaries, uterus, and fallopian tubes can be evaluated. A small incision is made at the level of the umbilicus with the patient under local or general anesthesia. A special needle is inserted, and approximately 2 L of carbon dioxide or nitrous oxide is instilled into the abdominal cavity to distend the abdominal wall and provide organfree space to aid in visualization. The laparoscope is then advanced into the peritoneal cavity. The gas is removed after the examination is completed. If fallopian tube patency is being evaluated, a dye is injected through the cervix and observed before gas removal.

Purpose

- Perform procedures such as lysis of adhesions, ovarian biopsy, tubal ligation, removal of foreign bodies, or cholecystectomy.
- Detect ectopic pregnancy, endometriosis, pelvic inflammatory disease, or appendicitis.
- Evaluate pelvic masses.
- Examine the fallopian tubes of infertile women.
- Harvest eggs (ovum) for in vitro fertilization.
- Evaluate ascites of unknown origin.
- Evaluate liver disease of unknown cause. This can add diagnostic accuracy to a blind liver biopsy.
- Evaluate abdominal trauma.

Findings
Normal

Uterus, ovaries, and fallopian tubes are of normal size and shape without adhesions, cysts, or presence of endometriosis. Normally appearing liver, spleen, and peritoneum.

Abnormal

Presence of cysts, adhesions, fibroids, endometriosis, ectopic pregnancy, infection, abscess, or trauma.

Pharmacy Implications

- The patient should not eat or drink after midnight the night before the procedure.
- The patient should avoid aspirin for 7 to 10 days before the procedure and should avoid NSAIDs 2 to 4 days before the procedure.
- Pelvic or abdominal postoperative discomfort may require analgesics.

Mammography[4,7,64]

Description

A mammogram is a radiograph of the breast. A low-energy x-ray beam (0.1–0.8 rads) delineates the breast on mammograms. A frontal view and a lateral view are taken.

Purpose

- Screen for breast cancer and investigate or detect masses missed during physical examination of the breast.
- Help differentiate benign from malignant masses identified by other means.

Findings

Normal

No calcification, no abnormal mass, and normal duct contrast with narrowing of ductal branches.

Abnormal

A poorly outlined, irregularly shaped, and opaque lesion suggests malignancy. Malignant cysts are usually solitary and unilateral and contain an increased number of blood vessels. Benign cysts are usually round and smooth with definable edges.

Pharmacy Implications

- No medications/preparations are needed.
- The American Cancer Society recommends for women ages 20 to 39 to have a clinical breast exam by a health professional every 3 years, and for women ages 40 years and older to have an annual mammogram. Routine breast self-examination is recommended.

Ultrasonography of Pelvis, Uterus, and Ovaries
See General Procedures, Ultrasound.

Hematology

Bone Marrow Aspiration and Biopsy[4,7,8]
Description
Aspiration
The preferred site is the posterior superior iliac spine (PSIS), but this may also be performed at the sternum. The skin is prepared with povidone-iodine, and the area is anesthetized with lidocaine including deeper structures down to the periosteum. A small incision is made over the PSIS extending down to the periosteum. A special aspiration needle (Illinois) is directed into the cortex of the PSIS. Once in the marrow, a sample of 4 to 5 mL is aspirated for microscopic examination.

Biopsy
A biopsy of the bone marrow is most commonly obtained from the posterior superior iliac spine (preferred site), the spinous process, or the tibia. Preparation of the site follows the same procedure as aspiration biopsy. A large-bore hollow needle (Jamshidi) is then inserted through the skin, through the subcutaneous fatty tissues, and into the cortex of the bone being sampled. With this large-bore needle, a back and forth rotary motion is used to harvest a bone marrow core from the cortex of the bone. Unlike aspiration, biopsy preserves the marrow architecture for histologic evaluation.

Purpose
- Diagnose disorders such as anemias, thrombocytopenia, leukemias, and granulomas.
- Distinguish between primary and metastatic tumors.
- Determine the cause of bone infection.
- Aid in the staging of neoplastic disease.
- Evaluate the effectiveness of chemotherapy and monitor myelosuppression.

Findings
Normal
Normal hematologic analysis with differential count. Normal relative amounts of fat and hemopoietic cells and normal number of megakaryocytes, immature platelets, plasma, and mast cells.

Abnormal

Detection of osteoclasts or osteoblasts, groups of malignant cells in the marrow, granulomas, and cells with indistinct margins indicating marrow necrosis.

Pharmacy Implications

Patients may require sedation before bone marrow aspiration or biopsy with an IM or IV narcotic analgesic and/or an IM or IV benzodiazepine.

Infectious Disease

Gram Stain[11,12,65]

Description

Gram stain is a procedure whereby a specimen or sample of a body fluid (e.g., blood, sputum, urine, or wound aspirate) is fixed to a slide stained with a crystal violet solution; rinsed, then flooded with Gram iodine solution; rinsed, decolorized with a mixture of ethanol and/or acetone; rinsed, then counterstained with safranin; rinsed, and then allowed to dry. This is a relatively quick screening method for identifying infecting bacteria. The composition of the cell wall appears to be the key element in the staining and differentiation of organisms.

Purpose

Classify bacterial organisms into gram-positive or gram-negative cocci or rods.

Findings

- Gram-positive organisms retain the primary dye and appear dark purple.
- Gram-negative organisms will appear pinkish-red following decolorization and counterstaining.

Pharmacy Implications

The ability to differentiate Gram-positive and Gram-negative organisms and the knowledge of their antibiotic sensitivity patterns aids in the selection of appropriate empiric antibiotic therapy until the final identification of the organism occurs.

Indium-Labeled WBC Scan (Indium-111 Leukocyte Total Body Scan)[4,7,11,12,16]

Description

Approximately 40 mL of blood is taken from the patient for labeling of the WBCs with radioactive Indium-111. The labeled WBCs are intravenously reinjected into the patient. The radioisotope-labeled WBCs concentrate in areas of inflammation or infection. At 6 and 24 hours after reinjection, imaging studies are performed on the patient. The scanner detects radiation that is emitted from the radioisotope-tagged WBCs. It takes approximately 1 hour for each imaging study. The radiation from this test is equivalent to one abdominal radiograph.

Purpose

Diagnose infectious and inflammatory processes.

Findings
Normal

Results will show high concentrations of the labeled WBCs in the liver, spleen, and bone marrow.

Abnormal

Results will show high concentrations of the labeled WBCs outside the liver, spleen, and bone marrow, such as in an abscess formation, acute and chronic osteomyelitis, orthopedic prosthesis, infection, and active inflammatory bowel disease.

Pharmacy Implications

Hyperalimentation, steroid therapy, and long-term antibiotic therapy can produce false-negative results because of their ability to change the chemotactic response of WBCs.

 Nephrology

Renal Biopsy[3,4]

Description

The safest method is percutaneous needle biopsy using a 6-inch, 20-gauge needle. After placing the patient in the prone position, US or anatomic landmark identification is used to locate the ideal site for biopsy. The skin is prepared with povidone iodine, and a local anesthetic is used to anesthetize the skin. A small incision is made,, and the deeper tissues are also anesthetized with a local anesthetic. The biopsy needle is then advanced toward the kidney, where a biopsy core is extracted and the needle is withdrawn. If a tissue sample from a solid lesion is necessary, an open biopsy may need to be performed.

Purpose

- Diagnose diseases that alter the structure of the glomerulus.
- Evaluate proteinuria of unknown origin.
- Determine the nature of a renal mass identified by other diagnostic techniques.
- Determine the cause of acute renal failure when other etiologic factors have been ruled out.
- Monitor the course of chronic renal disease.
- Evaluate suspected cases of renal dysfunction secondary to inflammatory vasculitides.
- Evaluate suspected rejection of a transplanted kidney.

Findings
Normal

Normal pathology and histology.

Abnormal

Presence of a tumor, clot, or renal stone. Presence of histologic changes characteristic of lupus erythematosus, amyloid infiltration, glomerulonephritis, renal vein thrombosis, pyelonephritis, and renal transplant rejection.

Pharmacy Implications

It is recommended that antiplatelet agents be stopped before open and needle biopsies. Aspirin should be discontinued 7 to 10 days before the procedure. NSAIDs (e.g., ibuprofen, naproxen) that inhibit the enzyme cyclooxygenase should be stopped 2 to 4 days before the procedure.

Renal Scan[4,7]

Description

A radioactive tracer, technetium-99m, is injected intravenously. A scanning camera then takes images of the blood flow to and through the kidneys. During the first stage of scanning, images are taken in rapid succession to evaluate renal perfusion. During the second stage, several still images are taken over a 30- to 45-minute period to evaluate renal function.

Purpose

- Detect or rule out masses.
- Investigate kidney function.
- Evaluate kidney transplant viability and renal blood flow.

Findings
Normal

Normal size, shape, position, and function of the kidneys.

Abnormal

Tumors (irregular masses) within the kidney, obstructions, decreased renal perfusion, abnormal kidneys (shape or size), and presence of rejection.

Pharmacy Implications

None.

Neurology

Brainstem Auditory Evoked Response (BAER)[7,66,67]

Description

Electrodes are placed on the scalp to obtain baseline electrical activity. An electrode is also placed on the earlobe of the ear to be tested. Then many click stimuli (10 clicks/second for about 1,000 clicks) are delivered to one ear and then the other by using earphones and a tone stimulator. White noise is presented to the ear that is not being tested to isolate the ear that is being tested. The clicks induce electrical activity (evoked response) in the auditory pathways, which is then detected by the electrodes. A computer enhances the electrical activity and records it as wave activity. This activity is translated into seven discrete waves (I–VII) that correspond to specific anatomic structures.

Purpose

- Diagnose cerebral deficiencies of the eighth cranial nerve.
- Diagnose brainstem lesions such as multiple sclerosis, brainstem infarction, brainstem gliomas, and disorders of the central nervous system (CNS).
- Diagnose posterior fossa tumors and acoustic neuromas.
- Assess coma and cerebral death when electroencephalogram (EEG) findings are inconclusive.

- Assess a factitious hearing loss.
- Evaluate hearing loss in a child or newborn.

Findings
It takes about 10 ms for a sound stimulus to reach the cerebral cortex. Lesions at different sites in a tract along the eighth cranial nerve through the brainstem and into the cerebral cortex will alter these waves in different ways, providing a method of locating a suspected brainstem lesion.

Pharmacy Implications
None.

CT of the Head
See General Procedures, Computed Tomography (CT).

Electroencephalography (EEG)[4,7,16,68,69]
Description
Electrodes are placed on the scalp in the form of small discs. They are fastened to the scalp after an electrical conduction paste has been applied to the scalp/electrodes. The electrodes are connected by wires to an amplifier and are arranged in one of several patterns on the scalp. Electrical impulses from the brain (alpha, beta, and delta waves) are recorded on a moving paper tape. This tape is then compared against a standardized normal tape and against tapes showing patterns for specific pathologies. A period of hyperventilation and light stimulation at different frequencies is used to stimulate the brain. The EEG may be done under normal conditions in a sleep-induced state or in a sleep-deprived state. Both of these states have characteristic electrical patterns.

Purpose
- Measure and record electrical impulses in the brain to diagnose seizure disorders. An EEG should be performed while the patient is having a seizure or as soon after the seizure as possible. Simultaneous video monitoring and EEG monitoring may be necessary to classify the seizure.
- Evaluate suspected pseudoseizures.
- Aid in identifying brain tumors, abscesses, and subdural hematomas.
- Ascertain information about the possibility of other cerebrovascular diseases, such as cerebral infarcts and intracranial hemorrhage, and cerebral diseases, such as advanced cases of multiple sclerosis, narcolepsy, and acute delirium.

- Diagnose infections of the CNS such as herpes simplex encephalitis, and Creutzfeldt-Jakob disease.
- Determine brain death.
- Aid in the diagnosis and characterization of sleep apnea or other sleep disorders.

Findings
Normal
The EEG tracing produces a tape that is consistent with normal electrical brain activity in the awake and sleep state.

Abnormal
Brain wave activity consistent with a seizure disorder or other cerebral disease or lesion. A flat EEG results from cerebral hypoxia or ischemia from which there is no neurologic recovery.

Pharmacy Implications
- A sleep EEG patient receives chloral hydrate, 1–2 g PO, before the test to promote rest and sleep.
- Caffeine-containing drinks should be withheld for 8 hours before the test.
- Drugs altering brain wave activity (e.g., anticonvulsants, sedatives, tranquilizers) will interfere with an accurate tracing. A physician may choose to stop anticonvulsant therapy before the EEG.

Electromyography (EMG)[4,7,16,68,70]
Description
A needle electrode is inserted through the skin and into the muscle to measure the electrical activity of skeletal muscle. This electrical activity (muscle action potential) is amplified and displayed on a cathode-ray oscillograph, and a permanent record is obtained by recording on magnetic tape. To evaluate physiologic function fully, the electrical activity of the muscle is measured at three activity levels: rest, mild contraction, and maximal contraction. The muscle is not electrically stimulated during this test.

Purpose
The amplitude, duration, number, and configuration of the muscle action potentials aid in differentiating neurogenic pathology from myogenic

involvement. The procedure is used to evaluate the integrity of the nervous system, the neuromuscular junction, and the muscle itself. EMG by itself is not considered diagnostic for any specific disease.

Findings
Normal
A normally relaxed muscle is electrically silent at rest. During voluntary contraction, electrical activity increases significantly.

Abnormal
Waveforms that are different from normal muscle are evaluated to differentiate a muscle disorder from a denervation disorder. These results can aid in the diagnosis of muscular dystrophies, myopathies from various causes, amyotrophic lateral sclerosis, peripheral nerve disorders, myasthenia gravis, and certain corticospinal tract tumors.

Pharmacy Implications
Drugs that affect the nerve–muscle junction such as cholinergics, anticholinergics, and skeletal muscle relaxants can interfere with test results.

Lumbar Puncture (LP)[16,71]
Description
The patient lies on either side at the edge of a firm surface with knees drawn up and head bent forward to put the spine in hyperflexion. The usual site of puncture is between the 3rd and 4th (or 4th and 5th) lumbar vertebrae. The area is cleaned with an antiseptic and locally anesthetized. The lumbar puncture needle (3–4 in. long) is inserted through the skin in the midline between the vertebra, perpendicular to the surface of the back and diverted slightly upward toward the patient's head. When the needle penetrates the dura and enters the spinal canal, a slight decrease in resistance can be felt. Once the spinal canal has been penetrated, cerebrospinal fluid (CSF) is removed.

Purpose
- Obtain a CSF specimen for diagnostic study.
- Aid in the diagnosis of suspected meningitis, intracranial hemorrhage, and CNS involvement from malignant disease (e.g., leukemia, lymphoma).
- Determine the CSF pressure to document impairment of flow or to lessen pressure by removing a volume of fluid.

- Diagnose organic CNS disease (e.g., multiple sclerosis and Guillain-Barré syndrome).
- Evaluate certain electrolyte disturbances.
- Remove blood or exudate from the subarachnoid space.
- Administer x-ray contrast media (e.g., myelogram) or give drugs intrathecally (e.g., antibiotics and antineoplastic agents).

Findings
Normal
Normal appearance, consistency, expected cell composition, absence of bacteria, normal chemistry of the fluid, and normal pressure (see the section on cerebrospinal fluid examination in Chapter 5, Interpretation of Clinical Laboratory Results).

Abnormal
See Table 6.5.

Pharmacy Implications
- Patients may experience a headache after removal of CSF and require treatment with an analgesic.
- Patients should lie flat for up to 8 hours after the procedure.

MRI of the Head
See General Procedures, Magnetic Resonance Imaging (MRI).

Table 6.5 ABNORMAL CSF FLUID	
Appearance	Cloudy fluid
Protein content	>50 mg/dL
Glucose concentration	<30 mg/dL or >70 mg/dL
WBCs	>10/mm^3
pH of fluid	< or >7.3
Bacteria or virus	Present
RBCs	Present

Muscle Biopsy[11,12,73,74]

Description

A muscle biopsy can be performed by making a small incision through the skin and into the muscle. A sample of the desired muscle segment is excised (open biopsy). An alternate method is percutaneous by means of a biopsy needle. The needle is inserted into the muscle, and a small plug of muscle tissue is removed when the needle is withdrawn. In most cases the biopsy can be performed using a local anesthetic.

Purpose

- Investigate the origin of muscle weakness (neurogenic or myogenic).
- Diagnose localized or diffuse inflammatory disease of the muscle and suspected genetic diseases of the muscle.
- Assist in the diagnosis of diffuse vascular, connective tissue, and metabolic diseases.
- Evaluate suspected myopathy.

Findings
Normal
Presence of normal pathology and histology.

Abnormal
Presence of myogenic or myopathic changes.

Pharmacy Implications

- Antiplatelet agents should be discontinued before open and needle biopsies. Aspirin should be discontinued 7 to 10 days before the procedure. NSAIDs (e.g., ibuprofen, naproxen) that reversibly inhibit the enzyme cyclooxygenase should be stopped 2 to 4 days before the procedure.
- Preprocedure medications such as parenteral analgesics (e.g., meperidine, morphine) and parenteral sedatives/ anxiolytics (e.g., lorazepam, diazepam, midazolam) may be administered.
- A local anesthetic such as lidocaine may be necessary.

Myelography[4,7,72]

Description

Myelography is a radiographic examination of the cervical, thoracic, and/or lumbar spinal cord and the space around the spinal cord. A local anesthetic is administered at the needle insertion site. Using fluoroscopy, a spinal needle is guided into the subarachnoid space. A nonionic water-soluble contrast dye is then injected. With the patient tilted upward, x-ray films of the lumbar spine are taken. The patient is tilted downward to take x-ray films of the thoracic and cervical spine. Generally, a sample of spinal fluid is collected before administration of the contrast media and is sent for laboratory analysis.

This test is sometimes followed or replaced by CT scanning, which can improve visualization.

Purpose
Visualize spinal cord abnormalities.

Findings
Normal
Normal outline of spinal cord and normal nerve structures. Contrast medium flows freely through the subarachnoid space. No evidence of spinal cord abnormalities.

Abnormal
Presence of a herniated disc, spinal cord compression, nerve root injury, degenerative spur, vascular abnormalities, CSF leakage, dural tear, traumatic injury, neoplasm, or mass.

Pharmacy Implications
- The patient should have no food or fluids 4 hours before the examination.
- A local anesthetic, such as lidocaine, is used to anesthetize the area at the site of spinal needle insertion.
- The procedure should not be performed if the patient is receiving anticoagulants.
- Medications that can lower the seizure threshold, such as phenothiazines, monoamine oxidase inhibitors (MAOIs), tricyclic antidepressants, and CNS stimulants, should be discontinued ≥ 48 hours before and ≥ 24 hours after myelography.
- The use of phenothiazine antiemetics should be avoided.

Nerve Biopsy[11,12,75]
Description
The sural nerve (situated in the lower leg near the Achilles tendon), the deep peroneal nerve (located in the area of the calf below the knee), or the superficial radial nerve are the sites most commonly used for nerve biopsy. An incision is made, the nerve is exposed, and by sharp dissection

a 3- to 4-cm length of nerve or nerve tissue is removed for evaluation. A nerve deficit may be a complication resulting from the biopsy.

Purpose
Diagnose neuropathic disorders and distinguish between demyelinating disease versus axon degeneration disease.

Findings
Normal
Presence of normal pathology and histology.

Abnormal
Presence of polyarteritis nodosa, amyloidosis, sarcoidosis, vasculitis, various neuropathies, mononeuritis multiplex, specific nerve (radial, distal median, tibial) dysfunction, leprosy, metachromatic leukodystrophy, Krabbe disease, ataxia telangiectasia, giant axonal neuropathy, and genetically determined pediatric neurologic disorders.

Pharmacy Implications
It is recommended that antiplatelet agents be stopped before open and needle biopsies. Aspirin should be stopped 7 to 10 days before the procedure. NSAIDs (e.g., ibuprofen, naproxen) that reversibly inhibit the enzyme cyclooxygenase should be discontinued 2 to 4 days before the procedure.

Nerve Conduction Study[7]
Description
Peripheral nerves are electrically stimulated using EMG equipment in combination with a nerve stimulator. This produces action potentials that travel through the nerve to distant sites and are detected by surface electrodes. These evoked action potentials are displayed on an oscilloscope screen, which enables the investigator to see the amplitude and duration of the action potential. By knowing the time interval between applying the electrical stimulus and the initiation of the action potential along with the maximum nerve conduction velocity, objective information about nerve conduction can be obtained. Nerve conduction testing is the preferred test for evaluating patients with peripheral nerve dysfunction. This testing may be done at the same time as EMG to differentiate peripheral nerve disease from myogenic disease. Nerves commonly tested include the median, ulnar, radial, peroneal, tibial, superficial peroneal, and sural.

Purpose

- Confirm a sensory deficit and distinguish from a motor deficit.
- Evaluate the extent and severity of polyneuropathy.
- Differentiate muscle disease from neuropathic disease, and demyelinating disease from axonal disease.
- Confirm the diagnosis of Guillain-Barré syndrome, mononeuritis multiplex, and other demyelinating diseases.
- Assess nerve entrapment, such as carpal tunnel syndrome, and differentiate from diffuse neuropathy.

Findings
Normal

Action potential amplitude, conduction velocity, and latency (nerve conduction time plus the time to muscle action potential after the distal electrode senses the electrical stimulus) are all within normal ranges.

Abnormal

Slowing of conduction velocity, delayed distal latency, and decreased amplitude of the action potential compared with normal are signs of nerve dysfunction.

Pharmacy Implications

Cisplatin, carboplatin, dapsone, vincristine, paclitaxel, docetaxel, metronidazole, foscarnet, ganciclovir, isoniazid, lamivudine, didanosine, ritonavir, and stavudine are known causes of neuropathy (this list is not inclusive).

Visual Evoked Response (VER)[7,66,67]
Description

EEG electrodes are placed on the scalp over the occipital or visual cortex area. Baseline electrical activity is recorded. The patient is instructed to fix on a point. A visual stimulus such as flashes of light or a sudden change of a checkerboard pattern is administered. First one eye is stimulated, then the other. The time interval between the stimulus and the response is recorded and displayed.

Purpose

VER aids in diagnosing lesions of the optic nerve or confirming the diagnosis of multiple sclerosis. It may also be used to rule out hysterical blindness, to monitor surgery of the optic nerve, and to assess visual acuity in special circumstances.

Findings
Normal
No evidence of optic nerve damage.

Abnormal
A difference in the responses between the left and right eye, with an increased latency and duration in one eye, indicates a lesion in that optic nerve. Both optic nerves can be involved. VER is abnormal with optic neuritis, pseudotumor cerebri, toxic amblyopias, nutritional amblyopias, neoplasms interfering with the optic pathway, sarcoidosis, pernicious anemia, and Friedreich ataxia.

Pharmacy Implications
None.

Ophthalmology

Ophthalmoscopy[11,12,76,77]
Description
The inner eye is viewed using an ophthalmoscope, an instrument with a special illumination system. A strong light is directed into the patient's eye by reflection from a small mirror. The light is reflected from the fundus of the eye back through the ophthalmoscope to the examiner. The opening of the instrument is held as close as possible to the patient's and the examiner's eyes.

Purpose
Examine the fundus of the eye including the optic disk, macula, retina, retinal vessels, choroid, and sclera. Baseline and follow-up ophthalmoscopy is recommended when hypertension or diabetes is present or when certain drugs are being taken.

Findings
Normal
Optic disk is normal size, color, and vascularity. Macula is devoid of blood vessels and darker than surrounding retina. Retina is attached and has normal vascularity and color. Choroid and sclera should not be visualized.

> ## Table 6.6   RETINAL VASCULAR GRADING SYSTEMS
>
> ### *Hypertensive retinopathy (Keith-Wagner Method)*
>
> | | |
> |---|---|
> | Grade I | Constriction of retinal arterioles only |
> | Grade II | Constriction and sclerosis of retinal arterioles |
> | Grade III | Hemorrhages and exudates in addition to vascular changes |
> | Grade IV | Papilledema (edema of the optic disk) |
>
> ### *Diabetic retinopathy (retinal changes fall into two categories)*
> *Background retinopathy*
> - Multiple microaneurysms appear
> - Veins dilate, multiple dot and blot hemorrhages occur, and hard waxy white and yellow exudates may leak from the retinal vasculature in the area of the macula.
> - Cotton-wool patches (microinfarcts of the retinal nerve fiber layer) appear in the superficial retina; hard exudates may form what is described as the macular star.
>
> *Proliferative retinopathy*
> - Neovascularization occurs.
> - Neovascularization of the optic disk occurs.
> - End-stage of retinopathy occurs with organized vitreous hemorrhage, fibrosis, and retinitis proliferans (detached retina) leading to blindness.

Abnormal

- Two descriptive approaches for staging or grading of retinopathy are used. The choice of grading methods for retinal vascular changes is influenced by the underlying disease (Table 6-6).
- Optic disk has abnormal vascularity, elevation (bulging), small hemorrhages, and abnormal color. The macula is edematous and ischemic with degeneration appearing as a round white mass. Blood vessels of the choroid and sclera can be visualized. Malignant melanoma appears as a pigmented elevated mass.

Pharmacy Implications

- Drugs affecting the retina include chloroquine, hydroxychloroquine, phenothiazines, penicillamine, isoniazid, ethambutol, and indomethacin.
- Dilating eye drops may be used to improve visualization of eye structures.

Slit Lamp Examination[76,78]

Description

Slit lamp examination involves the combination of a light and microscopic examination of the eye. Dilation of the pupil using a mydriatic and cycloplegic agent facilitates viewing.

Purpose

The slit lamp allows for examination of the lids, cornea, anterior chamber of the eye, and transparent and nearly transparent ocular fluids and tissues.

Findings
Normal

Clear, avascular vitreous fluid.

Abnormal

Vitreous disease including retraction, condensation, and shrinkage. Presence of blood and floaters. Presence of cataracts or corneal deposits.

Pharmacy Implications

Slit lamp examination may be needed to evaluate drug-induced ocular toxicity associated with indomethacin, clofazimine, allopurinol, corticosteroids, gold salts, chloroquine, hydroxychloroquine, griseofulvin, chlorambucil, cytosine arabinoside, mitotane, tamoxifen, amiodarone, quinidine, phenothiazines, phenytoin, and isotretinoin.

Tonometry[7,76,77,79]

Description

There are three types of tonometers: indentation, applanation, and noncontact. In the case of indentation and applanation, these tonometers make contact with the eye. The most commonly used contact tonometer is the applanation (Goldman) tonometer. After first anesthetizing the eye with a topical anesthetic, fluorescein is dripped in the eye to outline the corneal rings (standard area of the cornea). The applanating prism mounted at the end of an arm projecting vertically from a black box is placed in contact with the patient's cornea. A knob on the black box actuates a spring-loaded device that allows the examiner to increase or decrease the pressure necessary to flatten a standard area of cornea. The pressure needed for flattening to occur is read off a scale on the knob.

Noncontact tonometry is performed by directing a puff of air at the cornea to determine eye pressure. This method is less reliable when the pressure in the eye is at a higher pressure range, when the cornea is abnormal, or when the patient is unable to establish visual fixation.

Purpose

Measure the eye's intraocular pressure.

Findings
Normal

Ten to 20 mm Hg (16 mm average).

Abnormal

Greater than 24 mm Hg is diagnostic for glaucoma.

Pharmacy Implications

Drugs that may increase intraocular pressure include anticholinergics, corticosteroids, and sympathomimetics.

Orthopedics

Arthroscopy[4,8,11,12,16]
Description

Arthroscopy is visual examination of a joint (most commonly the knee and less commonly the shoulder) using a special fiber-optic endoscope called an arthroscope. Arthroscopy is performed using a local anesthetic. However, general or spinal anesthesia may be used if surgery is anticipated. For knee arthroscopy, approximately 75 to 100 mL of normal saline solution is injected into the joint to distend it. The arthroscope is then inserted close to the knee tendon and upper tibia. All parts of the knee are examined at various degrees of flexion and extension, and joint washings are examined. Arthroscopy usually follows arthrography, because arthroscopy is an invasive procedure.

Purpose
- Diagnose athletic injuries.
- Differentiate and diagnose acute and chronic disorders of the knee and other large joints.
- Perform joint surgery.
- Monitor progression of disease and effectiveness of therapy.

Findings
Normal

Normal joint vasculature, normal color of synovium, normal ligaments, normal cartilage, and undamaged suprapatellar pouch.

Abnormal

Torn and displaced cartilage and meniscus, trapped synovium, loose fragments of bone or cartilage, torn ligaments, chronic inflammatory arthritis, chondromalacia of bone, secondary osteoarthritis, presence of cysts or foreign bodies, torn rotator cuff, or rotator cuff tendonitis.

Pharmacy Implications

- Patient should take nothing by mouth from midnight the night before the procedure.
- A sedative is usually given before the examination.
- Analgesics may be given after the procedure as needed for pain. NSAIDs are commonly used along with narcotic analgesics.

Arthrography[4,7,80]

Description

An arthrogram is a radiograph of a joint following injection of contrast media into the synovium. If fluid is present in the joint space, a sample is aspirated and sent to the laboratory to detect the presence of bacteria and/or chemicals. The aspiration is performed before injecting the contrast medium into the joint. Using a fluoroscope, contrast material and air are injected into the joint space. The joints most often examined in this manner are the knee, hip, and shoulders.

Purpose

Elucidate soft tissue injury in cartilage and ligaments surrounding the joint that cannot be seen with conventional x-ray techniques.

Findings
Normal

Normal anatomy and condition of the joint supportive tissues.

Abnormal

Ligamentous and cartilaginous tears or injuries.

Pharmacy Implications

Hypersensitivity reactions to the iodine dye are less likely to occur due to the small amount of iodine present in the synovial space.

Bone Densitometry[7,81]

Description

Several noninvasive techniques are used to measure bone density. They include single photon absorptiometry (SPA), dual photon absorptiometry (DPA), dual-energy x-ray absorptiometry (DEXA), and quantitative computed tomography (QCT). DPA, DEXA, and QCT can be used to measure the bone density of the femoral neck and the lumbar spine. However, SPA can only measure bone mineral density of the radius. Unlike SPA, DPA, and DEXA, QCT can be used to measure bone density in other peripheral bones. All the techniques measure cortical and trabecular bone. Because the bone density of the radius may not accurately reflect the density of the femur or spine, SPA has limited usefulness. DEXA is considered the gold standard for bone mineral density measurement.

SPA, DPA, and DEXA use much less radiation than QCT and can be performed in a shorter period. Furthermore, the non-QCT techniques use a narrow beam of radiation.

METHOD RADIATION SOURCE

SPA	I-125
DPA	Gd153
DEXA	X-ray
QCT	X-ray

With recent advances in bone mineral density equipment, two types of portable equipment are now available that measure the bone mineral density of the heel. One of these technologies uses radiation, whereas the other uses ultrasound.

The T-score (number of standard deviations the bone density is above or below the mean for young, normal subjects) is used to determine fracture risk and the need for treatment. There is approximately a 10% reduction or increase in bone mineral density for each standard deviation below or above zero.

Purpose

Bone mineral density is the major determinant of fracture risk. Bone density studies are used to identify patients who are at risk for developing osteoporosis, to evaluate fracture risk, and to evaluate the patient's response to osteoporosis therapy.

Findings

Normal

A T-score greater than −1.

Abnormal

A T-score of −1 to −2.5 indicates osteopenia. A T-score less than −2.5 indicates osteoporosis.

Pharmacy Implications

- If a patient's T-score is less than −2, recommendations should be made about treatment.
- If a patient's T-score is less than −1.5 and the patient smokes tobacco, has had a fracture, has a first-degree relative with a fracture history, or is of low body weight (<57.7 kg), treatment should be initiated.
- For those patients undergoing treatment, follow-up bone scans should be performed on an annual or biannual basis.

Bone Scan?

Description

A bone scan is a radiograph of the whole body after IV injection of Tc-99m methylene diphosphate. The radionuclide has particular affinity for bone and collects in areas of abnormal metabolism. There is a 2- to 3-hour waiting period after injection of the tracer to allow for full concentration in the bone.

Purpose

- Determine the site of bone and bone marrow biopsy.
- Diagnose myeloproliferative disorders.
- Identify focal defects in bone and bone marrow.
- Stage lymphoma or Hodgkin disease or find cancer metastases.
- Aid in the diagnosis of bone pain and inflammatory processes (e.g., infection or osteomyelitis).

Findings

Normal

The radioisotope is distributed evenly throughout the bone. No "hot spots" (concentrated areas of uptake) are noted.

Abnormal

Presence of hot spots indicating increased concentration of the radioactive compound at sites of abnormal metabolism (e.g., infection, fracture, degenerative bone disease, failing bone grafts). Bone marrow depression following radiation or chemotherapy. Nonvisualization in myelofibrosis. Sites of primary bone tumors and bone metastases from other malignancies.

Pharmacy Implications
None.

Otolaryngology

Laryngoscopy[82,83]

Description
Three types of examination can be performed:

- *Indirect.* This involves the placement of a laryngeal mirror in the mouth and a light source to visualize the back of the tongue, the epiglottis, valleculae, the pyriform fossae, and the structures of the larynx.
- *Direct, involving the use of a flexible fiber-optic nasolaryngoscope.* The scope is passed through the locally anesthetized nasal cavity and then suspended above the larynx to provide a direct view of the nose, nasopharynx, larynx, and adjacent structures.
- *Direct, involving the use of a rigid lighted laryngoscope.* This technique requires the patient to undergo general anesthesia. The scope is inserted through the mouth and passed through the throat to expose the larynx and its structures.

Purpose
- Examine the visible structures for disease, trauma, and strictures.
- Detect and remove foreign bodies.
- Perform tissue biopsies of suspicious lesions to aid in the diagnosis of cancer.

Findings
Normal
Normal position, color, and anatomy of the examined area. Absence of lesions, strictures, inflammation, and foreign bodies.

Abnormal
Color changes of laryngeal and adjacent structures. Position changes, presence of lesions, strictures, or foreign bodies.

Pharmacy Implications
Indirect Laryngoscopy
None.

Direct Fiber-Optic Laryngoscopy

A sedative/anxiolytic (e.g., midazolam, diazepam) may be administered before the procedure.

Direct Rigid Laryngoscopy

An IM anticholinergic (e.g., atropine or glycopyrrolate) and an IM sedative/anxiolytic (e.g., midazolam) may be administered 30 minutes before the procedure.

Pulmonology

Bronchial Alveolar Lavage (BAL)

See Pulmonology, Bronchoscopy.

Bronchoscopy[7,84]

Description

Bronchoscopy is the examination of the inside of the tracheobronchial tree by direct visualization. After first anesthetizing the throat, and possibly the nasal passage, with a local anesthetic, a flexible fiber-optic lighted bronchoscope (tube) is inserted through an oral endotracheal tube and advanced into the tracheobronchial tree. An eyepiece at the proximal end of the bronchoscope allows viewing of the fourth to sixth division of the bronchi, the upper airway, and the vocal cords. A camera can also be attached to the eye piece.

If bronchial alveolar lavage is to be performed, 100 mL of normal saline is instilled into the lung through the bronchoscope. Approximately 30 to 60 mL of fluid is aspirated for cytologic, microbiologic, and cell count analysis.

If brush biopsy is to be performed, the brush is passed through the bronchoscope to the lesion to be biopsied. The lesion is brushed, and the brush is withdrawn. An optional technique is to leave the brush in place at the tip of the bronchoscope and withdraw the bronchoscope slowly. With either technique, the material collected on the brush is transferred to glass slides where it is prepared for viewing under the microscope.

Purpose

- View nasopharyngeal and laryngeal lesions and visualize the source of hemoptysis.

- Further evaluate a patient with positive sputum cytology and suspected interstitial lung disease.
- Perform transbronchial biopsy of the lung and bronchial alveolar lavage (BAL).
- Assess recurrent nerve paralysis.
- Identify cause of problems with airway (chronic cough).
- Remove airway obstructions.

Findings
Normal
No malignancies, lesions, source of bleeding, or infection.

Abnormal
Presence of malignancies, infections, or other abnormal findings as stated above.

Pharmacy Implications
- Patient should not eat or drink after midnight the evening before the procedure.
- A parenteral skeletal muscle relaxant (e.g., a benzodiazepine) and an anticholinergic (e.g., atropine) should be administered to dry up secretions 30 to 60 minutes before the procedure. A narcotic analgesic may also be administered IM or IV before the procedure.
- The patient should not eat or drink for 1 to 2 hours after the procedure to reduce the risk of aspiration. Clear liquids should be administered initially, and the patient should be observed for swallowing difficulties.

Chest Radiograph[4,7,16]
Description
A radiograph of the chest from the front, side, and sometimes back. It is best performed with the patient in the standing position.

Purpose
Chest radiographs are useful in the diagnosis of pulmonary, mediastinal, and bony thorax disease. The standing position demonstrates the presence of fluid levels.

Findings
Normal
Absence of fluids, masses, and infection. Air-filled spaces appear black.

Abnormal

The film will have opacities (shadowy or white areas) suggestive of the presence of fluid, tumors and other lesions, infectious processes, unusual air in the lungs, or a collapsed lung. Spinal deformities, bone destruction, and trauma can be observed.

Pharmacy Implications

None.

CT of the Chest

See General Procedures, Computed Tomography (CT).

Pulmonary Function Tests (PFTs)[85,86]

Description

Using spirometry, a patient is instructed to inhale and then exhale as rapidly as possible. As the patient exhales into the spirometer, he or she displaces a bell and the pen deflection records the volume of air entering or exiting the lung (Fig. 6.1).

The tidal volume or the volume of air being inhaled and exhaled during normal breathing can be recorded. The vital capacity (VC) is the amount of air being moved during maximal inhalation and exhalation. Residual volume (RV) reflects the volume of air left in the lung after maximal

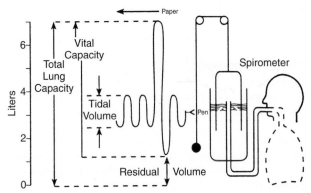

FIGURE 6.1 Spirometric graphics during quiet breathing and maximal breathing. (Reprinted from Young LY, Koda-Kimble MA. *Applied Therapeutics: The Clinical Use of Drugs.* 6th ed. Vancouver, WA: Applied Therapeutics, Inc.; 1995, with permission.)

expiration. Total lung capacity (TLC) is the sum of the vital capacity and the residual volume. Patients with restrictive lung disease often display a decrease in all lung volumes, whereas those individuals with obstructive disease often have normal TLC but decreased VC and increased RV.

In evaluating the performance of the lung, forced expiration techniques together with a spirometer can measure lung volumes and airflow, providing useful information in graphic form (Figs. 6.2 and 6.3). The forced expiratory volume (FEV) measures the amount of air the patient can exhale after a maximal inhalation, often over a set period such as 1 second (FEV_1). Together with the forced vital capacity (FVC), which measures the maximum volume of air exhaled with maximally forced effort after a maximal inhalation effort, these values can provide important performance measures of the lung. The peak expiratory flow rate (PEFR) measures the maximal flow that can be produced during the forced expiration. Generally, this measurement provides similar information as

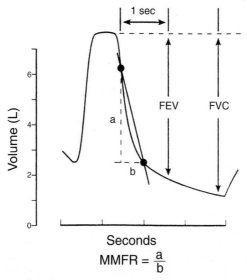

FIGURE 6.2 Volume versus time curve resulting from a forced expiratory volume (FEV) maneuver. FVC, forced vital capacity; MMFR, maximal midexpiratory flow rate. (Reprinted from Young LY, Koda-Kimble MA. *Applied Therapeutics: The Clinical Use of Drugs.* 6th ed. Vancouver, WA: Applied Therapeutics, Inc.; 1995, with permission.)

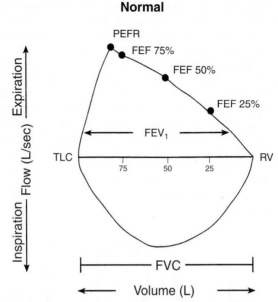

FIGURE 6.3 A normal flow/volume curve resulting from a forced expiratory maneuver. FEF, forced expiratory flow; FEV, forced expiratory volume; FVC, forced vital capacity; PEFR, peak expiratory flow rate; RV, residual volume; TLC, total lung capacity. (Adapted from Young LY, Koda-Kimble MA. *Applied Therapeutics: The Clinical Use of Drugs*. 6th ed. Vancouver, WA: Applied Therapeutics, Inc.; 1995, with permission.)

the FEV_1 but is less reproducible. Portable peak flow meters are in common use by patients with reactive airway disease to assist patients and medical providers in following variations in airway tone throughout the day. Another measurement is the forced expiratory flow, which occurs during the middle 50% of the expiratory curve ($FEF_{25\%-75\%}$, $FEF_{50\%}$ or maximal midexpiratory flow rate [MEFR]). This measure is helpful for patients with emphysema, because it represents the elastic recoil force of the lung and is less dependent on the patient's expiratory effort.

Spirometry can also be used to establish the reversibility of airway disease. The use of bronchodilators can be administered after baseline pulmonary function tests to determine the degree of reversibility. Generally, a significant clinical reversibility is defined as a 15% to 20% improvement in the FEV_1 after administration of the bronchodilator.

Arterial blood gases ($PaCO_2$, pH, PaO_2) are often measured at the same time as spirometry to assess the degree of blood oxygenation. The use of the carbon monoxide diffusing capacity (D_{co}) can help determine whether the ventilatory change is due to poor diffusion or ventilation. This test involves the inspiration of a small amount of carbon monoxide (CO) that is then held for 10 seconds while the blood CO test is measured. A reduction is seen in emphysema, pulmonary edema, and pulmonary fibrosis and is normal in asthma and pneumonia. For a more complete discussion, see Chapter 5, Interpretation of Clinical Laboratory Results.

Purpose

The respiratory system is responsible for the exchange of carbon dioxide (CO_2) and oxygen (O_2). Together with the circulatory system, body tissues can exchange CO_2 and receive adequate O_2. Various disease processes alter the exchanges of these gases between the alveoli and the bloodstream. Pulmonary function tests are performed to provide an objective measurement of the respiratory system.

Pulmonary disorders are often classified as restrictive or obstructive. Typical airflow and volume curves can assist in classifying a disorder, as shown in Figure 6.4.

Findings
Normal
FEV_1/FVC, 75% to 80%.

Abnormal

- In the obstructive pattern that reflects limitations to airflow during expiration, the expiratory flow rate is decreased. In later stages of the disease, the FEV_1/FVC and $FEF_{25\%-75\%}$, are also reduced. The TLC may be normal or increased and the RV is elevated due to trapping of air during expiration. The ratio of RV/TLC is often increased.
- A restrictive pattern of lung disease that closely corresponds to impairment in inhalation (e.g., bronchitis, asthma) will present as a decrease in lung volumes, primarily TLC and VC.

Pharmacy Implications

- Bronchodilators should be administered before the procedure to evaluate the degree of reversibility.

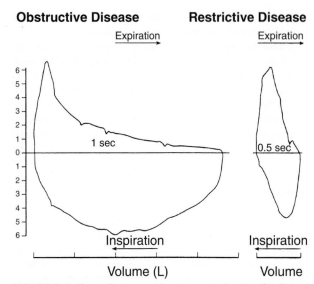

FIGURE 6.4 Flow/volume curve showing a typical pattern for obstructive and restrictive diseases. (Adapted from Young LY, Koda-Kimble MA. *Applied Therapeutics: The Clinical Use of Drugs.* 6th ed. Vancouver, WA: Applied Therapeutics, Inc.; 1995, with permission.)

- No preparation is needed before or after the procedure, unless bronchodilators are used.

Pulse Oximetry[7]

Description

A spectrophotometric sensor is placed (clipped) on the finger, toe, ear, or bridge of the nose. Light at two different wavelengths are passed through the pulsing capillary bed. The light sensed on the other side of the site is proportional to the amount of oxyhemoglobin present in the arterial capillary bed relative to the amount of hemoglobin available for binding with oxygen. The test may not be as sensitive as arterial blood gas because it does not take into consideration total hemoglobin, carboxyhemoglobin, or methemoglobin. Consequently, pulse oximetry may overestimate the oxygen content of the blood. Poor circulation to the tested area will produce an inaccurate result. Skin pigmentation can also affect the measurement. Advantages of the test include noninvasiveness, portability, and an immediate result.

Purpose

Measure the level of arterial oxygenation at rest, during exercise, when undergoing a surgical procedure, during bronchoscopy, when providing ventilator support, and when evaluating the need for and flow rate of supplemental oxygen therapy.

Findings
Normal
Oxyhemoglobin saturation $\geq$95%.

Abnormal
Oxyhemoglobin saturation <93%.

Pharmacy Implications
None.

Sweat Test[4,11,12,87]

Description
Pilocarpine solution is applied topically to the forearm. Three mA of current applied for 5 to 12 minutes cause the pilocarpine to penetrate into the skin, thus stimulating the sweat glands. The area is then washed with distilled water. Preweighted filter paper is placed over the area, covered with paraffin to prevent evaporation, and left in place for 30 to 60 minutes. The filter paper is removed, weighed, and diluted in distilled water. A chloridometer is used to determine the concentration of chloride. A minimum of 50 to 100 mg of sweat must be collected for an accurate result.

Purpose
Diagnose cystic fibrosis (CF) in conjunction with one or more other symptoms (i.e., documented exocrine pancreatic insufficiency, chronic obstructive airways disease, or a positive family history).

Findings
Normal
Chloride value in children is <40 mEq/L and in healthy adults may be $\leq$80 mEq/L.

Abnormal
- Chloride >60 mEq/L is diagnostic for CF if one or more of the above symptoms are present up to age of 20 years. Chloride levels of 40 to

60 mEq/L may be suggestive of CF in those patients who tend to have relatively normal pancreatic function.

- Other conditions that may cause elevations of sweat chloride include untreated adrenal insufficiency, ectodermal dysplasia, glucose-6-phosphatase deficiency, hypothyroidism, hypoparathyroidism, familial cholestasis, pancreatic insufficiency, mucopolysaccharidosis, fucosidosis, and malnutrition.

Pharmacy Implications
None.

Thoracentesis[4,7,61,88]

Description
Thoracentesis can be performed for diagnostic purposes (50- to 100-mL sample) or for therapeutic purposes (1,000- to 1,500-mL sample). It involves the insertion of a needle into the pleural space. The patient should be seated and leaning forward, with arms crossed in front and resting on an object such as a bedside table or back of a chair. If unable to sit and lean, the patient may lay supine in bed with the affected side elevated. A site at the fourth or fifth intercostal space along the posterior axillary line is generally selected. The intercostal space that is finally chosen should be one space below the highest level of pleural effusion. The skin is prepared with an antiseptic, and then the skin, subcutaneous tissues, and intercostal space are anesthetized with a local anesthetic. The type of equipment will dictate how a pleural fluid sample is collected. One option is to advance a large-gauge aspiration needle that has a catheter inside it. Once the pleura is penetrated and fluid can be aspirated, the inner catheter is advanced into the pleural space and the outer needle is withdrawn. The catheter is attached to a 50-mL syringe, and one or more 50-mL samples of fluid are collected. An alternate technique involves attaching the catheter to connecting tubing, which is in turn connected to glass vacuum bottles that can hold $\leq$1 L of fluid. As much as 1 L or more of fluid can be collected using this technique. Heparin must be added to glass tubes or bottles used for cytology samples.

Purpose
- Remove pleural fluid for culture, cell count, specific gravity, chemical analysis, and cytology for characterization as either a transudate (due to abnormalities of hydrostatic or osmotic pressure) or an exudate (due to increased vascular permeability or trauma). Transudate fluid can be

differentiated from exudate fluid by protein content, the ratio of pleural to serum protein, the LDH content, and the ratio of pleural LDH to serum content.

- Tap pleural effusions to make the patient more comfortable.
- Inject sclerosing agents such as antibiotics or cytotoxic agents into the pleural space to prevent further effusions.

Findings
Normal
No pleural fluid.

Abnormal
Blood in the pleural space (hemothorax) is generally a sign of a traumatic injury. Large volumes of pleural fluid due to inflammatory lung disease or neoplasms may be encountered. Cells may be found that will confirm the cell type of a malignancy. Infectious organisms may be found in the pleural fluid.

Pharmacy Implications
- Drugs such as bleomycin (60 U in 50 mL normal saline solution) or doxycycline (500 mg in 30 mL normal saline solution) may be instilled into the pleural space as sclerosing agents.
- Patients may require a sedative such as a benzodiazepine and/or an opiate analgesic 30 to 45 minutes before the procedure.
- A local anesthetic such as lidocaine should be available to anesthetize the skin and deeper tissues.
- Heparin, 5,000 to 10,000 units, must be added to containers used for cytology specimens.

Ventilation-Perfusion Scintigraphy (V-Q Scan)[4,89–91]
Description
The perfusion portion of the study requires aggregates of albumin labeled with technetium (Tc-99m) to be injected intravenously. These particles lodge in capillaries and precapillaries of the lung. The lungs are viewed with a gamma camera immediately after injection for perfusion. The ventilation portion of the study involves the breathing of air mixed with radioactive (xenon) gas. A nuclear scanner monitors the distribution of the gas in the lungs.

Purpose

Diagnose and monitor pulmonary embolism and to a lesser extent bronchiectasis, bronchial obstruction, and bronchopleural fistula. Ventilation by itself can be useful in quantifying ventilation status in patients with obstructive pulmonary disease. Ventilation-perfusion scans can also be used to assess pulmonary function in patients undergoing lung resection.

Findings
Normal

Normal perfusion and normal ventilation.

Abnormal

Normal areas of regional ventilation combined with segmental perfusion defects indicating pulmonary embolus.

Pharmacy Implications

Findings consistent with a diagnosis of pulmonary embolism will generally necessitate initiation of anticoagulants or fibrinolytic agents if no contraindications are present.

◼ Urology

Cystometrography (CMG)[4,7,11,12,92]
Description

A cystometrogram can be either simple or complex.

Simple

This version of the procedure can be completed at bedside. The patient is asked to empty his or her bladder. With a special device, the amount of urine, rate of flow of the urine, and time needed to void are all measured. Additional information gathered includes the time required to initiate voiding, the size of the urine stream, the continuity (single continuous stream versus interrupted stream), and the presence of urinary hesitancy, straining, or dribbling. A Foley or 14-French straight catheter is placed through the urethra into the bladder. Any remaining urine is measured. Thermal sensations are then measured by first instilling room temperature sterile water or sterile saline solution into the bladder followed by warm sterile water or saline. The patient is asked to report sensations such as discomfort, the need to void, flushing, sweating, or nausea. The fluid is then drained from the bladder and the catheter is connected to a cystometer used to measure pressure in the bladder. In small increments (approximately 50 mL) the bladder is filled with sterile water or normal saline. Alternatively, carbon dioxide gas can be used. The patient is instructed to report when the need to void is felt. Pressures and volumes are automatically recorded and plotted on a graph. When the patient's bladder becomes full, the patient must void and the pressures are recorded.

Complex

This procedure is usually performed in a urodynamics laboratory. A triple- or double-lumen Foley catheter is inserted into the bladder. Residual urine volume is measured in the same fashion as in simple cystometry. The patient is instructed to relax the bladder and avoid abdominal contractions. One lumen of the catheter is connected to an infusion pump and another lumen is connected to a microtip transducer or fluid-filled catheter/transducer setup. An anal probe is inserted, and intra-abdominal pressures are continuously recorded. The infusion pump instills room temperature sterile water into the bladder at a constant rate (slow, medium, or rapid). Simultaneously, bladder and anorectal pressures are recorded. The patient is instructed to report the first sensation of bladder fullness and the first strong urge to void. Filling of the bladder continues until the patient reports discomfort or an involuntary contraction is recorded. Alternatively, carbon dioxide gas can be substituted for fluid, but volume measurements may not be as accurate as fluid nor can gas be used for voiding cystometry. On some occasions the procedure continues by having the patient void as vigorously and as completely as possible. The catheter with the transducer measures bladder pressure during emptying. Variety of provocative tests can be performed to add to the diagnostic utility of the test. For example, cholinergic and anticholinergic drugs may be instilled into the bladder to assess its function by altering neurostimulation to the bladder.

Purpose

- Assess the integrity of neuroanatomic connections between the spinal cord and the bladder.
- Differentiate a flaccid bladder from an obstructed bladder.
- Document bladder muscle (detrusor) instability.
- Assess suspected bladder sensory or motor dysfunction.
- Evaluate postprostatectomy incontinence and possibly stress urinary incontinence.

Findings
Normal
Bladder wall activity demonstrates appropriate motor and sensory function with a normal bladder filling pattern.

Abnormal
Findings reveal either an uninhibited, reflex, or autonomous neurogenic bladder or a sensory or motor paralytic bladder. Each dysfunction is associated with specific neurons from the spinal cord.

Pharmacy Implications
All drugs that can affect bladder function or patient reporting (sedatives, cholinergic, anticholinergic, anxiolytics, or pain medications) should be withheld before the procedure.

Cystoscopy[4,11,12,82]
Description
Direct visual examination of the entire surface of the urethra, prostate (in men), and bladder by use of a rigid or flexible fiber-optic scope. This examination is also known as cystourethroscopy.

Purpose
- Evaluate patients with hematuria, voiding problems, history of bladder tumors, chronic urinary tract infections, or abnormalities revealed by other studies.
- Perform biopsies and extract stones from the lower ureters and from the bladder.
- Perform bladder irrigation and instill drugs.
- Perform resection and fulguration of bladder tumors and transurethral resection of the prostate.

Findings
Normal
Normal anatomy; absence of strictures, stones, and tumors.

Abnormal
Presence of stones, obstruction, stricture, tumors, signs of inflammation and infection, and sites of bleeding.

Pharmacy Implications
- Cystoscopy can be performed with a local anesthetic (e.g., lidocaine gel instilled into the urethra).
- A benzodiazepine such as diazepam, lorazepam, or midazolam may be administered before the procedure.
- Cystoscopy may be performed under general anesthesia, in which case an analgesic such as morphine and an anticholinergic such as atropine may be administered preoperatively.

Intravenous Pyelography (IVP)[4,7,93]
Description
IVP is visualization of the kidneys and collecting system both intrarenal (renal calices) and extrarenal (ureter and bladder) by administration of an iodine contrast dye through a vein, followed by radiographs taken at 5, 10, 15, and 20 minutes after the injection of dye. The term intravenous pyelography inaccurately describes the extent of this procedure because it limits the anatomy studied to the renal pelvis and calyceal system. The study examines anatomy beyond the scope of this term and should more appropriately be referred to as urography.

Purpose
- Detect congenital abnormalities, kidney obstruction, and changes in renal size.
- Determine the presence of renal masses (tumors, cysts, abscesses, or stones).
- Assess the extent of renal damage after traumatic injury.
- Evaluate a unilateral nonfunctioning kidney.

Findings
Normal
No anatomic defects, no obstructions, no masses, and a functional collecting system.

Abnormal
Presence of obstruction, masses, stones, signs of trauma to the kidney, or compromised function of the collecting system.

Pharmacy Implications
- Senna fruit concentrate (75 mL) should be administered at 4:00 PM the day before the procedure.

- The patient should have only clear liquids after the senna.
- The patient should not eat or drink on the morning of the examination.
- Patient allergies should be assessed due to the potential for hypersensitivity reactions to the contrast dye.
- IVPs should not be performed in patients whose creatinine clearance is <25 mL/minute.
- Adequate hydration (IV or PO) should be maintained after the procedure to prevent renal injury from the dye.

Kidneys, Ureters, Bladder (KUB)

See Gastroenterology, Abdominal Radiograph (KUB).

Retrograde Pyelography[4,7,16,94]

Description
A ureter is catheterized by means of a cystoscope, and dye is injected in a retrograde direction (opposite the normal flow of urine). A radiograph is taken to visualize the ureters.

Purpose
Retrograde pyelography allows visualization of the collecting structures of the kidney (renal pelvis) and ureters, which together compose the upper urinary tract. It is also used to confirm IVP findings.

Findings
Normal
Normal anatomy of the ureters and kidney pelvis.

Abnormal
Intrinsic disease of ureters and pelvis of the kidneys. Diseases of the ureters including obstructive tumors or stones.

Pharmacy Implications
See Urology, Cystoscopy.

Voiding Cystourethrography[4,7,95]

Description
Contrast medium is instilled into the bladder via a Foley catheter. Radiographs are taken as the bladder fills and when the patient voids.

Purpose
- Determine potential causes of chronic urinary tract infections (UTIs), bladder emptying dysfunction, and incontinence.
- Evaluate congenital abnormalities of the lower urinary tract.
- Evaluate and perform follow-up for patients with spinal cord injuries who have voiding difficulties.
- Evaluate prostatic hypertrophy in males and suspected strictures of the urethra.
- Evaluate a patient before renal transplantation.

Findings
Normal
Appropriate bladder and urethra structure and function.

Abnormal
Urethral strictures and diverticula, ureteroceles, prostatic enlargement, vesicoureteral reflux, or neurogenic bladder.

Pharmacy Implications
Iodine contrast medium may produce a hypersensitivity reaction. Special precautions should be taken in patients with known hypersensitivities to iodine compounds.

 Vascular

Arteriography/Venography[7,61]
Description
An iodine contrast dye is injected into an artery (arteriogram) or a vein (venogram) by means of a needle or catheter to outline and view a portion of the arterial or venous system. The arteries or veins are then observed using fluoroscopy and x-ray studies.

Purpose
Examine and evaluate the arterial or venous system of a particular organ or area of the body and evaluate the flow into or out of that area. This allows for the detection of lesions and abnormalities of flow. It can also allow for surgical correction if possible. Fluoroscopy is used to guide the catheter to the desired location for dye administration.

Findings
Normal
No flow abnormalities.

Abnormal
Presence of clots, strictures, obstructions, lesions, incompetent valves, aneurysms, embolism, thrombosis, fistulas, atherosclerosis, trauma, vasculitis, or congenital abnormalities.

Pharmacy Implications
- Iodine contrast dye may produce hypersensitivity reactions or anaphylaxis. Special precautions should be taken in patients with known hypersensitivities to iodine compounds.
- When necessary, diphenhydramine, ranitidine, and prednisone may be started ≥ 12 hours before the procedure to prevent or reduce the severity of the hypersensitivity reaction.
- A local anesthetic is used to anesthetize the area of the puncture site.
- Adequate IV hydration should be provided to reduce the risk of renal injury from the contrast media.

Doppler Studies[4,7,11,12,68,96]
Description
Doppler Ultrasound[11,12]
Doppler ultrasound is used as a blood flow detector that is sensitive to frequency shifts reflected from moving blood cells. The Doppler transducer is placed over the area to be evaluated (e.g., peripheral artery, peripheral vein, or the common carotid, internal carotid, and external carotid). The probe (transducer) directs high-frequency sound waves through tissue and hits RBCs in the bloodstream. The frequency of sound waves changes in proportion to the flow velocity of RBCs. The transducer then amplifies the sound waves, which permits direct listening. A graphic recording of the blood flow can be made from the sound waves.

Systolic pressures using compression maneuvers are also measured. To evaluate arterial disease in the lower extremities, a pressure cuff is placed around the calf and inflated. A systolic pressure over the dorsalis pedis and posterior tibial arteries is obtained, and waveforms are recorded. The cuff is then wrapped around the thigh, and the procedure is repeated over the popliteal artery. The entire process allows segmental evaluation of the arterial tree in the lower extremities to aid in localizing the area of disease. An evaluation of the upper extremities can be performed in a similar fashion using forearm and upper arm compression taking ulnar, radial, and brachial artery readings. The transducer is placed near the cuff. The pressure in the cuff is slowly released. When a swishing noise is heard, the pressure is recorded as the systolic blood pressure.

The pressures and waveforms from the ankle and brachial arteries can be compared in the tested individual, and an ankle-arm pressure index is calculated. Pulse volume recording (PVRs) can be done concurrently to quantitate blood volume or flow in an extremity.

Duplex Doppler Ultrasound[7,11,12]

The technique is the same as standard Doppler ultrasound. However, with the duplex method, the sound waves can be used to create an image that is recorded on x-ray film.

Colorflow Doppler Ultrasound[7,11,12]

Colorflow Doppler enhances standard Doppler ultrasound by providing flow data from the studied vessel. Various colors displayed on a screen represent different velocities and direction of blood flow.

Purpose

Doppler studies allow the detection of arterial or venous obstruction or thrombi. They are also used to monitor patients who have had reconstructive or peripheral artery bypass surgery.

Findings
Normal

Veins will make a swishing sound, and there is no evidence of narrowing. Flow should be spontaneous and phasic with respiration (venous). For arteries, blood pressure is normal and has a multiphasic signal with prominent systolic sound and one or more diastolic sounds. Signals should fluctuate with respiration, not heart beat. The ankle-arm pressure index (API), the ratio between ankle systolic pressure and brachial systolic pressure, is >1. Proximal thigh pressure is greater than arm pressure by 20 to 30 mm Hg. There is increased flow velocity with compression of vessels.

Abnormal

- Evidence of arterial or venous occlusion or blood clots.
- API is <1 (see Table 6-7 for severity ranking). Arm pressure is changed. Diminished or absent blood flow velocity signal. Calcified and noncompressible vessels produce unreliable measurements.

Table 6.7 RELATIONSHIP OF ANKLE-ARM PRESSURE INDEX (API) AND DISEASE SEVERITY

API	Severity of Disease
1–0.7	Mild ischemia
0.75–0.5	Claudication
0.5–0.25	Pain at rest
0.25–0	Pregangrene

Pharmacy Implications
None.

Impedance Plethysmography (Occlusive Cuff)[4,97]

Description
Plethysmography is a noninvasive test that detects blood volume changes in the leg. A pneumatic cuff is placed around the midthigh and inflated to occlude venous return. Occlusion is maintained for a minimum of 45 seconds, and the cuff is then rapidly deflated. Electrodes placed around the calf detect changes in electrical resistance (impedance) due to alteration in blood volume distal to the cuff. The impedance changes occurring during inflation and deflation of the cuff are recorded on an ECG paper strip. The changes in impedance during cuff inflation and deflation are compared against a discriminant line that separates the normal from the abnormal graph.

Purpose
Detect thrombi that produce obstruction to venous outflow. The test is sensitive and specific for occlusive thrombosis of the popliteal, femoral, or iliac veins. The test is relatively insensitive to calf vein thrombosis. Diagnostic accuracy nears 90%. The test is unable to distinguish between thrombosis and nonthrombotic obstruction.

Findings
Normal
The graph for the patient will fall above the discriminant line (i.e., the test will be negative for proximal vein thrombi). However, false-negative

results can occur in patients with extensive collateral circulation, which allows for adequate venous outflow, and in patients in whom proximal vein thrombosis is not occlusive.

Abnormal

The graph will fall below the discriminant line (i.e., positive for proximal vein thrombosis). False-positive results can occur when nonthrombotic occlusion (mechanical) is present and when arterial inflow disease limits the amount of venous filling, decreasing venous return.

Pharmacy Implications

None.

Lymphangiography (Lymphography)[8,11,12,98]

Description

Lymphography is the radiographic examination of the lymphatic system after radioactive material is injected into a lymphatic vessel in each foot (alternately, the hand, mastoid area, or spermatic cord can be used). Fluoroscopy is used to monitor the spread of the contrast media through the lymphatic system of the legs, groin, and the back of the abdominal cavity. Radiographs are taken of the legs, pelvis, abdomen, and chest. Twenty-four hours later, additional radiographs are taken to compare and evaluate contrast distribution.

Purpose

- Detect obstruction, disease, or neoplasm in the lymphatic system.
- Stage lymphoma.
- Distinguish between primary and secondary lymph edema.
- Evaluate the need for surgical treatment.
- Assess the results of previous chemotherapy or radiation therapy.

Findings
Normal

Homogeneous and complete filling of the lymphatic system with the radioactive contrast material on the initial films.

Abnormal

Presence of enlarged, foamy-looking nodes indicate lymphoma. Filling defects or lack of opacification of vessels indicate metastatic involvement of nodes by neoplasm. The number of nodes, the unilateral versus bilateral location of the nodes, and the extent of extranodal involvement determine staging of neoplastic disease.

Pharmacy Implications
The patient should be evaluated for hypersensitivity to iodine or other contrast media.

Magnetic Resonance Angiography (MRA)[7,99]
Description
MRA uses the same hardware technology as standard MRI (see Magnetic Resonance Imaging [MRI]). Large magnets and radio waves are used to create an image of the vascular anatomy being investigated. This non-invasive test can produce information about the vascular system (head and neck, abdomen, chest, and peripheral) comparable to the information provided by standard angiography. Although MRA can generally be performed without the use of a contrast agent, gadolinium may need to be administered to increase the accuracy of the test. The patient must remain very still during MRA and is placed in a narrow tube to perform the test. Patients who are unable to lie still or who are claustrophobic may require sedation. Certain implanted metallic objects are absolute or relative contraindications for performing MRA.

Purpose
Diagnose vascular abnormalities such as vascular malformations, aneurysms, vertebrovascular and carotid atherosclerosis, thrombosis, and evidence of peripheral vascular disease.

Findings
Normal
Absence of atherosclerosis, aneurysm, AV malformation, or occlusive disease.

Abnormal
Presence of vascular malformation, occlusive vascular disease, aneurysm, and atherosclerosis.

Pharmacy Implications
- Use of a sedating benzodiazepine such as midazolam, lorazepam, or diazepam may be required to keep the patient still and to manage claustrophobia.

- Patients receiving gadolinium should be monitored for hypersensitivity reactions.

References

1. Kline TS, ed. *Handbook of Fine Needle Aspiration Biopsy Cytology*. 2nd ed. New York, NY: Churchill Livingstone; 1988:9–16.

2. Teplick SK, Haskin PK. Imaging modalities. In: Kline TS, ed. *Handbook of Fine Needle Aspiration Biopsy Cytology*. 2nd ed. New York, NY: Churchill Livingstone; 1988:17–48.

3. Michaels D, ed. Procedures requiring the use of contrast media. In: *Diagnostic Procedures: The Patient and the Health Care Team*. New York, NY: John Wiley and Sons; 1983:274–279.

4. Ford RD, ed. *Diagnostic Tests Handbook*. Springhouse, PA: Springhouse Corporation; 1987.

5. Taub WH. Relative strengths and limitations of diagnostic imaging studies. In: Straub WH, ed. *Manual of Diagnostic Imaging*. Boston, MA: Little, Brown and Company; 1989:13–15.

6. Grossman ZD, et al., eds. *The Clinicians Guide to Diagnostic Imaging Cost Effective Pathways*. 2nd ed. New York, NY: Raven Press; 1987.

7. Golish JA, ed. *Diagnostic Procedures Handbook*. Hudson (Cleveland), OH: Lexi-Comp, Inc.; 1994. Available at www.healthgate.com/dph/html. Accessed February 27, 2000.

8. Hamilton HK, Cahill M, eds. *Diagnostics*. Springhouse, PA: Springhouse Corporation; 1986.

9. Edelman RR et al. Basic principles of magnetic resonance imaging. In: Edelman RR, Hesselink JR, eds. *Clinical Magnetic Resonance Imaging*. Philadelphia, PA: WB Saunders; 1990:3–38.

10. Lufkin RB. *The MRI Manual*. Chicago, IL: Yearbook Medical Publishers; 1990:21–41.

11. Adam.com Encyclopedia. Available at www.adam.com/dir/Tests/Tests.htm. Accessed March 6, 2000.

12. Zaret BL, ed. *The Yale University School of Medicine Patient's Guide to Medical Tests*. Boston, MA: Houghton Mifflin; 1997. Available at health.excite.com/yale_books_a_to_z/asset/yale_books_a_to_z/a_to_z/A. Accessed March 6, 2000.

13. Wellness Web. Magnetic Resonance Imaging. Available at www.wellweb.com/diagnost/arnief/mri.htm. Accessed March 6, 2000.

14. Rodriguez P. *MRI Indications for the Referring Physician*. Garden City, KS: Aurora Publishing Company; 1995. Available at www.gcnet.com/maven/aurora/mri/mra.html. Accessed March 6, 2000.

15. Hagen–Ansert SL. *Textbook of Diagnostic Ultrasonography*. 3rd ed. St. Louis, MO: Mosby; 1989: 594–624.

16. Fischbach FT. *A Manual of Laboratory Diagnostic Tests*. 4th ed. Philadelphia, PA: JB Lippincott; 1992.

17. Webb DR. Diagnostic methods in allergy. In: Altman LC, ed. *Clinical Allergy and Immunology*. Boston, MA: GK Hall Medical Publishers; 1984:149–168.

18. Timmis A. *Essentials of Cardiology*. Oxford, UK: Blackwell Scientific Publications; 1988:40–45.

19. Gazes PC. *Clinical Cardiology*. 3rd ed. Philadelphia, PA: Lea & Febiger; 1990.

20. Conover MB. *Understanding Electrocardiography*. 3rd ed. St. Louis, MO: Mosby; 1980.

21. DaCunha JP, ed. *Diagnostics: Patient Preparation Interpretation Sources of Error, Post Test Care*. 2nd ed. Springhouse, PA: Springhouse; 1986:947–948.

22. Postgraduate Medicine: maximizing the exercise stress test. www.postgradmed. com/issues/1999/05_01_99/driggers.htm. Accessed January 15, 2008.

23. Zipe DP, Libby P, Bonow RO, et al., eds. *Branunwald's Heart Disease: A Textbook of Cardiovascular Medicine*. 7th ed. Philadelphia, PA: Elsevier Saunders; 2005:153–186.

24. Shors S, Cotts WG, Pavlovic-Surjancev B, et al. Non-invasive cardiac evaluation in heart failure patients using magnetic resonance imaging: a feasibility study. *Heart Fail Rev*. 2005;10(4):265–273.

25. Myerson SG, Bellenger NG, Pennell DJ. Assessment of left ventricular mass by cardiovascular magnetic resonance. *Hypertension*. 2002;39:750–755.

26. Michaels D, Willis K. Noninvasive cardiovascular procedures. In: Michaels D, ed. *Diagnostic Procedures: The Patient and The Health Care Team*. New York, NY: John Wiley & Sons; 1983:441–442.

27. Alpert JS, Rippe JM, eds. *Manual of Cardiovascular Diagnosis and Therapy*. 2nd ed. Boston, MA: Little, Brown and Company; 1985:21.

28. Tilkian AG, Daily EK. Endomyocardial biopsy. In: *Cardiovascular Procedures: Diagnostic Techniques and Therapeutic Procedures*. St. Louis, MO: Mosby; 1986:180–203.

29. Howard PA. Intravenous dipyridamole: use in thallous chloride TL 201 stress imaging. *Ann Pharmacother*. 1991;25:1085–1091.

30. Anonymous. Persantine IV. *Hosp Pharm*. 1991;26:356, 361–366.

31. Carpenter PC. Diagnosis of adrenocortical disease. In: Mendelsohn G, ed. *Diagnosis and Pathology of Endocrine Diseases*. Philadelphia, PA: JB Lippincott; 1988:179–197.

32. Stern N, Griffon D. Protocols for stimulation and suppression tests commonly used in clinical endocrinology. In: Lavin N, ed. *Manual of Endocrinology and Metabolism*. 1st ed. Boston, MA: Little, Brown and Company; 1986:703–720.

33. Merkle WA. Secretion and metabolism of the corticosteroids and adrenal function and testing. In: Degroot LJ, ed. *Endocrinology*. Philadelphia, PA: WB Saunders; 1989:2;1610–1632.

34. Fitzgerald PA. Pituitary disorders. In: Fitzgerald PA, ed. *Handbook of Clinical Endocrinology*. Greenbrae, CA: Jones Medical Publications; 1986:1–63, 450.

35. Carpenter PC. Cushing's syndrome: update of diagnosis and management. *Mayo Clin Proc*. 1986;61:49–58.

36. Larenzi M. Diabetes mellitus. In: Fitzgerald PA, ed. *Handbook of Clinical Endocrinology*. Greenbrae, CA: Jones Medical Publications; 1986:337–406.

37. Stern N, Griffin D. Protocols for stimulation and suppression tests commonly used in clinical endocrinology. In: Lavin N, ed. *Manual of Endocrinology and Metabolism*. Boston: Little, Brown and Company; 1986:703–719.

38. American Diabetes Association. Standards of Medical Care in Diabetes—2008. Diabetes care. 2008;31(suppl 1):S12–54.

39. Chemistry studies. In: Fischbach F, ed. *A Manual of Laboratory & Diagnostic Tests*. Crawfordsville: Lippincott Williams & Wilkins; 2000:375–380.

40. Drugs Affecting Laboratory Test Values (Appendix J). In: Fischbach F, ed. *A Manual of Laboratory & Diagnostic Tests*. Crawfordsville: Lippincott Williams & Wilkins; 2000:1214–1215.

41. Singer PA. Thyroid function tests and effects of drugs on thyroid function. In: *Manual of Endocrinology and Metabolism*. 1st ed. Boston, MA: Little, Brown and Company; 1986:341–354.

42. Safrit HF. Thyroid disorders. In: Fitzgerald PA, ed. *Handbook of Clinical Endocrinology*. Greenbrae, CA: Jones Medical Publications; 1986:122–169.

43. Field S. The acute abdomen—the plain radiograph. In: Grainger RG, Allison DJ, eds. *Diagnostic Radiology: An Anglo-American Textbook of Imaging*. Edinburgh, Scotland: Churchill Livingstone; 1986;2:719–742.

44. Rice RP. The plain film of the abdomen. In: Taveras JM, Ferrucci JT, eds. *Radiology: Diagnosis-Imaging-Intervention*. Philadelphia, PA: JB Lippincott; 1990:4;1–21.

45. Bartram CI. The large bowel. In: Grainger RG, Allison DJ, eds. *Diagnostic Radiology: An Anglo-American Textbook of Imaging*. Edinburgh, Scotland: Churchill Livingstone; 1986:2;859–895.

46. Kressel HY, Laufer I. Double contrast examination of the gastrointestinal tract. In: Taveras JM, Ferrucci JT, eds. *Radiology: Diagnosis-Imaging-Intervention*. Philadelphia, PA: JB Lippincott Co; 1990:4;1–21.

47. Nolan DJ. The small intestine. In: Grainger RG, Allison DJ, eds. Diagnostic Radiology: An Anglo-American Textbook of Imaging. Edinburgh: Churchill Livingstone; 1986:2;833–58.

48. Maglinte DDT. The small bowel: anatomy and examination techniques. In: Taveras JM, Ferrucci JT, eds. Radiology: Diagnosis-Imaging-Intervention. Philadelphia, PA: JB Lippincott; 1990:4;1–7.

49. Virtual Hospital: Iowa Health Book: Diagnostic Radiology: Enteroclysis. University of Iowa Health Care. Available at: http://www.vh.org/Patients/IHB/Rad/DRad/Enteroclysis.html. Accessed March 6, 2000.

50. Levinson SC. Percutaneous transhepatic cholangiography. In: Drossman DA, ed. Manual of Gastroenterologic Procedures. 2nd ed. New York, NY: Raven Press; 1987:162–168.

51. Bowley NB. The biliary tract. In: Grainger RG, Allison DJ, eds. Diagnostic Radiology: An Anglo-American Textbook of Imaging. Edinburgh: Churchill Livingstone; 1986:2;955–987.

52. Simeone JF. The biliary ducts: anatomy and examination technique. In: Taveras JM, Ferrucci JT, eds. Radiology: Diagnosis-Imaging-Intervention. Philadelphia, PA: JB Lippincott; 1990:4;1–11.

53. Drossman DA. Colonoscopy. In: Drossman, DA, ed. Manual of Gastroenterologic Procedures. 2nd ed. New York, NY: Raven Press; 1987:110–118.

54. Bozynski EM. Endoscopic retrograde cholangiopancreatography. In: Drossman DA, ed. Manual of Gastroenterologic Procedures. 2nd ed. New York: Raven Press; 1987:103–109.

55. Shapiro HA. Diagnostic and Therapeutic Procedures II. Endoscopic Retrograde Cholangiopancreatography (ERCP). Manchester, MA: American Society for Gastrointestinal Endoscopy. Available at: http://www.asge.org/resources/manual/185.html. Accessed March 6, 2000.

56. Sartar RB. Upper gastrointestinal endoscopy. In: Drossman DA, ed. Manual of Gastroenterologic Procedures. 2nd ed. New York, NY: Raven Press; 1987: 90–97.

57. Powell DW. Anoscopy and rigid sigmoidoscopy. In: Drossman DA, ed. Manual of Gastroenterologic Procedures. 2nd ed. New York, NY: Raven Press; 1987:125–132.

58. Sandler RS. Flexible sigmoidoscopy. In: Drossman DA, ed. Manual of Gastroenterologic Procedures. 2nd ed. New York, NY: Raven Press; 1987:119–124.

59. Drane WE. Radionuclide imaging of the liver, biliary system, and gastrointestinal tract. In: Chobanian SJ, Van Ness MM, eds. Manual of Clinical Problems in Gastroenterology. Boston, MA: Little, Brown, and Company; 1988:290–296.

60. Tao LC, Kline TS. Liver. In: Kline TS, ed. Handbook of Fine Needle Aspiration Biopsy Cytology. 2nd. ed. New York, NY: Churchill Livingstone; 1988:343–363.

61. Corbett JV. Diagnostic Procedures in Nursing Practice. Norwalk, CT: Appleton and Lange; 1987.

62. Weinstein WM, Hill TA. Gastrointestinal mucosal biopsy. In: Berk JE, ed. Gastroenterology. 4th ed. Philadelphia, PA: WB Saunders; 1985:1;626–644.

63. Paulfrey ME. Histology: breast biopsy. In: Hamilton HK, Cahill M, eds. Diagnostics. Springhouse, PA: Springhouse Corporation; 1986:467–473.

64. American Cancer Society Rrecommendations for Early Breast Cancer Detection. http://www.cancer.org/docroot/PED/content/PED_2_3X_ACS_Cancer_Detection_Guidelines_36.asp?sitearea=PED. Accessed January 15, 2008.

65. Larson E. Clinical Microbiology and Infection Control. Boston, MA: Blackwell Scientific Publications; 1984: 527–577.

66. Adams RD, Victor M. Principles of Neurology. 3rd ed. New York, NY: McGraw-Hill; 1985:27–8.

67. Pryse-Phillips W, Murray TJ. Essential Neurology. 3rd ed. New York, NY: Medical Examination Publishing Co.; 1986:103–104.

68. Berkow R, ed. The Merck Manual of Diagnosis and Therapy. 14th ed. Rahway, NJ: Merck Sharp & Dohme Research Laboratories; 1982.

69. Coniglio AA, Garnett WR. Status epilepticus. In: Dipiro JT et al, eds. Pharmacotherapy: A Pathophysiologic Approach. New York, NY: Elsevier Science Publishing Company; 1989:599–610.

70. Vander AJ et al., eds. Human Physiology: The Mechanisms of Body Function. 4th ed. New York, NY: McGraw-Hill; 1985:690–691.

71. Rotschafer JC, Humphrey ZZ, Steinberg I. Central nervous system infection. In: Dipiro JT et al., eds. Pharmacotherapy: A Pathophysiologic Approach. New York, NY: Elsevier Science Publishing Co; 1989:1074–1088.

72. Virtual Hospital: Iowa Health Book: Diagnostic Radiology: Myelogram. University of Iowa Health Care. Available at: http://www.vh.org/Patients/IHB/Rad/Drad/Myelogram.html. Accessed March 6, 2000.

73. Kakulas BA, Adams RD, eds. Diseases of Muscle. Philadelphia, PA: Harper and Row; 1985:771–786.

74. Anderson JR. Atlas of Skeletal Muscle Pathology. Lancaster: MTP Press Limited; 1985:11–17.

75. Connolly ES. Techniques of diagnostic nerve and muscle biopsies. In: Wilkins RA, ed. Neurosurgery. New York: McGraw-Hill; 1985:2;1907–1908.

76. Vaughn D, Asbury T. General Ophthalmology. 10th ed. Los Altos, CA: Lange Medical Publications; 1983.

77. Peters HB, Bartlett JD. Optical fundus in diagnosis. In: Physifax: Physicians Pocket Compendium of Normal Values, Tests, Diagnostic Criteria, Drug Therapy, and Other Useful Data. Montclair: Medication International, Ltd; 1984:97–120.

78. Lesar TS. Drug-induced ear and eye toxicity. In: DiPiro JT et al. eds. Pharmacotherapy: A Pathophysiologic Approach. New York, NY: Elsevier; 1989:919–931.

79. Phillips CI. Basic Clinical Ophthalmology. London: Pitman Publishing; 1984:55–86.

80. Stoker DJ. Arthrography. In: Harris NH, ed. Postgraduate Textbook of Clinical Orthopaedics. Bristol: Wright-PSG; 1983:882–890.

81. Osteoporosis Education System. Bone mass measurement techniques (module 5). Whitehouse Station, NJ: Merck & Co., Inc. Available at: http://www.merck.com/pro/osteoporosis/inde113.htm. Accessed March 6, 2000.

82. Karmody CS. Textbook of Otolaryngology. Philadelphia, PA: Lea & Febiger; 1983.

83. Barton RP. Endoscopy. In: Keer Ag, Stell PM, eds. Scott-Brown's Otolaryngology: Laryngology. 5th ed. London: Butterworth's; 1987:31–41.

84. Ebadort AM. Bronchoscopy. In: Michaels D, ed. Diagnostic Procedures: The Patient and the Health Care Team. New York, NY: John Wiley and Sons; 1983:493–506.

85. Menendez R, Kelly HW. Pulmonary-function testing in the evaluation of bronchodilator agents. Clin Pharm. 1983;2:120–128.

86. Kelly HW. Asthma. In: Koda-Kimble MA, Young LY eds. Applied Therapeutics: The Clinical Use of Drugs. 5th Ed. Vancouver: Applied Therapeutics; 1992:15-1–4.

87. Behrman RE, Vaughn VC. Nelson Textbook of Pediatrics. 13th ed. Philadelphia, PA: WB Saunders; 1987:928–929.

88. Lim RC. Surgical diagnosis and therapeutic procedures. In: Dunphy JE, Way LW, eds. Current Surgical Diagnosis and Treatment. Los Altos, CA: Lange Medical Publications; 1981:1085–1097.

89. Sullivan D. Radionuclide imaging in lung disease. In: Putman C ed. Pulmonary Diagnosis: Imaging and Other Techniques. New York, NY: Prentice-Hall; 1981:67–78.

90. Bell WR, Simon TL. Current status of pulmonary thromboembolic disease: pathophysiology, diagnosis, prevention, and treatment. Am Heart J. 1982;103:239–262.

91. Hull DR et al. Pulmonary angiography, ventilation lung scanning, and venography for clinically suspected pulmonary embolism with abnormal perfusion lung scan. Ann Intern Med. 1983;98:891–899.

92. Blavis JG. Cystometry. In: deVere RW, Palmer JM, eds. New Techniques in Urology. New York, NY: Futura Publishing Corporation; 1987:193–219.

93. Friedenberg RM. Excretory urography in the adult. In: Pollack HM, ed. Clinical Urography. Philadelphia, PA: WB Saunders; 1990:101–243.

94. Imray TJ, Lieberman RP. Retrograde pyelography. In: Pollack HM, ed. Clinical Urography. Philadelphia, PA: WB Saunders; 1990:244–255.

95. Hertz M. Cystourethrography. In: Pollack HM, ed. Clinical Urography. Philadelphia, PA: WB Saunders; 1990:256–295.

96. Bastarche MM et al. Assessing peripheral vascular disease: noninvasive testing. AJN. 1983;85:1552–1556.

97. Hirsch J. Natural history and diagnosis of venous thrombosis. Paper presented at a symposium sponsored by the Page and William Black Post-Graduate School of Medicine of the Mount Sinai School of Medicine, New York, New York, October 30, 1981.

98. Bryan GT. Diagnostic Radiography: A Concise Practical Manual. 4th ed. Edinburgh: Churchill Livingstone; 1987:289–296.

99. Smith PL. Magnetic Resonance Angiography (MRA). Midsouth Imaging and Therapeutic, P.A. Memphis, TN. Available at: http://www.msit.com/ra-mra.htm. Accessed October 30, 2000.

7 Home Test Kits and Monitoring Devices

Ty Vo and Devon Flynn

Home self-test kits and monitoring devices are valuable tools and have become increasingly easier to use. The kits and devices provide patients with an opportunity to participate actively in early disease detection and monitoring. Pharmacists play an essential role in helping patients select the appropriate product, counseling them on appropriate use, interpreting results, and identifying limitations. Pharmacists should help patients make educated choices regarding product selection for home testing and monitoring. Product selection should be guided by accuracy, reliability, specificity, and sensitivity as well as professional judgment.

To achieve an appropriate rate of accuracy and to ensure safety and efficacy, the pharmacist should assess and counsel the patient on the following points:

1. General questions to consider in patient assessment include the following:[1]
   a. What is the purpose of using this product?
   b. What chronic medical conditions does the patient have?
   c. What prescription or nonprescription medications or herbal products is the patient taking?
   d. What limitations does the patient have including visual (i.e., poor vision, difficulty with color vision) or physical (i.e., limited dexterity, arthritis, peripheral neuropathies) that may affect the use of the product?
   e. What other health care practitioners have been consulted?
2. These products are for self-testing, not self-diagnosing. As a general principle, the patient should be advised to report positive results to the primary care clinician immediately and negative results should be

questioned if the patient is experiencing symptoms of a suspected condition. Some test results need to be reported whether they are positive or negative because they convey useful information.
3. A family member, friend, or caregiver may need to assist if it is determined that the patient is unable to perform and interpret the test results.

The following factors should be considered when selecting a product:

- Complexity of the test procedure.
- Ease of reading the results.
- Presence of a control to determine if the test is functioning appropriately.
- Cost.

The patient should be instructed on the following guidelines:[2]

- Check the test kit expiration date and follow the manufacturer's instructions for storage.
- Read the instructions entirely before attempting to perform a test. Note the time of day the test is to be conducted, necessary equipment, and length of time required.
- Use an accurate timing device that measures seconds if needed.
- Follow directions exactly and in sequence. A tollfree number is often available for assistance.

This chapter focuses on those products most commonly available: pregnancy tests, ovulation tests, thermometers, fecal occult blood tests, blood pressure monitors, blood glucose (diabetes) monitoring including ketones, cholesterol tests, human immunodeficiency virus (HIV) tests, illicit drug tests, and urinary tract infection tests. The products listed in this chapter are representative but not exhaustive of those currently available.

Pregnancy Tests[3,4]

Additional Questions to Ask the Patient

1. Have you used a pregnancy test?
   a. If so, which one did you use?
   b. Did you have difficulty with it?
2. How late is your menstrual period?

Home pregnancy tests are designed to detect the presence of human chorionic gonadotropic (hCG) hormone in the urine. This is detectable in the urine within 1 to 2 weeks after fertilization. The tests are indicated for use as early as the first day of a missed menstrual period but are most

Table 7.1 SELECTED PREGNANCY TESTS

Product Name	Sensitivity (mIU/mL)	Comments
First Response Early Result	25	Uses dipsticks
Clear Choice	25	Uses cup
Answer Early Result Quick & Simple	25	Uses dipsticks; no wick protection; possibly messy to use
e.p.t	40	Uses dipsticks; e.p.t. Certainty has digital display
Fact Plus Select	40	Uses dipsticks
ClearBlue Easy	50	Uses dipsticks; Clearblue Easy Digital displays "pregnant" or "not pregnant"

accurate by waiting ≥1 week after the first day of the missed period. The most current products available use monoclonal or polyclonal antibodies specific for detecting hCG hormone. Blood tests can detect a pregnancy earlier, usually 6 to 8 days after ovulation. They are useful for the health care provider in tracking certain problems of early pregnancy. However, urine pregnancy tests are the most common type and claim to have 99% accuracy. Most tests have sensitivity limits of 25 to 50 mIU/mL. Table 7.1 lists selected home pregnancy tests.

Considerations

- The numerous pregnancy tests, differ in reaction times and hCG sensitivity.
- Most pregnancy tests are one-step procedures.
- Some test have clear test sticks that allow the woman to see the reaction occuring as a check that sufficient urine was collected. Other tests include two devices, which can be helpful if a negative test is obtained first.
- The newest tests are digital and display the results as "pregnant" or "not pregnant" instead of colored lines, which eliminates the need to interpret the results, especially for patients with a color vision defect.
- False-positive results can occur if:
  - The patient has had a birth or miscarriage within the previous 8 weeks. This is due to residual levels of hCG hormone present in the body.
  - The patient is taking medications such as menotropins (Pergonal) injection and chroionic gonadotropin (Profasi) injection.

 ‣ Unreliable results may occur in patients with ovarian cysts or an ectopic pregnancy.
- False-negative results may occur if tests are performed on or before the first day of a missed period. This is a concern because of the delay in prenatal care and appropriate behavior modification.

Patient Education

- The most accurate results will be obtained by waiting ≥ 1 week after the first day of a missed period.
- Use the first morning urine because hCG hormone is most concentrated then.
- If testing at other times of the day, avoid fluid intake for 4 to 6 hours before urine collection to avoid dilution of the urine sample.
- Use the urine collection device provided in the kit.
- Apply urine to the testing device using one of the methods provided in package instructions:
  ‣ Hold the test stick in the urine stream for the designated time.
  ‣ Urinate into the testing well of the test cassette.
  ‣ Collect urine in a collection cup and keep the strip or use a dropper to apply the urine.
- After the urine is applied, lay the testing device on a flat surface. Wait for the recommended time of 1 to 5 minutes before reading results. Waiting the maximum allowed time may improve the sensitivity of the test.
- If the test result is negative, verify that the test was performed correctly and test again in 1 week if menstruation has not started. If the second test is negative and menstruation has not begun, a health care provider should be contacted.

◼ Ovulation Prediction Tests[3,5,6]

Additional Questions to Ask the Patient

1. Have you used an ovulation prediction test?
   a. If so, which one did you use?
   b. Did you have difficulty with it?
2. Have you consulted your primary care provider or a fertility specialist?
3. Are your menstrual cycles regular?

Ovulation prediction tests (Table 7.2) measure levels of luteinizing hormone (LH) in the urine. Current products available on the market

Table 7.2 SELECTED OVULATION PREDICTION TESTS AND DEVICES

Product Name	Reaction Time	Product Features
ClearBlue Easy Ovulation Test	3 min	5-Day kit; uses urine test sticks; predicts ovulation within 24–36 h; most sensitive product in the Consumer Reports test
ClearBlue Easy Fertility Monitor	3 min	Reusable monitor; uses urine test sticks; predicts 1- to 5-day window of peak fertility
Answer 1-Step Ovulation	5 min	5-Day kit; uses urine test sticks; predicts ovulation within 24–36 h
Conceive Ovulation Test	3 min	5-Day kit; uses urine test cassette; predicts ovulation within 24–40 h
First Response 1-Step Ovulation Predictor Test	5 min	5-Day kit; uses urine test sticks; predicts ovulation within 24–36 h
OvuQuick One Step	4 min	6-Day or 9-day kit; uses urine test pads; predicts ovulation within 24–40 h
OvaCue Fertility Monitor	3 s	Monitor; reusable saliva electrolyte sensor and optional vaginal sensor; predicts ovulation within 5–7 days; tracks cycle data; can upload results to free software for graphing
Mini-Microscope Saliva Ovulation Tester	10–15 min	Reusable microscope; lipstick size; uses saliva; predicts ovulation within 5–7 days
Ovulook Ovulation Tester	5–20 min	Reusable microscope; uses saliva; round compact-disk size device with 12 tracking disks; 31 days of samples per disk; battery-operated light
BD Basal Thermometer	1 min	Digital thermometer; auto memory for last reading; continuous beep to indicate it is working; signals when done; large lighted display
Geratherm Basal Thermometer	3 min	Mercuryfree thermometer; magnified case for easier reading

Reprinted with permission from Rosenthal WM, Briggs GC. Home testing and monitoring devices. In: Berardi RR, Kroon LA, McDermott JH, et al., eds. *Handbook of Nonprescription Drugs: An Interactive Approach to Self-Care.* 15th ed. Washington, DC: American Pharmacists Association; 2006:1052.

include basal thermometers, urine tests, and saliva tests. Each detection method has a different mechanism of action and method of use.

Urinary Hormone Tests

Urinary hormone tests use monoclonal antibodies specific to the detection of the surge of LH. The LH surge is noted by changes in the color or color intensity directly proportional to the LH concentration in the urine sample.

Considerations

- Fertility medications, polycystic ovary syndrome, menopause, and pregnancy can cause false-positive results for ovulation.
- Patients receiving clomiphene should not test until the second day after drug therapy ends when the true LH surge can be detected.
- Recent pregnancy, discontinuation of oral contraceptives, or breast-feeding will delay ovulation for one or two cycles. Start testing after two natural menstrual cycles have occurred.

Patient Education

Ovulation Prediction Tests Excluding ClearBlue Easy Fertility Monitor

- Test 2 to 3 days before ovulation is expected.
- Early morning urine collection is recommended because the LH surge occurs early in the day and the urine concentration is relatively consistent at this time.
- If using a kit designed to be passed through the urine stream, either hold a test stick in the urine stream for the specified time or collect urine in a collection cup and dip the stick in the urine.
- If using a kit designed to collect urine in a collection cup, dip the stick in the urine.
  - If immediate testing is not feasible, refrigerate the urine sample for the length of time specified in the directions for each product. Allow the sample to stand at room temperature for 20 to 30 minutes before beginning the test.
- Wait for the time recommended by the manufacturer.
- The test's first significant increase in color intensity indicates that the LH surge has occurred, and ovulation will occur within a day or two.
- Once the surge is detected, verify that the test was performed correctly.
  - If the testing procedure was accurate, discontinue testing.
  - Discard the test stick after use.
  - Remaining tests can be used later, if necessary.

- If the LH surge is not detected and the test procedure was correct, ovulation may not have occurred or testing may have occurred too late in the cycle. Consider testing for a longer duration next cycle to increase the chances of detecting the LH surge.

ClearBlue Easy Fertility Monitor Test
- For the first month, test on the sixth day after beginning menstruation and test for 20 days.
- For subsequent months, test the number of days indicated by the monitor manufacturer.
- Remove the test stick from its packaging before use and hold in the urine stream.
- Insert the stick in the monitor.
- Discard the test stick after use.

Basal Thermometry

Basal body temperature (BBT) is the temperature of the body at rest. A "normal" oral BBT is 98.6°F or 37°C. For years, women have measured BBT to predict the time of ovulation. Usually, resting BBT is below normal during the first part of the female reproductive cycle and rises to normal temperature.

Considerations
- Fertility specialists require a woman to chart her BBT for at least 3 consecutive months or menstrual cycles to identify cyclic patterns.
- Basal digital thermometers do not require the patient to interpret the reading, they track multiple temperature readings, and they are more expensive.
- Eating, drinking, talking, and smoking should be postponed until after taking each temperature reading as they can influence the basal metabolic temperature.

Patient Education
- Before using the basal thermometer, read the instructions thoroughly.
- Choose one method of taking temperatures—orally, vaginally, or rectally—and use the same method consistently.
- If using a nondigital basal thermometer, it should be shaken down to ≤96°F or 35.6°C.
- Place the thermometer on the nightstand or within reach before going to bed.
- Take the temperature readings at approximately the same time each morning before rising after ≥5 hours of sleep.

- Plot the temperatures on a graph.
- A rise in BBT by approximately 0.4°F (0.2°C) to 1°F (0.5°C) indicates that ovulation has occurred. To maximize the chances of becoming pregnant, women should have intercourse as soon as the increase in BBT occurs.

Saliva Electrolyte Tests

Saliva electrolyte tests measure the concentration of electrolytes in saliva to predict ovulation. The fertility microscopes predict ovulation by ferning patterns, the crystallization of salts in dried saliva. Before, during, and after ovulation, the hormonal changes directly affect the saliva electrolyte concentrations.

Considerations

- Polycystic ovary syndrome (PCOS) and perimenopause may interfere with test results.
- The quality of saliva specimens can be affected by food consumption, smoking, alcohol, or anticholinergic medications.
- Saliva samples should not be collected within 2 hours of smoking, eating, or drinking.

Patient Education

- Wash and dry hands.
- Place saliva on the slide area of the microscope eyepiece.
- Allow saliva to dry for 5 to 7 minutes.
- Compare the observed saliva pattern with the pattern from the package insert to identify the fertile period.
- Clean the round slide surface after each use with a cotton swab soaked with water or alcohol.
- Do no wash or soak the eyepiece because water may be trapped between the lens of the microscope and the slide.

■ Thermometers[6]

A normal temperature is 98.6°F or 37°C (Box 7.1). Each person has his or her own normal temperature, which may be slightly higher or lower than average (Table 7.3). Rectal temperature is not affected by environmental factors. It is accurate, reproducible, and considered the gold standard. Rectal temperatures are approximately 1° higher than oral temperatures and 2° higher than axillary temperatures.

Box 7.1	Conversion of Temperatures (°F to °C)

Celsius	Fahrenheit
37°	98.6°
38°	100.4°
39°	102.2°
40°	104°

Celsius = 5/9 (°F −32); Fahrenheit = (9/5 × °C) + 32

Temperatures can be measured in different ways with different types of thermometers. Product selection considerations include ease of use, safety, accuracy, reliability, and cost. Types of thermometers include mercury-free-glass thermometers, digital thermometers, infrared thermometers, and color-change thermomters.

Mercury-Free-Glass Thermometers

- Alternative to mercury-in-glass thermometer to measure body temperature.
- Prevents environmental mercury contamination and exposures.
- Are available for oral and rectal use.

Table 7.3 BODY TEMPERATURE RANGE DEPENDING ON SITE OF MEASUREMENT

Route	Normal	Fever
Rectal	97.9°F–100.4°F (36.6°C–38°C)	>101.8°F (38.8°C)
Oral	95.9°F–99.5°F (35.5°C–37.5°C)	>100°F (37.8°C)
Axillary	94.5°F–99°F (34.7°C–37.2°C)	>99°F (37.2°C)
Tympanic	96.4°F–100.4°F (35.8°C–38°C)	>100.4°F (38°C)

Reprinted with permission from Takiya L. Fever. In: Berardi RR, Kroon LA, McDermott JH, et al., eds. *Handbook of Nonprescription Drugs: An Interactive Approach to Self-Care.* 15th ed. Washington, DC: American Pharmacists Association; 2006:94.

- Are low cost, light weight, and of compact size.
- Are difficult to read and take $\leq$5 minutes for an accurate reading.
- Are subject to breakage and risk of injuries.

Digital Thermometers

- Are easier and quicker to use than glass thermometers.
- Are available for oral, rectal, and axillary use.
- Provide a temperature reading in about 30 to 60 seconds.
- Eliminate the risk of glass breakage, mercury toxicity, and cuts.
- Are easier to read with digital temperature displays.
- Require batteries and need to be calibrated periodically.

Infrared Thermometers

- Are very accurate, if used appropriately.
- Are available for tympanic and temporal temperature measurements.
- Measure the emitted infared energy from the surface of the tympanic membrane and temporal artery.
- Measure body temperature in <5 seconds.
- Are relatively expensive.
- Require batteries and routine calibration.

Color-Change Thermometers

- Are less accurate or reliable than other available devices.
- Have a heat-sensitive adhesive strip that changes color in response to different temperature gradients.
- May be placed anywhere on the skin but show less variation in temperature on the forehead.

■ Fecal Occult Blood Tests[3]

Additional Questions to Ask the Patient

1. What is the purpose of your using this product?
2. Have you ever used a product like this? If so, which product have you used?
3. What type of diet do you follow?

The fecal occult blood test (FOBT) detects blood in the stool with a colorimetric assay for hemoglobin. It is nonivasive and easy to use in the privacy of the patient's home. Detection of blood in the stool may signify several conditions that include but are not limited to Crohn disease,

Table 7.4 SELECTED FECAL OCCULT BLOOD
TESTS

Category	Product Name
Toilet test	AccuStat Colorectal Disease Test EZ-Detect Stool Blood Test ww.ezdetect.com
Stool wipes	LifeGuard www.orderlifeguard.com
Manual stool application device	ColonTest-Sensitive

colitis, anal fissures, diverticulitis, hemorrhoids, or colon or rectal cancer.
The blue-green color indicates a positive test. Currently, three categories
of FOBTs are available—the toilet test, stool wipes, and manual stool
application device. Table 7.4 lists selected fecal occult blood tests.

Considerations

- EZ-Detect Stool Blood test does not require a diet or medication change.
- ColonTest-Sensitive has a card for recording results to give to the primary care clinician.
- Avoid nonsteroidal anti-inflammatory drugs, aspirin, antiplatelet drugs, steroids, vitamin C >250 mg per day, and red meat for ≥2 to 3 days before and during testing period because they can interfere with test results.
- Increase dietary fiber intake for several days before testing to stimulate bleeding from lesions that might not otherwise bleed and to increase the frequency of bowel movements.
- The patient should consult his or her health care provider before discontinuing any prescribed medication.

Patient Education

EZ-Detect and Accustat

- Before testing, remove toilet tank cleansers and deodorizers and flush toilet twice.
- Use one test pad to perform a water quality test. If any trace of blue appears in the cross-shaped area, use another toilet to test and perform a water quality test on the second toilet.
- After a bowel movement, place a pad printed side up in the toilet bowl. Check for the appearance of a blue cross on the test pad (positive result).
- Repeat the test on the next two bowel movements.

LifeGuard

- Wipe with test pad after a bowel movement.
- Peel and flush biodegradable tissue liner. Fold test in half to seal sample.
- Add 4 drops of developer to test pad. The blue color change indicates a positive result. The patient can wait ≤14 days to add the developer.
- Add one drop of the developer between the positive and negative lines on the control side of pad.
- Add controls after the stool sample is developed.
- If the positive control line (+ • + • +) turns blue and the negative control line (− • − • −) stays red, the test is working properly.
- Repeat the test on the next two bowel movements.

ColonTest-Sensitive

- Open the test lid device and apply stool sample to wells A and B.
- Close the lid and press on the "press last" space to break the test ampule.
- Turn the test device over and hold vertical for 15 seconds.
- The test is positive if wells are partially or completely blue.
- The test is negative if wells are beige or brown.
- Repeat the test on the next two bowel movements.

Notify the primary care clinician if any of the three tests is positive.

Blood Pressure Monitors[3,7,8]

Hypertension is a risk factor for many serious conditions including coronary heart disease, congestive heart failure, stroke, kidney disease, and eye problems. It is asymptomatic and often called a "silent killer." Monitoring blood pressure is indicated for patients with hypertension or who are at risk. Refer to Table 7.5 for the classification of blood pressure by

Table 7.5 CLASSIFICATION OF BLOOD PRESSURE FOR ADULTS

Category	Systolic (mm Hg)		Diastolic (mm Hg)
Normal	<120	and	<80
Prehypertension	<120–139	or	80–89
Hypertension, stage 1	140–159	or	90–99
Hypertension, stage 2	≥160	or	≥100

Box 7.2	Hypertension Treatment Goals
Uncomplicated hypertension	<140/90 mm Hg
Diabetes or renal disease	<130/80 mm Hg
Renal disease with >1 g/24 h proteinuria	<125/75 mm Hg

the Joint National Committee on Prevention, Detection, Evaluation, and Treatment of High Blood Pressure (JNC 7). Patients should know their treatment goals for hypertension (Box 7.2). The JNC 7 guideline is available online at www.nhlbi.nih.gov/guidelines/index.htm.

There are three types of blood pressure measuring devices: mercury, aneroid, and automatic. Mercury column devices are expensive and not recommended for home use because they pose a potential risk of mercury toxicity should the glass tubing break. Aneroid devices are light, portable, and affordable. Many come with a stethoscope attached to the cuff, which frees the patient from having to hold the bell of the stethoscope in place. Good eyesight and hearing are necessary for accurate readings. Digital blood pressure monitors have become more accurate, reliable, and easy to use but are most expensive. They require less manual dexterity. Digital displays are easy to read for patients with visual impairments. In addition to the standard monitors, finger and wrist monitors are available. Wrist monitors are accurate as long as the cuff size is appropriate and the wrist is at the heart level during measurement. Finger monitors are considered inaccurate and are not recommended.

It is important to choose an appropriate cuff size for accurate blood pressure measurement. To determine the proper cuff size, measure the circumference of the arm. Arm cuff sizes are available in child/small adult (7–10.25 in.), standard (9–13 in.), and large (13–17 in.). Refer to the product package for specifications to help determine the appropriate size for the patient. Table 7.6 lists selected blood pressure monitors.

General guiding principles for patients when measuring blood pressure include the following:

- Sit comfortably with the back supported.
- Keep arms free of constrictive clothing.
- Keep legs uncrossed and feet flat on floor.

Table 7.6 SELECTED BLOOD PRESSURE MONITORS

Manufacturer	Model	Automatic/ Manual	Arm/ Wrist
Health o meter www.healthometer.com	7630	Manual	Arm
	7631	Automatic	Arm
	7632	Automatic (two-person feature)	Wrist
	7633	Automatic	Wrist
Lumiscope www.lumiscope.net	1100	Manual	Arm
	1130	Automatic	Arm
	1140	Automatic	Wrist
Omron	HEM-432	Manual	Arm
	HEM-711AC	Automatic	Arm
	HEM-712C		
	HEM-629	Automatic	Wrist
	HEM-637		
	HEM-650		
LifeSource www.lifesourceonline.com	UA-704	Manual	Arm
	UA-705		
	UA-767	Automatic	Arm
	UA-767PC		
	UA-851		
	UA-853AC		
	UB-328	Automatic	Wrist
	UB-511		

- Sit for a minimum of 5 minutes before the first reading.
- Avoid talking while taking blood pressure.
- Avoid physical activity, alcohol, caffeine, or nicotine consumption for 30 minutes before taking blood pressure.

Diabetes (Blood Glucose) Monitoring[9-12]

A home glucose monitoring system is essential to assist patients with managing and achieving glycemic goals in conjunction with pharmacotherapy. Routine monitoring of blood glucose is an integral component of diabetes self-care. The knowledge of current glycemic status provides patients with immediate feedback on their disease-control status. Patients are encouraged to keep a daily record of all monitoring results. The American

---

Box 7.3 **ADA Glycemic Recommendations for Adults**

Hemoglobin A1c	<7%
Fasting plasma glucose	70–130 mg/dL
Postprandial plasma glucose	<180 mg/dL

Diabetes Association glycemic recommendations for adults with diabetes are summarized in Box 7.3. The Standards of Medical Care in Diabetes—2008 is available online at www.diabetes.org. Most glucose monitors report the concentrations of plasma glucose, which is about 10% to 15% higher than whole blood. Refer to Table 7.7 for a selected list of blood glucose monitors.

Considerations

- Determine the best monitor for patients based on size, visual display, blood sample size, time to results, alternate testing site capabilities, calibration, memory, price, and so on.
- Require a single finger stick to obtain a blood sample.
- The range of glucose detection varies with each monitor from 0 mg/dL to 500 or 600 mg/dL.
- Some insurance plans cover all or part of the cost of monitors and/or strips under prescription or durable medical supply deductibles.

Patient Education

- Supplies needed include strips, a lancet, and lancing device as well as a glucose meter.
- Calibrate the glucose meter if required.
- Perform quality control as recommended by the meter manufacturer.
- Wash the hand properly and dry thoroughly before obtaining a blood sample.
- Lance the side of the fingertip to obtain the blood sample, and rotate the sites. (Avoid the pad of the finger because there are more nerves in this area, which may cause pain.)
- Place the blood sample on the strip as recommended by the manufacturer.

Table 7.7   SELECTED GLUCOSE MONITORS

Product	Test Strip	Range (mg/dL)	Time(s)
Accu-Chek Active	Accu-Chek Active	10–600	5
Accu-Chek Advantage	Accu-Chek Comfort Curve	10–600	26
Accu-Chek Aviva	Accu-Chek Aviva	10–600	5
Accu-Chek Compact Plus	Accu-Chek Compact	10–600	5
Breeze 2	Breeze 2	20–600	7
Contour	Contour	10–600	5
Freestyle	Freestyle	20–500	7
Freestyle Flash	Freestyle	20–500	7
Freestyle Freedom	Freestyle	20–500	5
Freestyle Lite	Freestyle Lite	20–500	5
One Touch Basic	One Touch	0–600	45
One Touch Ultra 2	One Touch Ultra	20–600	5
One Touch UltraSmart	One Touch Ultra	20–600	5
One Touch UltraMini	One Touch Ultra	20–600	5
Precision Xtra	Precision Xtra	20–500	5 (glucose); 10 (ketone)

- Dispose of lancets and strips properly.
- Store monitor at room temperature.

Urine Ketone Testing

Home blood ketone monitoring is used to detect or predict ketoacidosis. When the body is lacking insulin, the uptake of glucose into the cells for energy and storage is inhibited. During these times, the liver breaks down fat as an alternative source of energy and produces ketone bodies and acetone as byproducts. An accumulation of ketones in the blood can result in diabetic ketoacidosis, a potentially fatal condition if not treated. The excess ketones in the blood that spill into the urine can be detected. Table 7.8 lists selected urine ketone testing products.

Table 7.8 SELECTED URINE KETONES TESTING PRODUCTS

Product	Measures Glucose/Ketones
Acetest Tablets	Ketones
Chemstrip uGK	Glucose and ketones
Chemstrip K	Ketones
DiaScreen 1K	Ketones
DiaScreen 2GK	Glucose and ketones
Ketostix	Ketones
Keto-Diastix	Glucose and ketones

Patient Education
- Patients with type I diabetes should test for ketones when plasma glucose is ≥240 mg/dL.
- All patients should test for ketones when experiencing any of the following: extreme stress, illness, pregnancy, and symptoms such as diarrhea, vomiting, loss of appetite, increased urine production, fruity-smelling breath, high fever, or when ketoacidosis is suspected .
- If ketones are present on two or more consecutive times, the patient should report to the primary care provider.

Hemoglobin A1c Testing

Hemoglobin A1c testing provides useful information about a patient's glycemic control over the past 3 months. The American Diabetes Association recommends testing every 3 months for patients not at goal and every 6 months for patients who are stable and meeting glycemic goals. The goal for most patients with diabetes is <7%, and the normal range is 4% to 6%. Many A1c kits require patients to mail the samples to the clinical laboratory for analysis. A new monitor, ChoiceDM A1c Home Test (A1c Now) for home and office use provides results in approximately 8 minutes. Table 7.9 lists selected hemoglobin A1c kits.

Patient Education
- Testing hemoglobin A1c should not replace daily glucose testing.
- Discuss the use and results with the primary care provider.

Table 7.9	SELECTED HOME HEMOGLOBIN A1c TESTS

AccuBase A1c Glycohemoglobin Testing System
(www.diabetestechnologies.com)

A1c At Home
(www.flexsite.com)

Appraise A1c Diabetes Monitoring System
(www.matria.com)

Biosafe Hemoglobin A1c Test Kit
(www.ebiosafe.com)

ChoiceDM A1c Home Test (A1c Now)
(Bristol-Myers Squibb www.bms.com)

- Perform quality control and procedures as recommended by the manufacturer.

Additional Patient Information

Patients with diabetes should wear an identification bracelet, necklace, or tag. Additional information may be found for MedicAlert at www.medicalert.com or by calling 800-432-5378. Patients should carry an identification card including their name, address, phone number, medications, and name of the primary care clinician and phone number.

Cholesterol Tests[3,5]

Additional Questions to Ask the Patient

1. What is the purpose of your using this product?
2. Which product have you used?
3. Have you consulted the primary care clinician?
4. What are your current medications?

Many current home cholesterol tests measure only total cholesterol. However, a few tests also measure low-density lipoprotein cholesterol (LDLc), high-density lipoprotein cholesterol (HDLc), and triglycerides. With the exception of BIOSAFE products requiring patients to mail the samples to the clinical laboratory, cholesterol kits allow them to perform the tests and receive the results at home. Patients should be informed that home cholesterol tests should not replace a complete lipid panel and the

Table 7.10 SELECTED HOME CHOLESTEROL TESTS

Product	Measures
CholesTrak AccuMeter Home Cholesterol Test AccuStat Home Cholesterol Test Home Access Instant Cholesterol Test Personal Cholesterol Monitor	Total cholesterol
Cardiochek	Total cholesterol, HDLc, triglycerides Can also measure glucose and ketone
BIOSAFE Total Cholesterol	Total cholesterol. Mail sample to clinical laboratory
BIOSAFE Total Cholesterol Panel	Total cholesterol, triglycerides, HDLc, LDLc. Mail sample to clinical laboratory

Reprinted with permission from Rosenthal WM, Briggs GC. Home testing and monitoring devices. In: Berardi RR, Kroon LA, McDermott JH, et al., eds. *Handbook of Nonprescription Drugs: An Interactive Approach to Self-Care*. 15th ed. Washington, DC: American Pharmacists Association; 2006:1061.

results should be shared with the primary care clinician. Refer to Table 7.10 for a list of selected home cholesterol tests.

Patient Education

- Patients who have coagulation disorders or take anticoagulants should not self-test.
- Home cholesterol testing should not replace a complete lipid panel.
- Proper finger-sticking technique is important for accurate results.
- Read the instructions thoroughly before performing the test.
- Report test results to the primary care clinician.

HIV Testing[13,14]

The only Food and Drug Administration (FDA)-approved home HIV-1 testing kits are the Home Access HIV-1 Test System and the Home Access Express HIV-1 Test System (both manufactured by Home Access Health Corporation). Both of these testing kits have been shown to be 99.9% accurate. They do not test for HIV-2 (a much less common cause of AIDS).

Table 7.11	POTENTIAL ADVANTAGES AND DISADVANTAGES OF AT-HOME HIV-1 TESTING
Advantages	**Disadvantages**
Anonymous	Requires relatively high level of health literacy to navigate the large amount of written materials
Widely available and easily accessible	Patient does not receive behavior risk assessment and counseling
Results within 3–7 business days	Expensive ($40–$60 usually)

Included in the test kits are the following:

- Anonymous and confidential pretest and posttest counseling, available via the tollfree phone number and written materials that are provided.
- A patient personal identification number (PIN) for obtaining anonymous testing results via the tollfree phone number.
- Materials for obtaining and packaging the patient's blood sample (a lancet device, collection paper, and mailing envelope).
- Technical support via the tollfree phone number.

Other Considerations

- Is the patient physically able to perform a finger stick and collect his or her own blood sample on a small piece of paper?
- Was the patient's potential exposure to HIV ≥3 months before he or she will take the test? (See Chapter ___ section on HIV/AIDS for explanation of the window period of false-negative HIV test results.)
- The test systems are not recommended for use by patients with hemophilia.

Table 7.11 summarizes some of the potential advantages and disadvantages of at-home HIV testing.

 Illicit Drug Use Tests[3]

Home drug tests are marketed as an aid to alleviate concerns from parents who suspect illicit drug use in their children and those seeking employment. It is not meant to be substituted for open communication betweens the parents and their children regarding drug use. Samples of urine, hair, or saliva may be used to test. Hair and some urine tests are required to be mailed to a clinical laboratory for analysis. Results are obtained by telephone using the code accompanying the test kit. Other urine and saliva tests can be performed at home. Currently, saliva tests are marketed only to drug testing programs and employers. Table 7.12 lists selected home drug abuse tests available.

Considerations

- Each kit varies by drug(s) that is/are suspected.
- The urine test detects drug use within hours to several days.
- The hair test detects drug use within 5 to 90 days.

Patient Education

- Read directions carefully before collecting samples.
- Urine samples report positive or negative results.
- Collect the urine sample using the collection devices included.
- The temperature of the urine sample should be between 90°F (32°C) and 100°F (38°C).
- Hair samples report a low, medium, or high level of drug use.
- Obtain a $1/2$-in. hair sample and one strand deep from the crown of the head and place in the collection package included.
- Hair from a hairbrush, comb, or clothing is not recommended.
- Medications such as codeine, decongestants, antidiarrheals, and possibly poppy seeds may cause false-positive test results.
- Open communication and discussion of test results are best conducted in a nonthreatening manner.

Additional Information

Information on FDA approval of a test for illicit drugs for home use is available at www.accessdata.fda.gov/scripts/cdrh/cfdocs/cfIVD/Search.cfm.

█ Urinary Tract Infection Tests[3]

Home urinary tract infection (UTI) tests are used for detection of such infection and confirmation of the resolution of infection after treatment. Symptoms of UTI include frequency, urgency, and burning with urination. Two types of UTI tests are available (Table 7.13), and the primary difference is mechanism of action. TECO Nitrite and UTI Home Screening

Table 7.12 SELECTED HOME DRUG ABUSE TESTS

Product	Time to Result	Testing Location	Specimen	Detection
At Home Drug Test Single Drug and Multiple Drugs	3–15 Min for initial screen; 5–7 Days for laboratory confirmation	Home and send away for confirmation	Urine	Amphetamine Methamphetamine Ecstasy Marijuana Cocaine Opiates
First Check Home Drug Test	5 Min for initial screen; 5–7 Days for laboratory confirmation	Home and end away for confirmation	Urine	Panel 1: marijuana Panel 2: marijuana and cocaine Four-drug test: marijuana, cocaine, opiates, methamphetamine Seven-drug test: marijuana, cocaine, opiates, ecstasy, methamphetamine, PCP, amphetamine Twelve-drug test: five prescription drugs: tricyclic antidepressants, barbiturates, methadone, benzodiazepines, oxycodone; seven illicit drugs: marijuana, cocaine, opiates, ecstasy, methamphetamine, PCP, amphetamine

(continued)

Table 7.12 SELECTED HOME DRUG ABUSE TESTS (continued)

Product	Time to Result	Testing Location	Specimen	Detection
AccuStat Home Drug Test	3–8 Min for initial screen; 5–7 Days for laboratory confirmation	Home and send away for confirmation	Urine	Panel 1: marijuana Panel 2: marijuana, cocaine Panel 3: marijuana, cocaine, methamphetamine Panel 4: marijuana, cocaine, methamphetamine, morphine/opiates
Parent's Alert Home Drug Testing Service	3–5 Days	Send away	Urine	Marijuana, cocaine, opiates, methamphetamine, ecstasy, barbiturates, benzodiazepines, LSD
Quick Screen Pro Multi-Drug Screening	3–15 Min; 5–7 Days for laboratory confirmation	Home and send away for confirmation	Urine	Amphetamine, cocaine, marijuana, opiates, phencyclidine
PDT-90 Personal Drug Testing Service	5–7 Days	Send away	Hair	Marijuana, cocaine, opiates, methamphetamine amphetamine, phencyclidine, barbiturates, benzodiapines

Reprinted with permission from Rosenthal WM, Briggs GC. Home testing and monitoring devices. In: Berardi RR, Kroon LA, McDermott JH, et al., eds. *Handbook of Nonprescription Drugs: An Interactive Approach to Self-Care.* 15th ed. Washington, DC: American Pharmacists Association; 2006:1068.

Table 7.13	SELECTED URINARY TRACT INFECTION TEST	
Product	**Reaction Time**	**Positive Indicator**
AZO Strips	30–60 s	Color change to dark tan to purple
TECO Nitrite Test	30–60 s	Color change to pink
UTI Home Screening Test	30–60 s	Color change to pink

Test detect nitrites in the urine reduced from nitrate by Gram-negative bacteria. AZO Strips detect nitrite and leukocyte esterase.

Patient Education

- Testing the first urine of the morning is preferred. If tested later, urine must dwell in the bladder for at least 4 hours.
- Pass the test pad or stick through the urine stream.
- Wait for 30 to 60 seconds and compare the color on the sensor pad with the color chart provided.
  - ‣ Pink indicates a positive result for the TECO and UTI Home Screening Test.
  - ‣ Dark tan to purple indicates a positive result for the AZO Test.
- If the test result is positive, contact the primary care provider immediately.
- If symptoms of UTI are present, contact the primary care provider immediately.
- If the test result is negative but UTI symptoms persist, contact the primary care provider immediately.

References

1. Limon L, Cimmino A, Lakamp J, eds. *APhA Nonprescription Products: Patient Assessment Handbook.* Washington, DC: American Pharmaceutical Association; 1997:25, 201.
2. Munroe WP. Home diagnostic kits. *Am Pharm.* 1994;34:50–59.
3. Rosenthal WM, Briggs GC. Home testing and monitoring devices. In: Berardi RR, Kroon LA, McDermott JH, et al., eds. *Handbook of Nonprescription Drugs: An Interactive Approach to Self-Care.* 15th ed. Washington, DC: American Pharmacists Association; 2006.
4. Cole LA, Khanlian SA, Sutton JM, et al. Accuracy of home pregnancy tests at the time of missed menses. *Am J Obstet Gynecol.* 2004;190:100–105.

5. Facts and Comparisons 4.0 (online). Available at www.efactsonline.com. Accessed January 2, 2008.

6. Takiya L. Fever. In: Berardi RR, Kroon LA, McDermott JH, et al., eds. *Handbook of Nonprescription Drugs: An Interactive Approach to Self-Care.* 15th ed. Washington, DC: American Pharmacists Association; 2006.

7. National Heart Lung and Blood Institute. Clinical Practice Guidelines on Hypertension. Available at www.nhlbi.nih.gov/guidelines/hypertension/jnc7full.pdf. Accessed January 18, 2008.

8. National Kidney Foundation. K/DOQI Clinical Practice Guidelines on Hypertension and Hypertensive Agents in Chronic Kidney Disease. Available at www.kidney.org/professionals/KDOQI/guidelines_bp/index.htm. Accessed January 18, 2008.

9. Assemi M, Morello CM. Diabetes mellitus. In: Berardi RR, Kroon LA, McDermott JH, et al., eds. *Handbook of Nonprescription Drugs: An Interactive Approach to Self-Care.* 15th ed. Washington, DC: American Pharmacists Association; 2006:955–994.

10. American Diabetes Association Diabetes Forecast 2008 Resource Guide. Blood Glucose Monitoring and Data Management Systems. Available at www.diabetes.org/uedocuments/df-rg-monitors-0108.pdf. Accessed February 1, 2008.

11. American Diabetes Association Diabetes Forecast 2008 Resource Guide. Urine Testing. Availalble at www.diabetes.org/uedocuments/df-rg-urine-testing-0108.pdf. Accessed February 1, 2008.

12. American Diabetes Association. Standard of Medical Care in Diabetes—2008. Diabetes Care 2008;31:S12–S54.

13. FDA Center for Biologics Evaluation and Research (CBER). Vital Facts About HIV Home Test Kits. January 29, 2008. Available at www.fda.gov/consumer/updatesh/hivtestkit012908.htm. Accessed February 5, 2008.

14. FDA Center for Biologics Evaluation and Research (CBER). Premarket Approval Information—Devices. Updated September 24, 1999. Available at www.fda.gov/cber/PMAltr/P950002L.htm. Accessed February 5, 2008.

Drug Administration

Susan M. Stein

Advances in technology continually provide greater variety for administration of drugs. New delivery systems can expand the therapeutic indication or decrease the adverse effects of an older drug. This chapter presents
various routes of drug administration and provides a selection process to
determine the most appropriate drug/dosage formulation and route.

Common routes of drug administration are oral and parenteral. Topical and rectal administration are used less often. Site-specific routes also
exist, such as ophthalmic and otic administration. The nature of the drug
will dictate the dosage form and route available. For example, a drug
will initially be available parenterally to avoid complications involving
metabolism or may only be available orally as a tablet due to solubility
complications.

Patient Assessment

When determining an appropriate route of administration, assessing the
patient's clinical health status provides valuable information. The seri-
ousness of the condition being treated can assist in selection of the most
effective route of administration. Examples of patient conditions and recommended administration routes are described in Table 8.1.

Routes of Administration

When selecting an appropriate route of administration, available forms
of the desired drug should be reviewed. Various references may be used,
including Drug Facts and Comparisons, Lexi-Comp, Micromedex, and
American Hospital Formulary Service (AHFS). In addition, it may be

Table 8.1 EXAMPLES OF RECOMMENDED ROUTES OF ADMINISTRATION FOR VARIOUS PATIENT CONDITIONS

Patient Status	Recommended Route
Oral intake	Oral, topical
Nothing by mouth (NPO)	Parenteral, rectal, topical
Critical condition	Parenteral
Chronic condition	Oral, rectal, topical
Severe hypokalemia (potassium level <3 mEq/L)	Parenteral
Nausea, vomiting	Parenteral, rectal

Table 8.2 ISSUES RELATING TO VARIOUS DOSAGE FORMULATIONS

Route	Dosage Form	Comments
Oral	Solid—capsule, tablet, powder packet, lozenge, troche, pastille	Limited dosing
	Solution	Titratable dose
	Suspension	Titratable dose, shake well to resuspend
	Emulsion	Oil-in-water more palatable
Parenteral	Solution (drug source)	Fewer stability issues, sterility issues
	Lyophilized (drug source)	Reconstitution, diluent, stability issues, sterility issues
	Dispersion (liposomal)	Limited availability, sterility issues
Topical	Bulk—cream, lotion, ointment, emulsion, gel, powder	Compounding flexibility
	Transdermal	Controlled release, adhesive irritation
Rectal/vaginal	Suppositories	Good absorption, compounding flexibility, temperature dependent
	Cream	Applicator for administration
Ophthalmic	Solution	Sterility issues
	Suspension	Shake well to resuspend, sterility issues
	Ointment	Difficult to apply
Otic	Solution	Sterility issues
	Suspension	Shake well to resuspend, sterility issues

feasible to prepare a commercially unavailable formulation. A literature review is useful to locate compounded drug formulations. Maintaining this information for future reference is advised. Issues relating to various dosage formulations are described in Table 8.2.

Other limitations should be considered when determining the most appropriate dosage form. Factors involving these choices are shown in Table 8.3.

Monitoring Parameters

It is vital to monitor the patient's condition to evaluate the effectiveness of drug therapy (see Chapter 13, Clinical Drug Monitoring, for a more

Table 8.3 COMPARISON OF ADVANTAGES AND DISADVANTAGES OF VARIOUS DOSAGE FORMULATIONS

Route	Advantages	Disadvantages
Oral	Functional gastrointestinal maintained Ease of administration Less expensive	Slower to effect First-pass metabolism Bioavailability issues
Parenteral	Rapid time to effect No bioavailability issues Ability to titrate dose	Expensive preparation Expensive administration Sterility and stability issues Compatibility issues Safety issues (related to administration) Painful administration
Topical	Localized effect Little systemic absorption Few adverse reactions Controlled absorption (transdermal) No first-pass metabolism	Inaccurate dosing Irritation at application site Response altered with physiologic changes (blood pressure, fever) Drug diversion (transdermal) Increased absorption (elderly patients, exposed skin) May stain clothing
Rectal/vaginal	Well-absorbed No first-pass metabolism Generally inexpensive	Socially unacceptable Limited availability May stain clothing Indication/route potentially unrelated
Ophthalmic	Localized effect Little systemic absorption	Difficult self-administration Contamination possible
Otic	Localized effect Little systemic absorption	Difficult self-administration

Table 8.4 EXAMPLES OF MONITORING PARAMETERS PERTAINING TO MAJOR ROUTES OF ADMINISTRATION

Route	Monitoring Parameters	Examples
Oral	Nausea, pain relief, respiratory rate	Acetaminophen with codeine
Parenteral	Redness at site, line infiltration	Azithromycin infusion
Topical	Skin irritation, blood pressure	Clonidine transdermal patch

detailed discussion). Parameters can include indications from the signs of an infection (redness, warmth, fever) to the appearance of an allergy to the medication (rash). Table 8.4 contains a sample of monitoring parameters that relate to routes of administration.

Oral Medications

Oral administration is often the most desired route of administration despite limitations. Additional considerations involving oral medications pertain to the ability to crush or divide a tablet to increase dosing flexibility. Due to continually changing formulations, it is vital to clarify this information for each manufacturer and formulation. Box 8.1 and Table 8.5 provide information regarding these issues.[1,2]

Box 8.1 **Types of Medications That Should Not Be Divided or Crushed**

Extended release or enteric coated tablets: examples long-acting (LA), sustained-release (SR), controlled-release (CR), extended-release (XL or XR), sustained action (SA), time delay (TD), time release (TR)

    Sublingual tablets

    Buccal tablets

From McPherson ML. Don't crush that tablet! Am Pharm. 1994;NS34:57–58; and Mitchell JF. Oral dosage forms that should not be crushed: 2000 update. Hosp Pharm. 2000;35:553–557, with permission.

Table 8.5 ORAL DOSAGE FORMS THAT SHOULD NOT BE CRUSHED

Drug Product	Dosage Forms	Dosage Reasons/Comments[2]
Accutane	Capsule	Mucous membrane irritant
Aciphex	Tablet	Slow-release
Actiq	Lozenge	Slow-release **Note:** this lollipop delivery system requires the patient to slowly allow dissolution
Actonel	Tablet	Irritant **Note:** chewed, crushed, or sucked tablets May cause oropharyngeal irritation
Adalat CC	Tablet	Slow-release
Adderall XR	Capsule	Slow-release[a]
AeroHist Plus	Tablet	Slow-release[h]
Afeditab CR	Tablet	Slow-release
Aggrenox	Capsule	Slow-release
Alavert Allergy Sinus 12 Hour	Tablet	Slow-release
Allegra-D	Tablet	Slow-release
Allfen Jr	Tablet Capsule	Slow-release Slow-release[a]
Alpophen	Tablet	Enteric-coated
Alprazolam ER	Tablet	Slow-release
Altoprev	Tablet	Slow-release
Ambien CR	Tablet	Slow-release
Amrix	Capsule	Slow-release
Aptivus	Capsule	**Note:** oil emulsion within spheres; taste
Aquatab C	Tablet	Slow-release[h]
Aquatab D	Tablet	Slow-release[h]
Arthrotec	Tablet	Enteric-coated
Asacol	Tablet	Slow-release

(continued)

Table 8.5 ORAL DOSAGE FORMS THAT SHOULD NOT BE CRUSHED *(continued)*

Drug Product	Dosage Forms	Dosage Reasons/Comments[2]
Ascriptin A/D	Tablet	Enteric coated
Azulfidine EN-tabs	Tablet	Enteric-coated
Augmentin XR	Tablet	Slow-release[b,h]
Avinza	Capsule	Slow-release (a; not pudding)
Avodart	Capsule	**Note:** drug may cause fetal abnormalities; women who are, or may become, pregnant, should not handle capsules; all woman should use caution in handling capsules, especially leaking capsules
Bayer Enteric-coated	Caplet	Enteric-coated
Bayer Low Adult	Tablet	Enteric-coated
Bayer Regular Strength	Caplet	Enteric-coated
Bellahist-D LA	Tablet	Slow-release
Biaxin-XL	Tablet	Slow-release
Bidhist	Tablet	Slow-release
Bidhist-D	Tablet	Slow-release
Biltricide	Tablet	Taste[h]
Biohist LA	Tablet	Slow-release[h]
Bisac-Evac	Tablet	Enteric-coated[c]
Bisacodyl	Tablet	Enteric-coated[c]
Bisa-Lax	Tablet	Enteric-coated[c]
Boniva	Tablet	Irritant: do not chew or suck **Note:** Potential for oropharyngeal ulceration
Bromfed PD	Capsule	Slow-release
Budeprion SR	Tablet	Slow-release
Calan SR	Tablet	Slow-release[h]
Carbatrol	Capsule	Slow-release[a]
Cardene SR	Capsule	Slow-release

(continued)

Table 8.5 ORAL DOSAGE FORMS THAT SHOULD NOT BE CRUSHED *(continued)*

Drug Product	Dosage Forms	Dosage Reasons/Comments[2]
Cardizem	Tablet	**Note:** although not described as slow release in the PI, the drug has a coating that is intended to release the drug over a period of approximately 3 hours
Cardizem CD	Capsule	Slow-release
Cardizem LA	Tablet	Slow-release
Cardura XL	Tablet	Slow-release
Cartia XT	Capsule	Slow-release
Cefaclor Extended-Release	Tablet	Slow-release
Ceftin	Tablet	Taste[b] **Note:** use suspension for children
Cefuroxime	Tablet	Taste[b] **Note:** use suspension for children
CellCept	Capsule, Tablet	Teratogenic potential[i]
Charcoal Plus	Tablet	Enteric-coated
Chlor-Trimeton 12-Hour	Tablet	Slow-release[b]
Cipro XR	Tablet	Slow-release
Claritin-D 12 Hour	Tablet	Slow-release
Claritin-D 24 Hour	Tablet	Slow-release
Colace	Capsule	Taste[e]
Colestid	Tablet	Slow-release
Concerta	Tablet	Slow-release
Commit	Lozenge	**Note:** integrity compromised by chewing or crushing
Cotazym-S	Capsule	Enteric-coated[a]
Covera-HS	Tablet	Slow-release
Creon 5, 10,20	Capsule	Slow-release[a]

(continued)

Table 8.5 ORAL DOSAGE FORMS THAT SHOULD NOT BE CRUSHED *(continued)*

Drug Product	Dosage Forms	Dosage Reasons/Comments[2]
Crixivan	Capsule	Taste **Note:** capsule may be opened and mixed with fruit puree (e.g., banana)
Cymbalta	Capsule	Slow-release[a]; may add to apple juice
Cytoxan	Tablet	**Note:** drug may be crushed but company recommends using injection
Cytovene	Capsule	Skin irritant
Dallergy	Tablet	Slow-release[b,h]
Dallergy-JR	Capsule	Slow-release
Deconamine SR	Capsule	Slow-release[b]
Depakene	Capsule	Slow-release mucous membrane irritant[b]
Depakote	Tablet	Slow-release
Depakote ER	Tablet	Slow-release
Detrol LA	Capsule	Slow-release
Dilacor XR	Capsule	Slow-release
Dilatrate-SR	Capsule	Slow-release
Dilt-CD	Capsule	Slow-release
Dilt-XR	Capsule	Slow-release
Diltia XT	Capsule	Slow-release
Ditropan XL	Tablet	Slow-release
Doxidan	Tablet	Enteric-coated[c]
DriHist SR	Tablet	Slow-release[h]
Drisdol	Capsule	Liquid filled[d]
Drixoral Allergy Sinus	Tablet	Slow-release
Drixoral Cold/Allergy	Tablet	Slow-release
Drixoral Nondrowsy	Tablet	Slow-release

(continued)

Table 8.5 ORAL DOSAGE FORMS THAT SHOULD NOT BE CRUSHED (continued)

Drug Product	Dosage Forms	Dosage Reasons/Comments[2]
Droxia	Capsule	**NOTE:** exposure to the powder may cause serious skin toxicities; healthcare workers should wear gloves to administer
Drysec	Tablet	Slow-release[h]
Dulcolax	Tablet	Enteric-coated[c]
Dulcolax	Capsule	Liquid-filled
DuraHist	Tablet	Slow-release[h]
DuraHist D	Tablet	Slow-release[h]
DynaCirc CR	Tablet	Slow-release
Duraphen II	Tablet	Slow-release[h]
Duraphen II DM	Tablet	Slow-release[h]
Duraphen Forte	Tablet	Slow-release[h]
Duratuss	Tablet	Slow-release[h]
Duratuss A	Tablet	Slow-release[h]
Duratuss PE	Tablet	Slow-release[h]
Dynex	Tablet	Slow-release[h]
Easprin	Tablet	Enteric-coated
EC-Naprosyn	Tablet	Enteric-coated
Ecotrin Adult Low Strength	Tablet	Enteric-coated
Ecotrin Maximum Strength	Tablet	Enteric-coated
Ecotrin Regular Strength	Tablet	Enteric-coated
Ed A-Hist	Tablet	Slow-release[b]
E.E.S. 400	Tablet	Enteric-coated[b]
Effer-K	Tablet	Effervescent tablet[f]
Effervescent Potassium	Tablet	Effervescent tablet[f]
Effexor XR	Capsule	Slow-release

(continued)

Table 8.5 ORAL DOSAGE FORMS THAT SHOULD NOT BE CRUSHED *(continued)*

Drug Product	Dosage Forms	Dosage Reasons/Comments[2]
Efidac/24 Pseudoephedrine	Tablet	Slow-release
Efidac/24	Tablet	Slow-release
E-Mycin	Tablet	Enteric-coated
Enablex	Tablet	Slow-release
Entex LA	Capsule	Slow-release[b]
Entex PSE	Capsule	Slow-release
Entocort EC	Capsule	Enteric-coated[a]
Equetro	Capsule	Slow-release[a]
Ergomar	Tablet	Sublingual form[g]
Ery-Tab	Tablet	Enteric-coated
Erythrocin Stearate	Tablet	Enteric-coated
Erythromycin Base	Tablet	Enteric-coated
Erythromycin Delayed-Release	Capsule	Enteric-coated Pellets[a]
Evista	Tablet	Taste; teratogenic potential[i]
ExeFen PD	Tablet	Slow-release[h]
Extendryl DM	Tablet	Slow-release
Extendryl G	Tablet	Slow-release[h]
Extendryl H	Tablet	Slow-release
Extendryl JR	Tablet	Slow-release[h]
Extendryl SR	Tablet	Slow-release[b]
Extendryl PSE	Tablet	Slow-release
Feen-a-mint	Tablet	Enteric-coated[c]
Feldene	Capsule	Mucous membrane irritant
Fentora	Tablet	**Note:** buccal tablet; swallow whole
Feosol	Tablet	Enteric-coated[b]
Feratab	Tablet	Enteric-coated[b]

(continued)

Table 8.5 ORAL DOSAGE FORMS THAT SHOULD NOT BE CRUSHED *(continued)*

Drug Product	Dosage Forms	Dosage Reasons/Comments[2]
Fergon	Tablet	Enteric-coated
Fero-Grad 500 mg	Tablet	Slow-release
Ferro-Sequels	Tablet	Slow-release
Ftagyl ER	Tablet	Slow-release
Fleet Laxative	Tablet	Enteric-coated[c]
Flomax	Capsule	Slow-release
Focalin XR	Capsule	Slow-release[a]
Fosamax	Tablet	Mucous membrane irritant
Geocillin	Tablet	Taste
Gleevec	Tablet	Taste[h] **Note:** may be dissolved in water or apple juice
Glipizide	Tablet	Slow-release
Glucophage XR	Tablet	Slow-release
Glucotrol XL	Tablet	Slow-release
Glumetza	Tablet	Slow-release
Guaifed	Capsule	Slow-release
Guaifed-PD	Capsule	Slow-release
Guaifenesin/ Pseudoephedrine	Tablet	Slow-release
Guaifenex DM	Tablet	Slow-release[h]
Guaifenex GP	Tablet	Slow-release
Guaifenex PSE	Tablet	Slow-release[h]
GuaiMAX-D	Tablet	Slow-release
Halfprin 81	Tablet	Enteric-coated
Heartline	Tablet	Enteric-coated
H 9600 SR	Tablet	Slow-release
Hista-Vent DA	Tablet	Slow-release[h]

(continued)

Table 8.5 ORAL DOSAGE FORMS THAT SHOULD NOT BE CRUSHED (continued)

Drug Product	Dosage Forms	Dosage Reasons/Comments[2]
Hydrea	Capsule	**NOTE:** exposure to the powder may cause serious skin toxicities; healthcare workers should wear gloves to administer
Imdur	Tablet	Slow-release[h]
Inderal LA	Capsule	Slow-release
Indocin SR	Capsule	Slow-release[a,b]
Innopran XL	Capsule	Slow-release
Intelence	Tablet	**Note:** tablet should be swallowed whole and not crushed; tablet may be dispersed in water
Invega	Tablet	Slow-release
Isochron	Tablet	Slow-release
Isoptin SR	Tablet	Slow-release[h]
Isordil Sublingual	Tablet	Sublingual form[g]
Isosorbide Dinitrate Sublingual	Tablet	Sublingual form[g]
Isosorbide SR	Tablet	Slow-release
Kadian	Capsule	Slow-release[a] **Note:** do give via N/G tubes
Kaletra	Tablet	Film-coated
Kaon CL-10	Tablet	Slow-release[b]
Keppra	Tablet	Taste **Note:** some extemporaneous formulas are Pharmacy prepared
Ketek	Tablet	Slow-release[b]
Klor-Con	Tablet	Slow-release[b]
Klor-Con M	Tablet	Slow-release[b,h]
Klotrix	Tablet	Slow-release
K-Lyte	Tablet	Effervescent tablet[f]

(continued)

Table 8.5 ORAL DOSAGE FORMS THAT SHOULD NOT BE CRUSHED (continued)

Drug Product	Dosage Forms	Dosage Reasons/Comments[2]
K-Lyte CL	Tablet	Effervescent tablet[f]
K-Lyte DS	Tablet	Effervescent tablet[f]
K-Tab	Tablet	Slow-release[b]
Lescol XL	Tablet	Slow-release
Levall G	Capsule	Slow-release
Levbid	Tablet	Slow-release[h]
Levsinex Timecaps	Capsule	Slow-release
Lexxel	Tablet	Slow-release
Lialda	Tablet	Slow-release
Lipram 4500	Capsule	Enteric-coated[a]
Lipram PN 10, 16, 20	Capsule	Enteric-coated, slow-release[a]
Lipram UL 12, 18, 20	Capsule	Enteric-coated, slow-release[a]
Liquibid-D 1200	Tablet	Slow-release[h]
Liquibid-PD	Tablet	Slow-release[h]
Lithobid	Tablet	Slow-release
Lodrane 24	Capsule	Slow-release
Lodrane 24D	Capsule	Slow-release
LoHist12 Hour	Tablet	Slow-release
Luvox CR	Capsule	Slow-release
Maxifed DM	Tablet	Slow-release[h]
Maxifed DMX	Tablet	Slow-release[h]
Maxiphen DM	Tablet	Slow-release[h]
Medent-DM	Tablet	Slow-release
Mestinon Timespan	Tablet	Slow-release[b]
Metadate ER	Tablet	Slow-release
Metadata CD	Capsule	Slow-release[a]
Methylin ER	Tablet	Slow-release
Metoprolol ER	Tablet	Slow-release

(continued)

Table 8.5 ORAL DOSAGE FORMS THAT SHOULD NOT BE CRUSHED *(continued)*

Drug Product	Dosage Forms	Dosage Reasons/Comments[2]
Micro K Extendcaps	Capsule	Slow-release[a,b]
Miraphen PSE	Tablet	Slow-release
Modane	Tablet	Enteric-coated[c]
Morphine sulfate extended-release	Tablet	Slow-release
Motrin	Tablet	Taste[e]
Moxatab	Tablet	Slow-release
MS Contin	Tablet	Slow-release[b]
Mucinex	Tablet	Slow-release
Mucinex DM	Tablet	Slow-release
Muco-Fen-DM	Tablet	Slow-release[h]
Myfortic	Tablet	Slow-release
Naprelan	Tablet	Slow-release
Nasatab LA	Tablet	Slow-release[h]
Nexium	Capsule	Slow-release[a]
Niaspan	Tablet	Slow-release
Nicotinic Acid	Capsule, Tablet	Slow-release[h]
Nifediac CC	Tablet	Slow-release
Nrfedical XL	Tablet	Slow-release
Nifedipine extended-release	Tablet	Slow-release
NitroQuick	Tablet	Sublingual route[g]
Nitrostat	Tablet	Subtingual route[g]
Norpace CR	Capsule	Slow-release form within a special capsule
Ondrox	Tablet	Slow-release
Opana ER	Tablet	Slow-release **Note:** tablet disruption may cause a potentially fatal overdose of oxymorphone
Oracea	Capsule	Slow-release

(continued)

Table 8.5 ORAL DOSAGE FORMS THAT SHOULD NOT BE CRUSHED (continued)

Drug Product	Dosage Forms	Dosage Reasons/Comments[2]
Oramorph SR	Tablet	Slow-release[b]
OxyContin	Tablet	Slow-release **Note:** tablet disruption may cause a potentially fatal overdose of oxycodone
Palcaps (all)	Capsule	Enteric-coated[a]
Pancrease MT	Capsule	Enteric-coated[a]
Pancrecarb MS	Capsule	Enteric-coated[a]
Pancrelipase	Capsule	Enteric-coated[a]
Panocaps	Capsule	Enteric-coated[a]
Panocaps MT	Capsule	Enteric-coated[a]
Paxil CR	Tablet	Slow-release
Pentasa	Capsule	Slow-release
PhenaVent D	Tablet	Slow-release[h]
PhenaVent LA	Capsule	Slow-release
Plendil	Tablet	Slow-release
Pre-Hist-D	Tablet	Slow-release[h]
Prevacid	Capsule	Slow-release
Prevacid SoluTab	Tablet	Orally disintegrating **Note:** do not swallow; dissolve in water only and dispense via dosing syringe or NG tube
Prevacid Suspension	Suspension	Slow-release **Note:** contains enteric-coated granules; mix with water only; not for use in NG tubes
Prilosec	Capsule	Slow-release
Prilosec OTC	Tablet	Slow-release
Pristiq	Tablet	Slow-release
Procardia XL	Tablet	Slow-release
Profen II	Tablet	Slow-release[h]
Profen II DM	Tablet	Slow-release[h]

(continued)

Table 8.5 ORAL DOSAGE FORMS THAT SHOULD NOT BE CRUSHED (*continued*)

Drug Product	Dosage Forms	Dosage Reasons/Comments[2]
Profen Forte	Tablet	Slow-release[h]
Profen Forte DM	Tablet	Slow-release[h]
Propecia	Tablet	**Note:** women who are, or may become, pregnant, should not handle crushed or broken tablets
Proquin XR	Tablet	Slow-release
Proscar	Tablet	**Note:** women who are, or may become, pregnant, should not handle crushed or broken tablets
Protonix	Tablet	Slow-release
Prozac Weekly	Tablet	Enteric-coated
Pseudo CM TR	Tablet	Slow-release[h]
Pseudovent	Capsule	Slow-release[a]
Pseudovent 400	Capsule	Slow-release[a]
Pseudovent DM	Tablet	Slow-release[h]
Pseudovent-PED	Capsule	Slow-release[a]
Pytest	Capsule	**Note:** radiopharmaceutical
QDALL	Capsule	Slow-release
QDALL AR	Capsule	Slow-release
Ralix	Tablet	Slow-release[h]
Ranexa	Tablet	Slow-release
Razadyne ER	Capsule	Slow-release
Renagel	Tablet	**Note:** tablets expand in liquid if broken or crushed
Rescon	Tablet	Slow-release[h]
Rescon JR	Tablet	Slow-release[h]
Rescon MX	Tablet	Slow-release[h]
Respa-1st	Tablet	Slow-release[h]
Respa-DM	Tablet	Slow-release[h]
Respahist	Capsule	Slow-release[a]

(*continued*)

Table 8.5 ORAL DOSAGE FORMS THAT SHOULD NOT BE CRUSHED (continued)

Drug Product	Dosage Forms	Dosage Reasons/Comments[2]
Respaire 120 SR	Capsule	Slow-release
Respaire 60 SR	Capsule	Slow-release
Resperdal M-Tab	Tablet	Orally disintegrating **Note:** do not chew or break tablet; after dissolving under tongue, tablet may be swallowed
Revlimid	Capsule	**Note:** Teratogenic potential; healthcare workers should avoid contact with capsule contents/body fluids
Ritalin LA	Capsule	Slow-release[a]
Ritalin SR	Tablet	Slow-release
R-Tanna	Tablet	Slow-release
Rythmol SR	Capsule	Slow-release
Seroquel XR	Tablet	Slow-release
Simcor	Tablet	Slow-release
Sinemet CR	Tablet	Slow-release[h]
SINUvent PE	Tablet	Slow-release[h]
Slo-Niacin	Tablet	Slow-release[h]
Solodyn	Tablet	Slow-release
Somnote	Capsule	Liquid filled
Sprycel	Tablet	film-coated **Note:** active ingredients are surrounded by a wax matrix to prevent healthcare exposure; women who are, or may become, pregnant, should not handle crushed or broken tablets
Stahist	Tablet	Slow-release
Strattera	Capsule	**Note:** capsule contents can cause ocular irritation
Sudafed 12 hour	Capsule	Slow-release[b]
Sudafed 24 hour	Capsule	Slow-release[b]

(continued)

Table 8.5 ORAL DOSAGE FORMS THAT SHOULD NOT BE CRUSHED (continued)

Drug Product	Dosage Forms	Dosage Reasons/Comments[2]
Sular	Tablet	Slow-release
Symax Duotab	Tablet	Slow-release
Symax SR	Tablet	Slow-release
Taztia XT	Capsule	Slow-release[a]
Tegretol-XR	Tablet	Slow-release
Temodar	Capsule	**Note:** If capsules are accidentally opened or damaged, rigorous precautions should be taken to avoid inhalation or contact of contents with the skin or mucous membranes[i]
Tessalon Perles	Capsule	**Note:** swallow whole; temporary local anesthesia of the oral mucosa and choking could occur
Theo-24	Capsule	Slow-release **Note:** contains beads that dissolve throughout the GI tract
Tiazac	Capsule	Slow-release[a]
Topamax	Tablet Capsule	Taste Taste[a]
Toprol XL	Tablet	Slow-release[h]
Touro CC-LD	Tablet	Slow-release[h]
Touro LA-LD	Tablet	Slow-release[h]
Tracleer	Tablet	**Note:** women who are, or may become, pregnant, should not handle crushed or broken tablets
Trental	Tablet	Slow-release
Tylenol Arthritis	Tablet	Slow-release
Ultram ER	Tablet	Slow-release **Note:** tablet disruption may cause a potentially fatal overdose of tramadol
Untphyl	Tablet	Slow-release

(continued)

Table 8.5   ORAL DOSAGE FORMS THAT SHOULD NOT BE CRUSHED (continued)

Drug Product	Dosage Forms	Dosage Reasons/Comments[2]
Urocit-K	Tablet	Wax-coated
Uroxatral	Tablet	Slow-release
Valcyte	Tablet	Teratogenic and irritant potential[i]
Verapamil SR	Tablet	Slow-release[h]
Verelan	Capsule	Slow-release[a]
Verelan PM	Capsule	Slow-release[a]
VesiCare	Tablet	Enteric coated
Videx EC	Capsule	Slow-release
Voltaren XR	Tablet	Slow-release
VoSpire ER	Tablet	Slow-release
Wellbutrin SR, XL	Tablet	Slow-release
Xanax XR	Tablet	Slow-release
Zolinza	Capsule	**Note:** irritant; avoid contact with skin or mucous membranes; avoid contact with crushed or broken tablets
ZORprin	Tablet	Slow-release
Zyban	Tablet	Slow-release
Zyflo CR	Tablet	Slow-release

[a]Capsule may be opened and the contents taken without crushing or chewing; soft food such as applesauce or pudding may facilitate administration; contents may generally be administered via nasogastric tube using an appropriate fluid provided entire contents are washed down the tube.

[b]Liquid dosage forms of the product are available; however, dose, frequency of administration, and manufacturers may differ from that of the solid dosage form.

[c]Antacids and/or milk may prematurely dissolve the coating of the tablet.

[d]The capsule may be opened and the liquid contents removed for administration.

[e]The taste of this product in a liquid form would likely be unacceptable to the patient; administration via nasogastric tube should be acceptable.

[f]Effervescent tablets must be dissolved in the amount of diluent recommended by the manufacturer.

[g]Tablets are made to disintegrate under the tongue.

[h]Tablet is scored and may be broken in half without affecting release characteristics.

[i]Skin contact may enhance tumor production; avoid direct contact.

Parenteral Administration

Parenteral delivery of medications is a common form of drug administration in hospitals, long-term care facilities, and the patient's home. Solutions delivered vascularly replenish fluid requirements, deliver medications, and supplement nutritional needs. Direct access, whether by bloodstream, spinal fluid, or peritoneal fluid, eliminates one of the human body's primary defense mechanisms. Therefore, sterility is of utmost importance when dealing with parenteral administration.

Medications intended for parenteral administration are most often delivered via subcutaneous (SC or SQ), intramuscular (IM), intradermal (ID), or intravenous (IV) route. Other less common methods of administration are also available. The following discussion describes these routes in more detail, and Figure 8.1 provides a visual display.

Not all parenteral drugs may be given by SQ, IM, ID, and IV routes. Table 8.6 lists examples of route limitations.

When using the SQ, IM, or ID route of administration, it is important to alleviate patient discomfort when possible. The smallest needle is used.

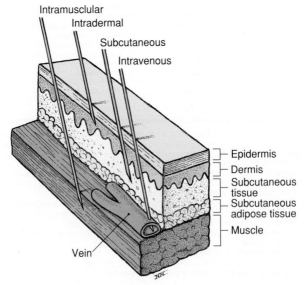

FIGURE 8.1 Diagram of various routes of drug administration.

Table 8.6 EXAMPLES OF DRUGS RESTRICTED TO SPECIFIC ROUTES OF ADMINISTRATION

Drug	SQ	IM	IV
Insulin	Yes	Yes	Yes
Midazolam	No	Yes	Yes
Erythropoietin	Yes	No	Yes
Heparin	Yes	No	Yes
Bleomycin	Yes	Yes	Yes

Needle sizes are characterized by bore size or gauge (abbreviated as "G") as well as length in inches. A smaller-gauge needle is reflected by a larger number size, with gauges ranging from 14 to 31. The length of the needle reflects the depth of the target tissue, with lengths ranging from 0.5 to 1.5 in.

Subcutaneous Routes

A SQ injection is delivered directly under the skin, between the dermal layer and the muscle. This route results in slow, steady drug absorption.[3] Absorption must occur prior to systemic circulation of the drug, which results in delayed effect.[4]

A shorter needle is used for a SQ injection. Often, a 24- to 27-G, 5/8- to 1/2-inch needle is used. The volume administered should be <1 to 2 mL. Shorter needles allow the injection to be administered at a 90-degree angle.[3] Additionally, continuous SQ infusion is possible with insulin using an insulin pump. Insulin can be delivered at a constant rate with the ability to bolus prior to a meal as needed.[5]

Intramuscular Route

An IM injection delivered directly into the muscle produces rapid drug absorption. IM injections also require a longer needle to access the muscle tissue. Again, patient comfort is of utmost importance. A typical needle used is 21- to 23-G, 1.5 in.[6] The volume of medication is determined by the age of the patient and the muscle selected. Table 8.7 specifies these limitations.[7,8]

When administering an IM injection, the needle should enter the muscle at a 90-degree angle.[3,9] If the bone is contacted, the needle should be withdrawn a small distance. Another concern regarding IM

Table 8.7 VOLUME LIMITATIONS OF INTRAMUSCULAR ADMINISTRATION

Muscle Group	Birth–1.5 y (mL)	1.5–3 y (mL)	3–6 y (mL)	6–15 y (mL)	15 y to Adult (mL)
Deltoid	Not recommended	Not recommended; if no other sites, 0.5	0.5	0.5	1
Gluteus maximus	Not recommended	Not recommended; if no other sites, 1	1.5	1.5–2	2–2.5
Ventrogluteal	Not recommended	Not recommended; if no other sites, 1	1.5	1.5–2	2–2.5
Vastus lateralis	0.5–1	1	1.5	1.5–2	2–2.5

From Howry LV, Bindler RM, Tso Y. *Pediatric Medications.* Philadelphia, PA: JB Lippincott Co; 1981:62; and Losek JD, Gyuro J. Pediatric intramuscular injections: do you know the procedure and complications? *Pediatr Emerg Care.* 1992 Apr;8(2):79–81, with permission.

administration involves the possibility of aspiration. This can be avoided by pulling the plunger of the syringe back slightly, piercing the tissue. If no blood is present, the needle is not in a vein and the medication may be administered. The typical rate of IM administration is approximately 1 mL every 10 seconds.[3]

A highly recommended method of IM administration is the Z-track method. Before injection, the skin is displaced downward approximately 1 to 2 cm. The injection is then given. After 10 seconds, the needle is removed and the skin is released. The skin movement allows the tissue to close over the site of entry after administration to decrease drug loss. This method decreases pain for the patient as well.[3]

Intradermal Route

An ID injection is delivered directly under the dermis layer of the skin resulting in a local effect. ID administration is often used for diagnostic skin testing. Selected vaccines may be administered ID as well. To administer an ID injection, a 25-G needle is inserted at a 10- to 15-degree angle into the dermis, the layer immediately below the epidermis. The volume administered is restricted to <0.5 mL for patient comfort.[3]

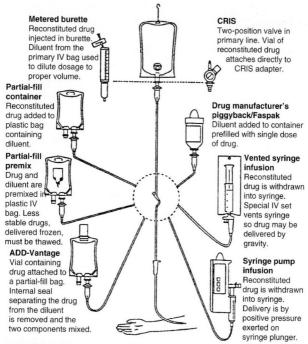

Metered burette
Reconstituted drug injected in burette. Diluent from the primary IV bag used to dilute dosage to proper volume.

Partial-fill container
Reconstituted drug added to plastic bag containing diluent.

Partial-fill premix
Drug and diluent are premixed in plastic IV bag. Less stable drugs, delivered frozen, must be thawed.

ADD-Vantage
Vial containing drug attached to a partial-fill bag. Internal seal separating the drug from the diluent is removed and the two components mixed.

CRIS
Two-position valve in primary line. Vial of reconstituted drug attaches directly to CRIS adapter.

Drug manufacturer's piggyback/Faspak
Diluent added to container prefilled with single dose of drug.

Vented syringe infusion
Reconstituted drug is withdrawn into syringe. Special IV set vents syringe so drug may be delivered by gravity.

Syringe pump infusion
Reconstituted drug is withdrawn into syringe. Delivery is by positive pressure exerted on syringe plunger.

FIGURE 8.2 Intravenous delivery systems. (Reprinted from Pleasants RA. *Intravenous Delivery Systems: Overview of Systems and Patient Care Implications.* Research Triangle Park, NC: Glaxo, Inc.; 1989, with permission.)

IV Administration

Administration of a medication directly into a vein is an IV infusion. Drug administered by rapid infusion will mix with the blood and reach maximum concentration in 4 minutes.[4]

IV administration delivers the medication into the bloodstream through direct push, intermittent, or continuous infusion methods. Direct push administration is a very short infusion, lasting a few minutes, with the intent of producing a high drug concentration swiftly. The drug is concentrated, often removed from the vial immediately before administration. Intermittent infusions involve dilute drug solutions, which are

Table 8.8 EXAMPLES OF VARIOUS METHODS OF IV INFUSION

Drug IV	Infusion	Concentration	Indication
Epinephrine	Push (1–2 min)	1 mg/mL	Cardiac emergency
Magnesium sulfate	Push (150 mg/min)	10%	Hypomagnesia
Sodium chloride	Continuous	0.9%	Hydration
Vancomycin	Intermittent (over 1 h)	≤5 mg/mL	Antibiotic
Rituximab	Intermittent (50–400 mg/h)	1–4 mg/mL	Chemotherapy

From Gahart BL, Nazareno AR. *Intravenous Medications.* 24th ed. St. Louis, MO: Mosby Elsevier; 2008, with permission.

given periodically throughout the day. These solutions may be infused over 30 to 120 minutes. Continuous infusion generally refers to large-volume (250–1,000 mL) solutions, with or without drug, running IV uninterrupted.[10] Figure 8.2 shows examples of various IV delivery systems available.

Multiple factors influence the most suitable method of infusion for a particular medication. Table 8.8 presents some examples of each method of IV infusion.[11]

Vascular Access

Vascular access for IV infusion is accomplished by using vascular access devices (VADs). Generally, either needles or catheters are used. Needles are placed peripherally and used short term. Catheters provide peripheral or central access and may be used short or long term. Peripheral catheters are placed in the dorsal metacarpal or cephalic vein in the arm, whereas central catheters span a small distance from the skin to the intravascular space. Entrance points for central catheters are usually the subclavian or external jugular vein. This additional distance from the point of entry to placement results in lower infections and longer patency. Figure 8.3 depicts catheter locations. Various types of catheters are available, each able to deliver medications and fluids to specific targets. These lines are flushed with dilute heparin or saline (0.9% sodium chloride sterile for injection) to maintain patency. Frequency of flushing catheters ranges

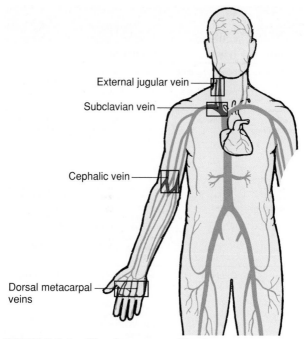

External jugular vein

Subclavian vein

Cephalic vein

Dorsal metacarpal
veins

FIGURE 8.3 Possible catheter access and location.

from twice daily to once weekly, and volumes administered range from 5 to 20 mL. Supplementary information regarding catheters is provided in Table 8.9.[6,12,13] Various catheter placements are shown in Figure 8.4.

Extravasation, which is unintentional leakage of IV fluid into interstitial tissue, is a major concern when dealing with IV administration of particular drugs. Box 8.2 lists drugs considered vesicants by many institutions. Vesicants require close monitoring due to their tendency to produce serious consequences such as necrosis and severe irritation on extravasation.[10,12,14]

Unconventional Routes

Available routes for parenteral administration of medications have evolved. In many cases, the drug can be delivered directly to the target tissue or organ. Table 8.10 describes some of these alternative routes of administration.[15,16]

Table 8.9 ISSUES RELATING TO VARIOUS TYPES OF CATHETERS

Access	Types	Comments	Use
Peripheral	Needle, butterfly needle, short plastic catheters	Catheters more comfortable than needles; flush every 6–8 h	Short-term IVs (<60 d)
Central— nontunneled	Subclavian	Short distance to exit site results in higher risk of infections; flush heparin every 12 h; single or multiple lumen	Short-term IVs (<60 d)
Central— tunneled (in-dwelling)	Hickman, Broviac, Corcath, Raaf, Hemed	Inserted centrally (surgically); long distance to exit site, lower infection; flush biweekly with heparin when not using daily; single or multiple lumen	Long-term IVs (1–2 y), total parenteral nutrition, chemotherapy
	Groshong	See above; also contains a three-position valve and closed tip; infrequent flushing; single or double lumen; flexible catheter	Infusions and blood draws
Central— PICC	Intrasil, C-PICs, Per-Q-Cath	Inserted peripherally (no surgery); increased phlebitis risk; flush every 12 h; single or multiple lumen	Long-term IVs (weeks to months)
Implantable (port)	Port-A-Cath, Infus-A-Port, Medtronic, Cath Link	Implanted SC (surgically—usually chest wall); low risk of infection; flush monthly or after draws	Long-term IVs

PICC, peripherally inserted central catheter.
From Lindley CM, Deloatch KH. *Infusion Technology Manual: A Self-Instructional Approach.* Bethesda, MD: ASHP Special Projects Division; 1993:37–50; LaRocca JC, Otto SF. *Mosby's Pocket Guide to Intravenous Therapy.* 3rd ed. St. Louis, MO: Mosby; 1997:42–60; And Abeloff MD, Armitage JO, Niederhuber JE, et al. *Clinical Oncology.* 3rd ed. Orlando, Fl: Churchill Livingstone; 2004, with permission.

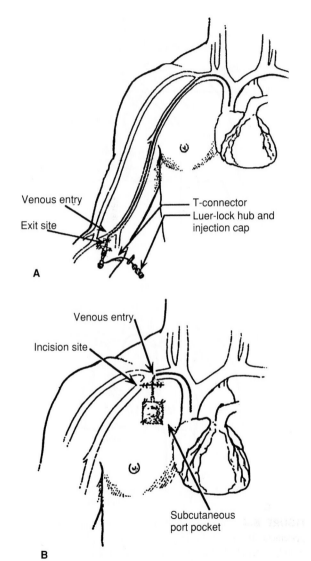

FIGURE 8.4 Catheter placements. **A:** PICC (peripherally inserted central catheter) placement. **B:** Subcutaneous port implanted in chest wall.

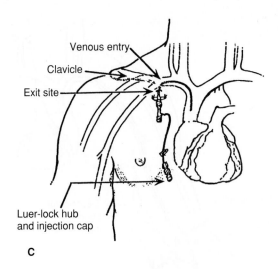

C

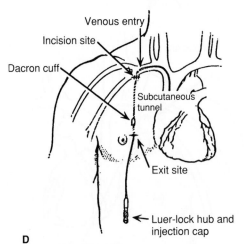

D

FIGURE 8.4 (*Continued*) **C:** Nontunneled central venous catheter placement. **D:** Tunneled central venous catheter placement. (Adapted from Wickham R. Techniques for long-term venous access. Presented at the Fifth National Conference on Cancer Nursing, ACS, with Association of Pediatric Oncology Nurses and Oncology Nursing Society, September 1987; 1988, with permission.)

> ### Box 8.2   Medications Known to Be Vesicants
>
> #### High Vesicant Potential
>
> Dactinomycin or actinomycin D   Mitomycin C
> Daunorubicin or daunomycin   Vinblastine
> Doxorubicin   Vincristine
> Epirubicin   Vindestine
> Idarubicin   Vinorelbine
> Mechlorethamine
>
> #### Low Vesicant Potential
>
> Cisplatin   Liposomal doxorubicin
> Dacarbazine   Menogaril
> Docetaxel   Mitoxantrone
> Etoposide   Oxaliplatin
> Fluorouracil   Paclitaxel
>
> *From Phillips LD. Manual of I.V. Therapeutics. 2nd ed. Philadelphia, PH: FA Davis Co; 1997: 513; LaRocca JC, Otto SF. Mosby's Pocket Guide to Intravenous Therapy. 3rd ed. St. Louis, MO: Mosby; 1997: 252; and Ener RA, Meglathery SB, Styler M. Extravasation of systemic hemato-oncological therapies. Ann Oncol. 2004;15:858–862, with permission.*

Flow Rate

When drugs are given by intermittent or continuous infusion, the flow of the solution is regulated. The rate at which the solution is administered to the patient is considered the flow rate. Flow rates vary depending on characteristics of the drug and drug concentration. It is imperative to calculate flow rates correctly to ensure that the medication is not delivered too quickly. See Chapter 12, A Pharmacy Calculations Anthology, for calculation tips. Specific information needed to calculate flow rate includes the following:

- Desired rate of infusion (mL/minute, mL/hour).
- Drug concentration (units/mL, mg/mL, g/mL).

Table 8.10 EXAMPLES OF UNCONVENTIONAL ROUTES OF ADMINISTRATION

Route	Location	Drug Treatment
Iontophoresis	Via electrical current into tissue	Corticosteroids
Intradermal	Superficial skin layer	Diagnostic test, vaccines
Intra-arterial catheter	Hepatic, celiac, or carotid artery	Chemotherapy
Intraosseous needle	Bone marrow	Emergency administration of IV drug
Intraperitoneal catheter	Peritoneal cavity	Chemotherapy
Intraspinal catheter	Epidural or intrathecal	Pain management, chemotherapy
Intraventricular catheter	Lateral ventricle of brain	Chemotherapy, antifungal, antibacterial

From West VL. Alternate routes of administration. *J Intraven Nurs*. 1998;21(4):221–231; and CDER Data Standard Manual, Route of Administration. Available at www.fda.gov/CDER/dsm/DRG/drg00301.htm. Accessed 01/10/08, with permission.

- Volume of the bag containing the drug (with or without overfill volume).
- Set size (the set is the tubing the medication flows through that is connected to the catheter inserted in the patient. It has a roller clamp and drip chamber, which control drug delivery. Set sizes are defined by drops/mL).

■ Pumps or Infusion-Controlled Devices

Parenteral infusion flow rates may be controlled by gravity or by an infusion-controlled device (pump).

- Gravity (without a controller).
  - System based on hydrostatic pressure, controlled by clamps.
  - Used for peripheral sites only.
  - Requires frequent monitoring to check drip rate.
- Infusion-controlled device.

Table 8.11 CHARACTERISTICS OF VARIOUS INFUSION-CONTROLLED DEVICES OR PUMPS

Pump Type	Mechanism	Comments	Volume	Variance
Gravity				
Controller	Gravity driven	Electronically measures and compensates drip rate; good for nonviscous solutions	No volume limits	5%–10%
Positive pressure				
Peristaltic	Tubing undergoes micropulses or constant massaging; linear or rotary pump	Inexpensive; use special sets to avoid tubing distortion	No volume limits	5%–10%
Cassette— piston	Piston actuated	Dual piston available also; special tubing required	50–100 mL	2%–5%
Cassette— syringe	Mechanical or electric	Programmable; special tubing required	≤60 mL	2–5%
Syringe	Programmable; good for slow flow rates, small volumes	≤60 mL	≤2%	
Elastomeric	Nonelectric; constant elastic pressure; flow-restricted rate	Limited pump volumes; small and portable; disposable	50–500 mL	10%–20%
Vacuum pressure	Nonelectric; constant vacuum pressure; flow-restricted rate	Specific flow rates; disposable	0.5–200 mL	Not available

From Lindley CM, Deloatch KH. *Infusion Technology Manual: A Self-Instructional Approach.* Bethesda, MD: ASHP Special Projects Division; 1993:37–50, 82–91; Capes DF, Asiimwe D. Performance of selected flow-restricting infusion devises. *Am J Health Syst Pharm.* 1998;55;351–59; and Schleis TG, Tice AD. Selecting infusion devices for use in ambulatory care. *Am J Health Syst Pharm.* 1996;53:868–877, with permission.

- Measured by various types of sensors.
- Used for central or peripheral infusion.
- Programmable, little monitoring.

Multiple forms of infusion-controlled devices are currently available. Recent technology has developed smaller, more accurate devices. Table 8.11 explains in further detail characteristics of each type of device.[6,17,18]

 Summary

As technology increases the availability of more effective and efficient dosage formulations and administration devices, the choices for delivering the right drug to the patient will expand. It is imperative to maintain a working knowledge of this area of pharmacy to ensure that patients receive high-quality care.

References

1. McPherson ML. Don't crush that tablet! *Am Pharm*. 1994;34:57–58.
2. Mitchell JF. Oral dosage forms that should not be crushed: 2000 update. *Hosp Pharm*. 2000;35:553–557.
3. Workman B. Safe injection techniques. *Nurs Stand*. 1999;13(39);47–53.
4. Turco SJ. *Sterile Dosage Forms: Their Preparation and Clinical Applications*. 4th ed. Philadelphia, PA: Lea & Febiger; 1994:7, 105.
5. Wallymahmed M. Insulin therapy in the management of type 1 and type 2 diabetes. *Nurs Stand*. 2006 Oct 18–24;21(6):50–56; quiz 58.
6. Lindley CM, Deloatch KH. *Infusion Technology Manual: A Self-Instructional Approach*. Bethesda, MD: ASHP Special Projects Division; 1993:37–50, 82–91.
7. Howry LV, Bindler RM, Tso Y. *Pediatric Medications*. Philadelphia, PA: JB Lippincott Co; 1981:62.
8. Losek JD, Gyuro J. Pediatric intramuscular injections: do you know the procedure and complications? *Pediatr Emerg Care*. 1992 Apr; 8(2):79–81.
9. Burden M. A practical guide to insulin injections. *Nurs Stand*. 1994;8(29);25–29.
10. Phillips LD. *Manual of I.V. Therapeutics*. 2nd ed. Philadelphia, PA: FA Davis Co; 1997:199–204, 208–213, 398–420, 513.
11. Gahart BL, Nazareno AR. *Intravenous Medications*. 24th ed. St. Louis, MO: Mosby Elsevier; 2008.
12. LaRocca JC, Otto SF. *Mosby's Pocket Guide to Intravenous Therapy*. 3rd ed. St. Louis, MO: Mosby; 1997:42–60, 252.
13. Abeloff MD, Armitage JO, Niederhuber JE, et al. *Clinical Oncology*. 3rd ed. Orlando, Fl: Churchill Livingstone; 2004.
14. Ener RA, Meglathery SB, Styler M. Extravasation of systemic hemato-oncological therapies. *Ann Oncol*. 2004;15:858–862.

15. West VL. Alternate routes of administration. *J Intraven Nurs*.1998;21(4);221–231.

16. CDER Data Standard Manual, Route of Administration. Available at www.fda.gov/CDER/dsm/DRG/drg00301.htm. Accessed January 10, 2008.

17. Capes DF, Asiimwe D. Performance of selected flow-restricting infusion devices. *Am J Health Syst Pharm*. 1998;55;351–359.

18. Schleis TG, Tice AD. Selecting infusion devices for use in ambulatory care. *Am J Health Syst Pharm*. 1996;53:868–877.

9 Fluid and Electrolyte Therapy

Pauline A. Cawley

This chapter provides reference information to assess each of the general approach elements included in Box 9.1. The information in this chapter must be used in the context of good clinical judgement.

Fluid Distribution within the Body

Total Body Water

- The amount of water present within the body is described as total body water (TBW). TBW for adults is estimated by using Equation 9.1.

$$\text{Total body water (L)} = \begin{array}{l} \text{Adult males: weight (kg)} \times 0.6 \\ \text{Adult females: weight (kg)} \times 0.4 \end{array} \quad (9.1)$$

- The percentage of body weight that is water declines as we age. Newborns typically have around 75% to 85% body weight as water, whereas adult males have 60% and females about 40% (variable; these estimations are not valid for obese patients or patients with larger than average muscle mass).[1]
- Most body water is housed within cells. Since adult males generally have a higher muscle cell mass than adult females, they will have a higher volume of body water (accounted for in the equation by applying a higher multiplication factor).
- TBW is used to help select an appropriate intravenous (IV) fluid as well as to provide information for fluid and electrolyte dosing.

> **Box 9.1** **General Approach to IV Fluid/Electrolyte Therapy**
>
> 1. Determine clinical goals based on specific patient.
> 2. Identify which IV fluids and/or electrolytes will assist with achieving clinical goals and make appropriate selection.
>   Consider the following:
>   - IV access (central or peripheral IV line).
>   - Oral intake capability of patient.
>   - All sources of fluids and/or electrolytes.
>   - IV fluid and electrolyte distribution characteristics.
> 3. For fluids: Determine volume needs and associated fluid rate.
>   - Consider maintenance fluid needs as well as replacement of excessive losses and requisite electrolyte content.
> 4. For electrolytes: Determine dose and administration method (oral, IV, other).
>   - Consider any electrolyte corrections necessary before assessing "true" electrolyte levels for dosing.
> 5. Monitor patient and reassess needs as clinical status changes.

Fluid Compartments and Determinants of Volume

- Figure 9.1 depicts the estimated typical distribution of TBW in the various body compartments of an adult. This information, together with an understanding of how different IV fluids distribute into different compartments, can be applied to determine the optimal fluid choices to meet particular clinical goals.
  - For example, a hypovolemic hypotensive patient requires fluid volume that will distribute by higher proportion into the intravascular space.

Determinants of Fluid Distribution
Osmolality, Osmolarity, Tonicity, and Free Water[1]

- *Osmolarity* is measured in mOsm/*kg solvent* whereas *osmolality* is measured in mOsm/*L solution*. The difference between these two terms is confusing and not consistently applied in the medical literature. Clinicians typically refer to the normal serum range for the pressure exerted across semipermeable membranes by particles in blood as 280 to 295 mOsm/L. Most commonly, this is calculated from the results of a basic metabolic panel or chem-7 using Equation 9.2, but direct lab measurement

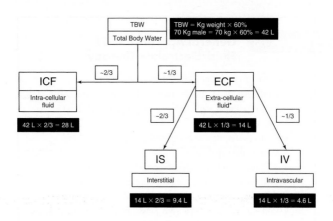

* Other extra-cellular fluid compartments not included, for diagramatic clarity; include:
connective tissues, bone water, glandular secretion, and cerebrospinal fluid [1].

FIGURE 9.1 Typical distribution of body water.

Serum osmolality (mOsm/L) $= 2 \times \text{Na} + (\text{BUN}/2.8) + (\text{Glucose}/18)$

$$\text{BUN, blood urea nitrogen; adult}$$
$$\text{reference range: } 280\text{--}295 \text{ mOsm/L}$$

(9.2)

may also be obtained. Figure 9.2 describes the mathematical interconversion between the different units that may be used clinically.

- *Tonicity* describes osmotic pressure exerted across a cell membrane by particles in plasma. Isotonicity describes equal osmotic pressure on both sides of a semipermeable membrane so there is no net movement of solvent across the membrane. Normal saline solution (NSS), 0.9% NaCl, is an isotonic solution, meaning that no net fluid is distributed into cells on administration.
  - Dextrose 5% in water (D5W) does distribute into cells (approximately two-thirds of the volume administered) and is therefore described as *free water*. Approximately 130 mL of a 1,000-mL infusion will remain in the intravascular compartment on administration.
  - NSS and lactated Ringer (LR) solution are both considered to be isotonic fluids. For each, approximately 300 to 340 mL of a 1,000-mL infusion will remain in the intravascular compartment on administration.
  - Hypotonic or hypertonic fluids may be uncomfortable or painful during the infusion and must be administered via central IV line.

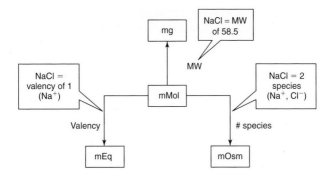

Key:
Going *with* direction of arrows: *multiply*
Going *against* direction of arrows: *divide*

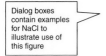

FIGURE 9.2 Unit interconversion. MW, molecular weight. (Adapted from Eric J. Mack, PhD, Loma Linda School of Pharmacy, with permission.)

- Equation 9.2 describes the major contribution of sodium toward serum osmotic pressure. The sodium load of intravenous fluids will therefore be a major determinant of the volume that remains in the IV space versus distributing to other body compartments.
- Free water describes the distribution of fluids that have neither oncotic nor colloidal pressure affecting compartment distribution. D5W is an example of a fluid that is 100% free water.

■ Intravenous Fluid Therapy

Types of IV Fluid

- Commonly used IV fluids can broadly be divided into three categories: colloids, crystalloids, and dextrose-containing fluids. Table 9.1 provides the definition of each, with example fluids. Various products containing a combination of crystalloids with dextrose are also commercially available. Fluid selection will depend on clinical goals, cost, institution formulary, and availability.

Table 9.1 COMMONLY USED IV FLUIDS

Colloid

Definition: IV fluids containing the dispersion of large molecular weight (MW) molecules

5% Albumin	• Iso-oncotic • Natural albumin product (possibility of sensitivity reaction) • Used for plasma volume expansion
25% Albumin	• Hyperoncotic • Natural albumin product • Used for fluid redistribution into the intravascular space
Hetastarch 6%	• Synthetic product • Used for plasma volume expansion • Can increase risk for bleeding • Less antigenic than dextran products
Dextran 6%	• Product derived from the bacterium *Leuconostoc mesenteroides* • Available as dextran 40, 70, or 75. Number refers to the average MW ($\times 1,000$ daltons) • Can increase risk for bleeding • Incidence of antigenic reactions increased with higher MW product

Crystalloid

Definition: IV fluids containing sodium

0.9% NaCl (normal saline solution, NSS)	• Isotonic • Used for plasma volume expansion • Can cause hyperchloremic metabolic acidosis if large volume is administered
Lactated Ringer solution (LRS)	• Isotonic • Used for plasma volume expansion • Contains lactate, which is converted by a healthy liver to bicarbonate • Contains potassium. Use with caution in patients with compromised renal function
3% NaCl	• Hypertonic • Used in patients with increased cerebral perfusion pressure due to traumatic brain injury or life-threatening hyponatremia • Extreme caution needed with this product since serum Na should not change by >10 mEq/d to avoid serious complications • Higher concentrations of NaCl solutions are available

(continued)

Table 9.1	COMMONLY USED IV FLUIDS *(continued)*
	Dextrose in water solutions
Dextrose 5% in water (D5W)	• Distributes 100% as free water • Weight per volume (w/v) solution containing 5 g dextrose in 100 mL water (or 50 g in 1 L) • Since 1 g dextrose contains 3.4 kcal, each 100 mL contains 17 kcal (or 170 kcal in 1 L)
Dextrose 10% in water (D10W)	• Distributes 100% as free water • Contains 10 g dextrose in 100 mL water (or 100 g in 1 L) • Each 100 mL contains 34 kcal (or 340 kcal in 1 L) • Often used as a step-up or step-down fluid to parenteral nutrition, or for patients who are consistently hypoglycemic

- Table 9.2 summarizes the fluid compartment distribution of various types of IV fluids.
- Figures 9.3 and 9.4 compare the compartment distribution of D5W and NSS, respectively (note that the D5W distribution figure matches Fig. 9.1 since D5W is 100% free water).
- Table 9.3 compares the healthy adult ranges for serum osmolilty and major electrolyte concentrations with those for selected IV fluids.
- Since in most cases biologic fluids can shift down concentration gradients across semipermeable membranes, the expected results from administration of a fluid containing higher concentrations of a given

Table 9.2	DISTRIBUTION OF IV FLUIDS		
Fluid	**% ICF**	**% ECF**	**Free water/L**
D5W	60	40	1,000 mL
0.45% NaCl	37	73	500 mL
D5W 0.45% NaCl	37	73	500 mL
0.9% NaCl	0	100	0 mL
154 mEq/L sodium bicarbonate (compounded solution)	0	100	0 mL
3% NaCl	0	100	−2,331 mL

ICF, intracellular fluid; ECF, extracellular fluid.

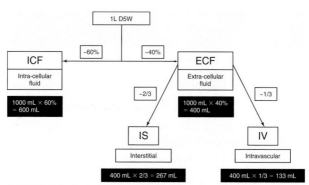

FIGURE 9.3 Typical distribution of 5% dextrose intravenous infusion.

electrolyte would include elevation of the serum electrolyte concentration. The opposite would typically occur if a relatively hypoconcentrated electrolyte-containing fluid was administered.

▸ For example, adminstration of LR, which contains 4 mEq/L potassium, to a patient with normal renal function and a serum potassium concentration of 3 mEq/L would typically result in an increase in serum potassium concentration until an equalibrium point serum concentration of around 4 mEq/L is reached (again, depending on rate of administration and clearance), with the rate of change depending on the rate of LR administration as well as the rate of potassium elimination. Giving LR to a patient with a serum potassium concentation of 5.4 mEq/L would typically result in a decrease in serum potassium until equilibrium is reached.

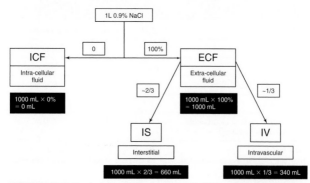

FIGURE 9.4 Typical distribution of 0.9% NaCl intravenous infusion.

Table 9.3 COMPARISON OF IV FLUID ELECTROLYTE CONTENT COMPARED TO SERUM

Fluid	Osm/L	Na$^+$ mEq/L	Cl$^+$ mEq/L	K$^+$ mEq/L	Ca2$^+$ mEq/L	Lactate[a] mEq/L
Serum	280–295	140	100	4	9	Bicarbonate 26
0.9% NaCl	308	154	154	0	0	0
LR	274	130	109	4	1.5	28
D5W	278	0	0	0	0	0

LR, lactated Ringer.
[a]Converted by healthy liver to bicarbonate.

Estimated Daily Fluid Requirements

- To estimate the daily fluid requirements for a patient, the clinical situation of the patient is the primary factor governing both volume and choice of fluid.
- General guidelines for patients without special need for fluid restriction or replacement of excessive loss are provided in Table 9.4.

Table 9.4 GENERAL GUIDELINES FOR PATIENTS WITHOUT SPECIAL NEED FOR FLUID RESTRICTION OR REPLACEMENT OF EXCESSIVE LOSS

Patient Population	Estimated Daily Fluid Requirements	Example(s)
Adults and pediatrics	Holliday Segar method[a] 100 mL/kg/d for the first 10 kg 50 mL/kg/d for the next 10 kg 20 mL/kg/d for additional weight >20 kg Add 10% for each degree of body temperature (Celsius) above normal Add extra for excessive fluid losses	8 kg child: 800 mL/d 17 kg child: 1,350 mL/d 50 kg adult: 2,100 mL/d
Adults	30–35 mL/kg/d	50 kg adult: 1,500–1,750 mL/d

[a]Segar WE, Holliday MA. The maintenance need for water in parenteral fluid therapy. *Pediatrics.* 1957;19:823–832.

Table 9.5 CALCULATING WATER DEFICIT OR EXCESS BASED ON TOTAL BODY WATER (TBW) AND SERUM SODIUM CONCENTRATION

Water Deficit	Water Excess
Water deficit (L) = normal TBW − present TBW Where normal TBW = wt in kg × 40% (female) or 60% (male) Present TBW = $\dfrac{\text{Desired Na}^+}{\text{Current Na}^+}$ × normal TBW **Note:** This equation does not account for ongoing losses such as insensible fluid loss and other sources of fluid loss.	Water excess (L) = TBW − (TBW × Observed Na$^+$/Desired Na$^+$)

From Lau A. Fluid and electrolyte disorders. In: Koda-Kimble MA, Young LY, Kradjan WA, et al., eds. *Applied Therapeutics: The Clinical Use of Drugs*. 8th ed. Philadelphia, PA: Lippincott Williams & Wilkins; 2005:12-1–12-33, with permission.

- For patients with demonstrated water deficit or excess, Table 9.5 provides associated equations to help guide volume therapy decisions.
- Estimated daily urine and insensible fluid losses are provided in Table 9.6.
- Table 9.7 includes common signs and symptoms of decreased versus increased fluid within each of the major body compartments. These can be used for both assessing the patient therapy needs and monitoring. Table 9.8 provides common renal markers of fluid status.

Table 9.6 ESTIMATED DAILY FLUID LOSS

Fluid Type	Adults	Pediatrics
Urine	• 0.5–1 mL/kg/h • ~30 mL/kg/d • ~50 mL/h	1 mL/kg/h
Insensible	~1,000 mL/d	Fever adjustment = 10% × maintenance fluid for each degree C >37°C[a]

[a]Chicella MF, Hak EB. Pediatric nutrition. In: Koda-Kimble MA, Young LY, Kradjan WA, et al., eds. *Applied Therapeutics: The Clinical Use of Drugs*. 8th ed. Philadelphia, PA: Lippincott Williams & Wilkins; 2005:97-1–97-22.

Table 9.7 ASSESSING AND MONITORING CLINICAL NEED FOR FLUID: COMMON SIGNS AND SYMPTOMS

Decreased Fluid	Increased Fluid
Total Body Water	
• Decreased body weight unrelated to changes in lean body mass • Intake and output records	• Increased body weight unrelated to changes in lean body mass • Intake and output records
Intracellular Fluid	
• Increased serum osmolality • Increased thirst sensation • Mental status changes	• Decreased serum osmolality • Decreased thirst sensation • Mental status changes
Extracellular Fluid—Interstitial	
• Dry skin and mucous membranes • Poor skin turgor • Sunken eyes • Depressed fontanelle in infants	• Peripheral or sacral edema • Pulmonary congestion (such as crackles, radiograph changes, dyspnea, hypoxia) • Ascites or other sequestered (third space) fluid
Extracellular Fluid—Intravascular	
• Decreased urine output: a sensitive indicator of intravascular volume if no organ failures are present • Oliguria • Urine chemistry: see Table 9-8 • Serum chemistry: increased values due to decreased intravascular water volume (concentration effect) • BUN:creatinine ratio >20 • Tachycardia • Signs of peripheral hypoperfusion such as increased nailbed capillary refill time • Cool temperature and color changes in extremities • Decreased level of consciousness • Orthostatic changes in pulse and blood pressure • Increased blood hematocrit and hemoglobin due to decreased intravascular water volume • Swan-Ganz catheter readings—decreased CVP, occlusion pressure, and cardiac output	• Increased urine output • Serum chemistry: decreased values due to increased intravascular water volume (dilutional effect) • S-3 heart sound • Increased CVP • Jugular venous distension • Hepatojugular reflux • Decreased blood hematocrit and hemoglobin due to increased intravascular water volume • Swan-Ganz catheter readings—increased CVP, occlusion pressure, and cardiac output

BUN, blood urea nitrogen; CVP, central venous pressure.

Table 9.8 ASSESSING FLUID STATUS WITH URINE MARKERS OF DECREASED RENAL PERFUSION

Urine specific gravity	>1.015
Urine Osm	>500
Urine Na mEq/L	<20
Fractional excretion of filtered Na (FENA) $FENA = 100 \times \dfrac{(Urine\ Na/Plasma\ Na)}{(Urine\ Cr/Plasma\ Cr)}$	<1

From Comstock TJ, Whitley KV. The kidneys. In: Lee M, ed. *Basic Skills in Interpreting Laboratory Data*. 3rd ed. Bethesda, MD: American Society of Health-System Pharmacists; 2004:233–262, with permission.

- If a patient has a large output of body fluids, it may be necessary to replace both fluid volume and the electrolytes these fluids typically contain.
- Table 9.9 provides typical volumes per day of various biologic fluids produced, with their major electrolyte concentrations. Typically, each 1 mL of fluid loss is replaced with 0.5 to 1 mL of replacement fluid.
  - For example, if a patient is experiencing large losses of fluid through vomiting, then it may be necessary to replace sodium and chloride,

Table 9.9 TYPICAL ELECTROLYTE COMPOSITION OF SELECTED BODY FLUIDS

Fluid	Volume mL/d	Na⁺ mEq/L	K⁺ mEq/L	Cl⁻ mEq/L	HCO₃⁻ mEq/L
Plasma	—	140	4	100	26
Gastric	1,500	60	10	130	0
Bile	800	145	5	100	35
Pancreatic	1,000	140	5	75	115
Small bowel	300–1,500	140	5	80	50
Sweat	500	45	4.5	60	0
Ileal	Variable; ~3,000	140	5	105	30
Cecal	Variable	60	30	40	20

Adapted from Chicella MF, Hak EB. Pediatric nutrition. In: Koda-Kimble MA, Young LY, Kradjan WA, et al., eds. *.Applied Therapeutics: The Clinical Use of Drugs*. 8th ed. Philadelphia, PA: Lippincott Williams & Wilkins; 2005:97-1–97-22, with permission.

and potentially potassium, since these three electrolytes are the major components lost. Keeping track of vomit volume may provide valuable information on replacement needs.

IV Fluids Associated with Metabolic Blood pH Alterations

- It is important to understand that IV fluid therapy can profoundly affect the blood gas status of a patient. This can be used to therapeutically treat a blood gas disorder or to prevent development or complication of an existing disorder.
- Figure 9.5 demonstrates the interelatonship between chloride and bicarbonate, as well as including the effects of an anion gap in metabolic blood gas disorders.
  - For example, an increase in chloride (from administration of a large volume of NSS, for example) will typically be reflected in a decreased bicarbonate concentration, described as a hyperchloremic metabolic acidosis).
- Table 9.10 includes the IV fluids that directly affect blood gas status. These fluids may be used therapeutically for this purpose, but they have the potential to cause or complicate an exisiting disorder.

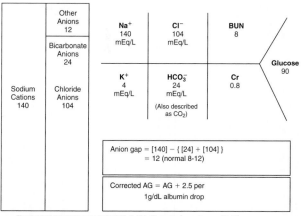

Plasma pH 7.4 (normal range: 7.35-7.45, P$_a$CO$_2$ 40 mm Hg (normal range: 35-45)

FIGURE 9.5 Diagrammatic relationship between serum chloride, bicarbonate and anion gap. BUN, blood urea nitrogen; AG, anion gap.

Table 9.10 IV FLUIDS THAT CAN AFFECT BLOOD GAS STATUS

	Affect on Metabobolic Acid-Base Status	Notes
Sodium chloride	• Can cause hyperchloremic metabolic acidosis	
Sodium bicarbonate	• Can cause metabolic alkalosis • Can be used to increase alkalinity of blood	• HCO_3^- deficit (mEq) = [24 − measured HCO_3^-] × TBW • Typically provide ~50% of the calculated deficit in first 24 h. Caution not to cause rapid changes in CNS pH and/or sodium concentration (not >12 mEq/L Na change in 24 h • Careful monitoring required • May induce intracellular acidosis. Not recommended for use when arterial pH is >7.15
Hydrochloric acid	• Can cause metabolic acidosis • Can be used to increase acidity of blood	• HCl (mmol) = [103 − measured Cl^- in mmol/L] × body weight in kg × 0.2 • Typically administer 50% over 12–24 h to lower pH by 0.2 • Alternative dosing: 0.1–0.2 mmol/kg/h, with frequent monitoring of ABG and electrolytes • Must administer via central line • Use 0.1 N solution (10 mmol HCl/L) in D5W
THAM (tromethamine; trihydroxymethyl-aminomethane)	• Can be used to buffer acidity of blood as an alternative to sodium bicarbonate • Does not increase serum sodium, bicarbonate, or PCO_2	• THAM mL = body weight in kg × base deficit (mEq/L) × 1.1 • Factor of 1.1 accounts for about a 10% reduction in buffering capacity due to the presence of sufficient acetic acid to lower pH of the 0.3 M solution to approximately 8.6 • Additional dosing is determined by serial measurement of base deficit

TBW, total body weight; M, molar solution; CNS, central nervous system; ABG, arterial blood gases.
From Lau A. Fluid and electrolyte disorders. In: Koda-Kimble MA, Young LY, Kradjan WA, et al., eds. *Applied Therapeutics: The Clinical Use of Drugs*. 8th ed. Philadelphia, PA: Lippincott Williams & Wilkins; 2005:12-1–12-33; Dellinger RP, Carlet JM, Masur H, et al. Surviving Sepsis Campaign guidelines for management of severe sepsis and septic shock. *Crit Care Med.* 2004 Mar;32(3):858–873; Metabolic Alkalosis: Acid-Base Regulation and Disorders: Merck Manual Professional Website. Available at www.merck.com/mmpe/sec12/ch157/ch157d.html. Accessed March 18, 2008; and Tham Solution [package insert]. Abbott Park, IL: Abbott Laboratories; 2000; with permission.

Table 9.11 GOAL-BASED APPROACH TO PATIENT FLUID THERAPY

What Is the Therapeutic Goal for Your Patient?	Possible Approach(es)
Restore circulating volume	• Provide fluid that will optimize intravascular volume (examples: NSS, LR)
Correct electrolyte disorders	• Treat life-threatening hyperelectrolyte or hypoelectrolyte disorders as first priority • Consider need for parenteral vs. enteral therapy depending on patient status • Treat any underlying causes including adjustment of any sources of exogenous electrolytes if elevated (such as electrolyte containing IV fluids), or agents contributing to hypo conditions (such as binding agents)
Correct acid-base disorder	• Treat the underlying cause (examples: Diarrhea can cause metabolic acidosis, vomiting can cause metabolic alkalosis, blunting of respiratory drive with agents such as benzodiazepines or opiates can cause respiratory acidosis) • Consider effects of any IV fluids administered (examples: NSS can contribute to hyperchloremic metabolic acidosis, sodium bicarbonate solutions can contribute to metabolic alkalosis) • THAM may be an option for patients with severe metabolic acidosis intolerant of sodium bicarbonate solution (due to high sodium load, increased PCO_2, or pH outside recommended range for use of this fluid)
Replace anticipated water and electrolyte losses	• Provide fluid and electrolyte therapy as necessary during the course of therapy • Consider options for fluid and electrolyte combination versus providing fluid separately from electrolyte therapy • Adjustments are based on repeated assessments of patient status
Remove excessive fluid	• Consider need for diuretic therapy, depending on renal function • Adjust any fluids currently being administered

Clinical Goals of IV Fluid Therapy

- The therapeutic plan relating to fluids for a patient will ultimately depend on the clinical goals.
- Table 9.11 identifies a goal-based approach to patient fluid therapy.

Electrolytes

Electrolyte Reference Ranges

- Figure 9.6 provides reference ranges for adult serum electrolytes in the commonly used medical format. Table 9.12 provides pediatric reference ranges for serum electrolytes.

Electrolyte Therapies

- Table 9.13 provides any correction factors that should be accounted for prior to providing pharmacotherapy, as well homeostasis factors to consider.
- Table 9.14 provides pharmacotherapy summaries for electrolyte level reduction and replacement.
- Table 9.15 contains selected medications associated with hypoelectrolyte or hyperelectrolyte disorders.

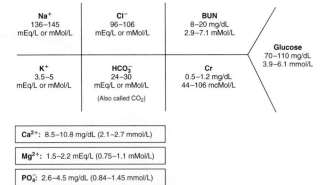

Na^+ 136–145 mEq/L or mMol/L	Cl^- 96–106 mEq/L or mMol/L	BUN 8–20 mg/dL 2.9–7.1 mMol/L	
			Glucose 70–110 mg/dL 3.9–6.1 mmol/L
K^+ 3.5–5 mEq/L or mMol/L	HCO_3^- 24–30 mEq/L or mMol/L (Also called CO_2)	Cr 0.5–1.2 mg/dL 44–106 mcMol/L	

Ca^{2+}: 8.5–10.8 mg/dL (2.1–2.7 mmol/L)

Mg^{2+}: 1.5–2.2 mEq/L (0.75–1.1 mMol/L)

PO_4^-: 2.6–4.5 mg/dL (0.84–1.45 mmol/L)

FIGURE 9.6 Adult reference ranges for serum electrolytes. BUN, blood urea nitrogen. (From Lau A. Fluid and electrolyte disorders. In: Koda-Kimble MA, Young LY, Kradjan WA, et al. eds. *Applied Therapeutics: The Clinical Use of Drugs.* 8th ed. Philadelphia, PA: Lippincott Williams & Wilkins; 2005:12-1–12-33, with permission.)

Table 9.12 INFANT AND PEDIATRIC ELECTROLYTE REFERENCE RANGES

	Premature Neonates	Newborns	Infants 1 mo–1 y	Children 1–12 y	Adults
Na^+	48 h life: 128–148 mEq/L or mol/L	133–146 mEq/L or mol/L	139–146 mEq/L or mol/L	138–145 mEq/L or mol/L	136–145 mEq/L or mol/L
K^+	48 h life: 3.0–6.0 mEq/L	3.7–5.9 mEq/L or mol/L	4.1–5.3 mEq/L or mol/L	3.4–4.7 mEq/L or mol/L	3.5–5 mEq/L or mol/L
Cr	0.3–1.0 mg/dL (27–88 μmol/L)		0.2–0.4 mg/dL (18–35 μmol/L)	0.3–0.7 mg/dL (27–62 μmol/L)	0.5–1.2 mg/dL (44–106 μmol/L)
Ca^{2+}	3–24 h life: 9.0–10.6 mg/dL (2.3–2.65 mol/L) 24–48 h life: 7.0–12.0 (1.75–3.0 mol/L) 4–7 d: 9.0–10.9 mg/dL (2.2–2.73 mol/L)	8.8–0.8 mg/dL (2.2–2.7 mol/L)	8.5–10.8 mg/dL (2.1–2.7 mol/L)		
Mg^{2+}	0–6 d: 1.2–2.6 mEq/L (0.48–1.05 mmol/L)	7 d–2 y: 1.6–2.6 mEq/L (0.65–1.05 mmol/L) 2–14 y: 1.5–2.3 mEq/L (0.6–0.95 mmol/L)	1.5–2.2 mEq/L (0.75–1.1 mmol/L)		
PO_4	4.8–8.2 mg/dL (1.55–2.65 mmol/L)	1–3 y: 3.8–6.5 mg/dL (1.55–2.1 mmol/L) 4–11 y: 3.7–5.6 mg/dL (1.2–1.8 mol/L) 12–15 y: 2.9–5.4 mg/dL (0.95–1.75 mol/L)	2.6–4.5 mg/dL (0.84–1.45 mmol/L)		

From Kraus, D. Interpreting pediatric laboratory data. In: Lee M, ed. *Basic Skills in Interpreting Laboratory Data*. 3rd ed. Bethesda, MD: American Society of Health-System Pharmacists; 2004;51–80, with permission.

Table 9.13 SELECT ADULT SERUM ELECTROLYTE RDI, REFERENCE RANGES, CORRECTION FACTORS, AND HOMEOSTASIS

	Serum Concentration	Lab Value Correction Factors	Recommended Daily Intake (RDI)	Homeostasis
Sodium (Na^+)	136–145 mEq/L or mmol/L	1. Correct for hyperglycemia (falsely low sodium due to lab error) 2. For every serum glucose of 100 >100, add 1.7 to the serum sodium $Na_{corr} = [(Glucose - 100)/100 \times 1.7$ mEq/L] + Na_{uncorr}	PO: • Variable; 50–100 mEq IV: • Per individual patient	• Antidiuretic hormone (ADH) • Renin-angiotensin-aldosterone system (RAAS)
Potassium (K^+)	3.5–5 mEq/L or mmol/L	• Correct for metabolic acidosis or alkalosis (pseudohyperkalemia as K^+ shifts from cells into the IV fluid (IVF) in exchange for hydrogen ions in acidemia; opposite effect seen with alkalemia) • For every 0.1 pH <7.4, deduct 0.6 from the lab reported K. For every 0.1 pH >7.4, add 0.6 to the lab reported K—see equation below: • $K_{corr} = [(7.4 - pH)/0.1 \times 0.6$ mEq/L] + K_{uncorr}	PO: • 50–100 mEq IV: • Per individual patient • Average 0.5–1.2 mEq/kg/d	• Renal elimination • Aldosterone • Transcellular distribution ($Na^+/K^+/$ ATPase pump) • Metabolic plasma pH changes • Beta-adrenergic (particularly beta-2) receptor stimulation • Insulin
Magnesium (Mg^{2+})	1.5–2.2 mEq/L (0.75–1.1 mmol/L)	N/A	Based on elemental magnesium PO: • 360 mg • 30 mEq • 15 mmol	Parathyroid hormone (PTH) • 1 Alpha, 25-dihydroxy-vitamin D • Renal elimination • Mineralocorticoids • Glucagon

Calcium (Ca^{2+})	8.5–10.8 mg/dL (2.1–2.7 mmol/L)	• Correct for hypoalbuminemia: • Most accurate: Obtain an ionized calcium	IV: • 120 mg • 10 mEq • 5 mmol • (~1/3 PO RDI) Based on elemental calcium PO: • 800–1,500 mg IV: • 200 mg • 10 mEq • 5 mmol • (~1/4 of PO RDI) calcium daily	• PTH • Vitamin D • Calcitonin
Phosphate ($PO4^-$)	2.6–4.5 mg/dL (0.84–1.45 mmol/L)	N/A	PO: • 1,000 mg • 30 mmol IV: • Same as PO	• Calcium concentration • PTH • Thyroid hormone • Vitamin D • Thyrocalcitonin • Dietary intake • Renal elimination

From Lau A. Fluid and electrolyte disorders. In: Koda-Kimble MA, Young LY, Kradjan WA, et al., eds. *Applied Therapeutics: The Clinical Use of Drugs.* 8th ed. Philadelphia, PA: Lippincott Williams & Wilkins; 2005:12-1–12-3; Lau A, Chan LN. Electrolytes, other minerals, and trace elements. In: Lee M, ed. *Basic Skills in Interpreting Laboratory Data.* 3rd ed. Bethesda, MD: American Society of Health-System Pharmacists; 2004:183–232; Dickerson RN. Guidelines for the intravenous management of hypophosphatemia, hypomagnesemia, hypokalemia, and hypocalcemia. *Hosp Pharm.* 2001;36:1201–1208; Baran DR, Aronin N. Disorders of mineral metabolism. In: Irwin RS, Rippe JM, eds. *Intensive Care Medicine.* 6th ed. Philadelphia, PA: Lippincott Williams & Wilkins; 2008:1287–1293; Cohen AJ. Physiologic concepts in the management of renal, fluid, and electrolyte disorders in the intensive care unit. In: Irwin RS, Rippe JM, eds. *Intensive Care Medicine.* 6th ed. Philadelphia, PA: Lippincott Williams & Wilkins; 2008:867–883; Black RM, Noroian GO. Disorders of plasma sodium and plasma potassium. In: Irwin RS, Rippe JM, eds. *Intensive Care Medicine.* 6th ed. Philadelphia, PA: Lippincott Williams & Wilkins; 2008:898–925; and Driscoll DF, Bistrian BR. Parenteral and enteral nutrition in the intensive care unit. In: Irwin RS, Rippe JM, eds. *Intensive Care Medicine.* 6th ed. Philadelphia, PA: Lippincott Williams & Wilkins; 2008:2186–2201, with permission.

Table 9.14 HYPERELECTROLYTE AND HYPOELECTROLYTE THERAPY

Dosing weight for electrolyte therapy:
- Use current body weight (CBW) unless patient is >130% ideal body weight (IBW), in which case, use adjusted body weight (AdjBW):
- $AdjBW = [0.25 \times (CBW - IBW)] + IBW$

Potassium (K$^+$)

Hyperkalemia (Assess for pseudohyperkalemia from metabolic acidosis or lab sample hemolysis.)

Signs and symptoms	• Parashthesias • Weakness • Peaked T waves on electrocardiogram (ECG)

Treatment	Shift K:
	1. Ca/glucose/insulin combination
	   a. 10 mL 10% calcium gluconate IV over 3 min (to antagonize cardiac cell effects of hyperkalemia, need cardiac monitoring), 50 mL of 50% glucose IV (unless hyperglycemic), 10 units SQ/IV fast-acting insulin
	2. Albuterol
	   a. (20 mg in 4 mL NSS inhaled nasally for 10 min, or 0.5 mg IV)
	3. Increase pH by providing bicarbonate
	   a. 45 mEq IV over 5 min (variable effect on pH)
	Remove from body
	1. Loop or thiazide diuretic
	   a. Unpredictable response, particularly in renal insufficiency. Not recommend as primary therapy
	2. Sodium polysterene sulfonate exchange resin
	   a. 1 g resin binds 0.5–1 mEq K$^+$ in exchange for Na$^+$
	   b. 20 g PO with 100 mL sorbitol solution (prevent constipation)
	   c. 50 g PR with 50 mL 70% sorbitol and 100 mL tap water. Retained in colon for 120–180 min
	3. Hemodialysis

Monitoring	• Patients require careful monitoring for hyperkalemia, including:
	  ○ Telemetry monitoring
	  ○ Serum potassium level monitoring
	  ○ Signs and symptoms such as weakness and parasthesias.

Notes	• Do not forget to discontinue all sources of potassium while treating a patient for hyperkalemia, such as:
	  ○ Lactated Ringer or other potassium-containing IV fluid
	  ○ Enteral or parenteral feedings
	                  (continued)

Table 9.14 HYPERELECTROLYTE AND HYPOELECTROLYTE THERAPY *(continued)*

Hypokalemia

Signs and symptoms	• ST-segment depression on ECG • QRS widening, PR prolongation • Hypotension • Decreased release of insulin • Decreased release of aldosterone • Cramps • Areflexia • Weakness • Increased risk of digoxin toxicity (for patients on digoxin)

Treatment	Serum K (mEq/L)	KCl Dose (mEq)	Monitoring
• Check Mg and treat any deficiency (often difficult to correct low potassium until Mg is corrected) • BMP, basal metabolic profile	3.5–3.9	Consider giving 40 mEq × 1	BMP and Mg next AM
	3.0–3.4	40 mEq × 2	BMP and Mg next AM Consider stat K 2 h after second dose
	2.0–2.9	40 mEq × 3	Stat K after second dose, reassess (may need an additional 1–2 doses. Check serum Mg

Notes	• Check Mg and treat any deficiency (often difficult to correct low potassium until Mg is corrected)
	• Reduce dose in renal impairment (usually by ~50% depending on renal function and need)
	• Potassium acetate and potassium phosphates are alternative salt forms to chloride for patients who are hyperchloremic. Each requires sterile preparation (not commercially available as premix)
	  ○ Acetate is converted to bicarbonate: 1 mEq acetate provides 1 mEq potassium
	  ○ 1 mmol phoshate provides 1.47 mEq potassium
	• Maximum rate of adminstration and concentration:
	  Peripheral IV—10 mEq/h; 0.1 mEq/mL
	  Central IV—20 mEq/h; 0.4 Eq/mL
	  Must be administered by IV infusion *(do not use IV push)*

(continued)

Table 9.14 HYPERELECTROLYTE AND
HYPOELECTROLYTE THERAPY
(continued)

	• Oral potassium replacement products:
	  ○ Potassium chloride powder for reconstitution: 20 mEq dissolved in 120 mL water
	  ○ Potassium bicarbonate effervescent tablet: 25 mEq dissolved in 120 mL water
	  ○ Potassium chloride liquid: 1.33 mEq/mL diluted in water or juice for palatability

Magnesium (Mg²⁺)

Hypermagnesemia

Signs and symptoms

Serum Magnesium Concentration	Possible Signs and Symptoms
2–5 mEq/L	• Bradycardia • Sweating • Nausea and vomiting • Decreased ability to clot
6–9 mEq/L	• Decreased deep tendon reflexes • Drowsiness
10–15 mEq/L	• Flaccid paralysis • Increased PR and QRS intervals
>15 mEq/L	• Respiratory distress • Asystole

Treatment	• 10 mL 10% calcium gluconate in 50 mL D5W IV • Repeat as needed, serum calcium not to exceed 11 mg/dL
Monitoring	• If patient has received exogenous source of magnesium, note that the true serum level may not be observed until ≤48 h after discontinuation due to tissue redistribution
Notes	• May not see clinical signs and symptoms of hypermagnesemia until level exceeds 5 mEq/L (2.5 mmol/L)

(continued)

Table 9.14 HYPERELECTROLYTE AND
HYPOELECTROLYTE THERAPY
(continued)

Hypomagnesemia	
Signs and symptoms	• Central nervous system (CNS) excitability • Hypokalemia

Treatment			
	Serum Mg (mg/dL):	**Magnesium IV Dose**	**Magnesium PO Dose**
	1.6–1.8 1–1.5	0.05 g/kg 0.1 g/kg	400–800 mg magnesium oxide daily—QID as tolerated
	<1	0.15 g/kg	Use IV

Monitoring	• Succesful treatment of hypomagnesemia typically takes several days since it usually takes ~48 h for Mg to redistribute in body tissues. Checking Mg level prior to 48 h should be undertaken with the understanding that the measured value will be falsely high until redistribution has been completed

Notes	• Reduce dose in renal impairment (usually by
	~50% depending on renal function and need)
	• Rate of administration for IV infusion: not to
	exceed 8 mEq/h (1g Mg sulfate per hour);
	otherwise the renal threshold will be
	exceeded, resulting in dispoportional
	excretion in patients with good renal function.
	• Suggested concentration: 10 mg/mL
	• Oral magnesium replacement products:
	  ○ Magnesium oxide: 400-mg tablets contain
	    241 mg elemental magnesium
	  ○ Magnesium gluconate: 1,000 mg/5 mL
	    contains 58.5 mg elemental magnesium
	  ○ Oral magnesium can cause diarrhea

Calcium (Ca^{2+})	

Hypercalemia	
Signs and symptoms	• Obtundation • Confusion • Lethargy • Decreased deep tendon reflexes • Myalgias • Decreased muscle strength • Shortened QT interval on ECG

(continued)

Table 9.14 HYPERELECTROLYTE AND HYPOELECTROLYTE THERAPY (continued)

Treatment	Increase renal elimination
	• Hydration with NSS to stimulate diuresis (4–6 L NSS to achieve goal urine output of 3–5 L in 24 h); can also administer furosemide, 40–80 mg IV every 1 to 2 h, to avoid fluid overload)
	Shift Ca^{2+} into bone
	1. Calcitonin
	2. Bisphosphonates
	  a. Etidronate disodium 7.5 mg/kg IV every 8 h (with NSS hydration)
	  b. Pamidronate disodium, 15 mg in 250 mL NSS once daily
	  c. Gallium nitrate, 200 mg/m² continuous infusion for 5 days (with NSS hydration; avoid aminoglycosides ≥48 h before or after administration)

Monitoring	• Serum calcium, magnesium, phosphorus, creatinine, albumin • Use of ionized calcium is preferred in acutely ill patients to corrected calcium calculations
Hypocalemia Signs and symptoms	• Parathesias • Tetany • Positive Chvostek/Trousseau (suggestive) • Increased QT interval on ECG

Treatment	Ionized Calcium (mmol/L):	Dose Calcium Gluconate IV
	1–1.12	1–2 g
	0.9–0.99	2 g
	0.89–0.89	3 g
	Administration: Mix in 100–250 mL NSS or D5W. Rate: 1–2 g/h	

Monitoring	• Check serum Mg since hypomagnesemia can induce hypocalemia • Recheck serum Ca 2–24 h after dose
Notes	• Serum calcium falls ~0.8 mg/dL for every 1 g/dL fall in serum albumin <4 • Use of ionized calcium is preferred in acutely ill patients to corrected calcium calculations

(continued)

Table 9.14 HYPERELECTROLYTE AND
HYPOELECTROLYTE THERAPY
(continued)

	• Doses are provided as calcium gluconate. For medication safety, it is important to note the different elemental calcium content between calcium gluconate and chloride:
	○ Gluconate: 1 g (10 mL) = 93 mg (4.65 mEq) Ca^{2+}
	○ Chloride: 1 g (10 mL) = 273 mg (13.6 mEq) Ca^{2+}
	• Oral calcium replacement products
	• Calcium carbonate tablet: 1,250 mg contains 500 mg elemental calcium (40%)
	○ Calcium carbonate chewable tablet: 750 mg contains 300 mg elemental calcium (40%)
	○ Calcium carbonate suspension: 1,250 mg/5 mL contains 500 mg elemental calcium/5 mL (40%)
	○ Calcium glubionate syrup: 1,800 mg/5 mL contains 126 mg elemental calcium/5 mL (6.5%)

Phosphate (PO_4^-)

Hyperphosphatemia

Signs and symptoms
Treatment (Based on end-stage renal disease [ESRD] studies; adjust dose to achieve goal level)

Increased risk of ectopic calcification when serum calcium and phosphorus exceed 55 mg^2/dL^2

Per Meal Initial Dose	Phos mg/dL		
	>5.5–<7.5	≥7.5–<9	≥9
Calcium acetate, 667 mg tab	1	2	3
Sevelemar, 400 mg tab	2	3	4
Sevelemar, 800 mg tab	1	2	2

Monitoring | Serum phosphorous, calcium, and creatinine

Hypophosphatemia

Signs and symptoms

• Decreased mentation
• Weakness
• Cardiomyopathy
• Tachypnea
• Osteomalacia
• Decreased insulin sensitivity
• Dysfunction of red blood cells, white blood cells, and platelets

(continued)

Table 9.14 HYPERELECTROLYTE AND HYPOELECTROLYTE THERAPY (continued)

Treatment	Serum Phosphorous (mg/dL):	Dose Sodium or Potassium Phosphate IV
	2.3–3	0.16 mmol/kg
	1.6–2.2	0.32 mmol/kg
	<1.6	0.64 mmol/kg
	Administration: Mix in 100–250 mL NSS or D5W. Rate: maximum of 7.5 mmol/h	
Monitoring	• Serum phosphorus, calcium, creatinine, potassium • 9.15 SSRI = selective serotonin reuptake inhibitor	

Notes	• Use sodium phosphate if serum K^+ is >4 mEq/L
	• Each 3 mmol IV phosphate salt contains either 4.4 mEq K^+ or 4 mEq Na^+
	• Reduce dose in renal impairment (usually by ~50% depending on renal function and need)
	• Oral phosphorous replacement products:
	  ○ Potassium and sodium phospate powder contains 8 mmol phosphorous, 7.1 mEq K, and 7.1 mEq Na per packet; dissolve in 75 mL water
	  ○ Potassium phosphate powder contains 8 mmol phosphorus and 14.25 mEq K per packet; dissolve in 75 mL water
	  ○ Sodium phosphate oral solution contains 4.14 mmol phosphorus/mL and 4.8 mEq of Na per mL; dilute in 120 mL water
	  ○ Oral phoshate can cause diarrhea	

Lau A. Fluid and electrolyte disorders. In: Koda-Kimble MA, Young LY, Kradjan WA, et al., eds. *Applied Therapeutics: The Clinical Use of Drugs.* 8th ed. Philadelphia, PA: Lippincott Williams & Wilkins; 2005:12-1–12-3; Lau A, Chan LN. Electrolytes, other minerals, and trace elements. In: Lee M, ed. *Basic Skills in Interpreting Laboratory Data.* 3rd ed. Bethesda, MD: American Society of Health-System Pharmacists; 2004:183–232; Dickerson RN. Guidelines for the intravenous management of hypophosphatemia, hypomagnesemia, hypokalemia, and hypocalcemia. *Hosp Pharm.* 2001;36:1201–1208; Brown KA, Dickerson RN, Morgan LM, et al. A new graduated dosing regimen for phosphorus replacement in patients receiving nutrition support. *JPEN J Parenter Enteral Nutr.* 2006;30:209–214; Baran DR, Aronin N. Disorders of mineral metabolism. In: Irwin RS, Rippe JM, eds. *Intensive Care Medicine.* 6th ed. Philadelphia, PA: Lippincott Williams & Wilkins; 2008:1287–1293; Cohen AJ. Physiologic concepts in the management of renal, fluid, and electrolyte disorders in the intensive care unit. In: Irwin RS, Rippe JM, eds. *Intensive Care Medicine.* 6th ed. Philadelphia, PA: Lippincott Williams & Wilkins; 2008:867–883; Black RM, Noroian GO. Disorders of plasma sodium and plasma potassium. In: Irwin RS, Rippe JM, eds. *Intensive Care Medicine.* 6th ed. Philadelphia, PA: Lippincott Williams & Wilkins; 2008:898–925; Driscoll DF, Bistrian BR. Parenteral and enteral nutrition in the intensive care unit. In: Irwin RS, Rippe JM, eds. *Intensive Care Medicine.* 6th ed. Philadelphia, PA: Lippincott Williams & Wilkins; 2008:2186–2201; and Renagel [package insert]. Cambridge, MA: Genzyme Corporation; 1998, with permission.

Table 9.15 SELECT MEDICATIONS ASSOCIATED WITH ELECTROLYTE DISORDERS

	Drugs Associated with Hyperelectrolyte Condition	**Drugs Associated with Hypoelectrolyte Condition**
Sodium (Na^+)	• Sodium polysterene sulfonate exchange resin • Sodium (in IV fluids, parenteral and enteral nutrition) • Sodium bicarbonate	• Diuretics—loops, thiazides SSRIs
Potassium (K^+)	• Angiotensin-converting enzyme inhibitors (ACEI) • Beta-adrenergic antagonists • Dapsone • Diuretics—K^+-sparing (amiloride, spirinolactone, triamterene) • Heparin • IV fluids containing K^+ • Nonsteroidal anti-inflammatory drugs (NSAIDs) • Penicillin (K^+ salt form) • Potassium (in IV fluids, parenteral and enteral nutrition) • Trimethoprim	• Acetazolamide • Amphotericin B • Beta-adrenergic agonists • Cisplatin • Corticosteroids • Diuretics—thiazides, loops • Insulin • Laxative abuse • Penicillins
Magnesium (Mg^{2+})	• Magnesium-containing antacids and bowel evacuant preparations	• Aminoglycosides • Cisplatin • Ethanol • Loop diuretics
Phosphate ($PO4^-$)	• Phosphate-containing bowel evacuation preparations	• Antacids (containing aluminum, magnesium, and calcium) • Epinephrine • Insulin • Loop diuretics • Sevalemer • Sucralfate • Thiazide diuretics
Calcium (Ca^{2+})	• Androgenic hormones • Calcium (in antacids and supplements) • Estrogen • Lithium • Progesterone • Tamoxifen • Thiazide diuretics	• Bisphosphonates • Calcitonin • Glucocorticoids • Loop diuretics • Plicamycin

Lau A. Fluid and electrolyte disorders. In: Koda-Kimble MA, Young LY, Kradjan WA, et al., eds. *Applied Therapeutics: The Clinical Use of Drugs.* 8th ed. Philadelphia, PA: Lippincott Williams & Wilkins; 2005:12-1–12-3; Lau A, Chan LN. Electrolytes, other minerals, and trace elements. In: Lee M, ed. *Basic Skills in Interpreting Laboratory Data.* 3rd ed. Bethesda, MD: American Society of Health-System Pharmacists; 2004:183–232; Dickerson RN. Guidelines for the intravenous management of hypophosphatemia, hypomagnesemia, hypokalemia, and hypocalcemia. *Hosp Pharm.* 2001;36:1201–1208; Baran DR, Aronin N. Disorders of mineral metabolism. In: Irwin RS, Rippe JM, eds. *Intensive Care Medicine.* 6th ed. Philadelphia, PA: Lippincott Williams & Wilkins; 2008:1287–1293; and Black RM, Noroian GO. Disorders of plasma sodium and plasma potassium. In: Irwin RS, Rippe JM, eds. *Intensive Care Medicine.* 6th ed. Philadelphia, PA: Lippincott Williams & Wilkins; 2008:898–925, with permission.

References

1. Lau A. Fluid and electrolyte disorders. In: Koda-Kimble MA, Young LY, Kradjan WA, et al., eds. *Applied Therapeutics: The Clinical Use of Drugs*. 8th ed. Philadelphia, PA: Lippincott Williams & Wilkins; 2005:12-1-12-33.

2. Lau A, Chan LN. Electrolytes, other minerals, and trace elements. In: Lee M, ed. *Basic Skills in Interpreting Laboratory Data*. 3rd ed. Bethesda, MD: American Society of Health-System Pharmacists; 2004:183–232.

3. Segar WE, Holliday MA. The maintenance need for water in parenteral fluid therapy. *Pediatrics*. 1957;19:823–832.

4. Chicella MF, Hak EB. Pediatric nutrition. In: Koda-Kimble MA, Young LY, Kradjan WA, et al., eds. *.Applied Therapeutics: The Clinical Use of Drugs*. 8th ed. Philadelphia, PA: Lippincott Williams & Wilkins; 2005:97-1-97-22.

5. Comstock TJ, Whitley KV. The kidneys. In: Lee M, ed. *Basic Skills in Interpreting Laboratory Data*. 3rd ed. Bethesda, MD: American Society of Health-System Pharmacists; 2004:233–262.

6. Dellinger RP, Carlet JM, Masur H, et al. Surviving Sepsis Campaign guidelines for management of severe sepsis and septic shock. *Crit Care Med*. 2004 Mar;32(3):858–873.

7. Metabolic Alkalosis: Acid-Base Regulation and Disorders: Merck Manual Professional Website. Available at www.merck.com/mmpe/sec12/ch157/ch157d.html. Accessed March 18, 2008.

8. Tham Solution [package insert]. Abbott Park, IL: Abbott Laboratories; 2000.

9. Kraus D. Interpreting pediatric laboratory data. In: Lee M, ed. *Basic Skills in Interpreting Laboratory Data*. 3rd ed. Bethesda, MD: American Society of Health-System Pharmacists; 2004:51–80.

10. Dickerson RN. Guidelines for the intravenous management of hypophosphatemia, hypomagnesemia, hypokalemia, and hypocalcemia. *Hosp Pharm*. 2001;36:1201–1208.

11. Brown KA, Dickerson RN, Morgan LM, et al. A new graduated dosing regimen for phosphorus replacement in patients receiving nutrition support. *JPEN J Parenter Enteral Nutr*. 2006;30:209–214.

12. Baran DR, Aronin N. Disorders of mineral metabolism. In: Irwin RS, Rippe JM, eds. *Intensive Care Medicine*. 6th ed. Philadelphia, PA: Lippincott Williams & Wilkins; 2008:1287–1293.

13. Cohen AJ. Physiologic concepts in the management of renal, fluid, and electrolyte disorders in the intensive care unit. In: Irwin RS, Rippe JM, eds. *Intensive Care Medicine*. 6th ed. Philadelphia, PA: Lippincott Williams & Wilkins; 2008:867–883.

14. Black RM, Noroian GO. Disorders of plasma sodium and plasma potassium. In: Irwin RS, Rippe JM, eds. *Intensive Care Medicine*. 6th ed. Philadelphia, PA: Lippincott Williams & Wilkins; 2008:898–925.

15. Driscoll DF, Bistrian BR. Parenteral and enteral nutrition in the intensive care unit. In: Irwin RS, Rippe JM, eds. *Intensive Care Medicine*. 6th ed. Philadelphia, PA: Lippincott Williams & Wilkins; 2008:2186–2201.

16. Renagel [package insert]. Cambridge, MA: Genzyme Corporation; 1998.

Gordon Sacks and Amy Hodgin

▣ Nutritional Assessment

Nutritional assessment consists of evaluations, including patient history, physical examination, and laboratory parameters. Alternative methods of evaluating nutritional status include use of subjective global assessment (SGA), muscle strength, and bioelectrical impedance (BIA) (Table 10.1, 10.2, and 10.3).[1–4] Physical findings of malnutrition are listed in Table 10.4. In pediatric patients, height/length ratios are compared to age-related percentiles to establish malnutrition. External head dimension is an additional parameter useful in evaluating the nutritional status of infants (Table 10.5).[5,6]

Laboratory Parameters to Monitor[7]

- Serum electrolytes.
- Blood glucose.
- Cholesterol panel, including triglycerides.
- Liver function tests.
- Renal function tests.
- Complete blood cell count (CBC).
- Prothrombin time (PT).
- Visceral proteins (Table 10.6)[8].

Serum albumin is most commonly used to assess protein nutritional status, but it is of limited usefulness in determining acute nutritional changes because albumin has a long half-life. Proteins with shorter half-lives are used increasingly for monitoring improvements in protein malnutrition.[8]

Table 10.1 NUTRITIONAL ASSESSMENT

Evaluation	Purpose
Medical and surgical history	Underlying pathology, medications, and risk factors related to nutritional status
Dietary history	Accurate food intake, weight changes, and possible food allergies
Physical examination	Lean body mass (LBM) and vitamin deficiencies
Laboratory parameters	Electrolyte abnormalities
Anthropometric measurements	Protein and fat stores
Subjective global assessment	Nutrition-related disease
Muscle strength	Functional ability
Bioelectrical impedance analysis (BIA)	Changes in LBM

From Hammond K. History and physical examination. In: Matarese LE, Gottschlich MM, eds. *Contemporary Nutrition Support Practice: A Clinical Guide.* Philadelphia, PA: WB Saunders; 1998:17–32; and ASPEN Board of Directors and the Clinical Guidelines Task Force. Guidelines for the use of parenteral and enteral nutrition in adult and pediatric patients. *JPEN J Parenter Enteral Nutr.* 2002;26(1 Suppl):1SA–138SA, with permission.

Table 10.2 ANTHROPOMETRIC MEASUREMENTS: BODY MASS INDEX

Body Mass Index[a] (kg/m²)	Classification
<18.5	Underweight
18.5–24.9	Normal
>25.0	Overweight
25.0–29.9	Overweight
30.0–34.9	Obesity class I
35.0–39.9	Obesity class II
>40.0	Obesity class III

[a]Body mass index = weight (kg)/height (m²)
Adapted from World Health Organization Technical Report Series; 894. Obesity: Preventing and Managing the Global Evidence: Report of a WHO Consultation. Geneva, Switzerland: World Health Organization; 2004 (reprint).

Table 10.3 ANTHROPOMETRIC MEASUREMENTS: BODY COMPOSITION

Body Composition[a]	Male	Female
Triceps skinfold (mm)	12.5	16.5
Midarm muscle Circumference (cm)	29.3	28.5

[a]Triceps skinfold measures fat reserve. Midarm muscle circumference measures protein reserve.
Reprinted with permission from Blackburn GL, Bistrian BR, Maini BS, et al. Nutritional and metabolic assessment of the hospitalized patient. *JPEN J Parenter Enteral Nutr.* 1977;1(1):11–22, with permission from the American Society for Parenteral and Enteral Nutrition (A.S.P.E.N.). A.S.P.E.N does not endorse the use of this material in any form other than its entirety.

Table 10.4 PHYSICAL FINDINGS OF NUTRIENT DEFICIENCIES

Finding	Nutrient Deficiency
Cheilosis	Niacin, riboflavin
Corkscrew hair (Menkes syndrome)	Copper
Dementia	Niacin, vitamin B_{12}
Enlarged parotids	Protein, bulimia
Enlarged thyroid	Iodine
Glossitis	Niacin, riboflavin, folic acid, iron, vitamin B_{12}
Growth retardation	Protein, calories, vitamin A
Heart failure	Thiamine
Hepatomegaly	Protein
Loss of weight, muscle mass, or fat stores	Protein, calories
Magenta tongue	Riboflavin
Nail plate and hair appear dull, lusterless	Protein
Poor wound/ulcer healing	Protein, vitamin C, zinc
Psychomotor decline/mental confusion	Protein
Rickets	Vitamin D, calcium
Swollen, painful joints	Vitamin C
Tetany	Calcium, magnesium

Adapted with permission from Hammond K. History and physical examination. In: Matarese LE, Gottschlich MM, eds. *Contemporary Nutrition Support Practice: A Clinical Guide.* Philadelphia, PA: WB Saunders; 1998:17–32.

Table 10.5 ANTHROPOMETRIC MEASUREMENTS: PEDIATRICS

Age	Weight (g/d)	Height (cm/mo)	Head Circumference (cm/wk)
0–3 mo	24–35	2.8–3.4	0.5
3–6 mo	15–21	1.7–2.4	0.5
6–12 mo	10–13	1.3–1.6	0.5
1–3 y	5–9	0.6–1.0	—
4–6 y	5–6	0.5–0.6	—
7–10 y	7–11	0.4–0.5	—

Adapted with permission from Chessman KH, Kumpf VJ. Assessment of nutrition status and nutrition requirements. In: DiPiro JT, Talbert RL, Yee GC, et al., eds. *Pharmacotherapy: A Pathophysiologic Approach*. 6th ed. New York, NY: McGraw-Hill; 2005:2559–2578; and Davis AM. Pediatrics. In: Matarese LE, Gottschlich MM, eds. *Contemporary Nutrition Support Practice: A Clinical Guide*. Philadelphia, PA: WB Saunders; 1998:347–364.

Table 10.6 LABORATORY PARAMETERS

Visceral Proteins

Serum Protein	Normal Range	Half-Life	Severe Malnutrition
Albumin[a]	3.5–5.0 g/dL	20 d	<2.1 g/dL
Fibronectin	220–400 mg/L	15 h	variable
Thyroxine-binding prealbumin[b]	15.7–29.6 mg/dL	2–3 d	<5 mg/dL
Retinol-binding protein	3–6 mg/dL	12 h	<2.4 mg/dL
Somatomedin C (insulinlike growth factor)	0.1–0.4 mg/L	2 h	Variable
Transferrin[c]	200–400 mg/dL	8–10 d	<100 mg/dL

[a]Decreased in the setting of infection, inflammation, fluid overload; increased in the setting of dehydration.
[b]Decreased in the setting of infection or inflammation; increased in the setting of renal failure or corticosteroid administration.
[c]Decreased in the setting of infection, inflammation, or iron-deficiency anemia.
From Russell MK, McAdams PM. Laboratory monitoring of nutritional status. In: Matarese LE, Gottschlich MM, eds. *Contemporary Nutrition Support Practice: A Clinical Guide*. Philadelphia, PA: WB Saunders; 1998:47–64, with permission.

Nitrogen balance may be an indicator of the patient's catabolic state (Eq. 10.1). It is often used to assess the efficacy of nutrition support.[9]

> Calculation of Nitrogen Balance[9]
> Nitrogen balance = nitrogen intake − nitrogen output
> Nitrogen intake = 24-hour protein intake/6.25
> Nitrogen output = (UUN g/24 hours) − 4   (10.1)

where the constant factor of 4 represents an estimated 2 g from gastrointestinal tract (GI) and respiratory losses and 2 g derived from nonurea nitrogen losses (i.e., ammonia, uric acid, creatinine).

- A 24-hour urine collection is often necessary to determine the amount of nitrogen excreted.
- Use this equation with caution because in some patient populations nitrogen excretion may be overestimated or underestimated.

Enteral Nutrition

Enteral nutrition (EN) is a method of providing nutritional support to patients with normal GI function who are unable to eat to meet metabolic demands.

- EN is preferred over parenteral nutrition because it is safe, effective, and economical for patients.[10]
- Administered by tube or mouth, enteral products can serve as the sole source of nutritional support, as a dietary supplement to oral intake, or as an adjunct during transition from parenteral to oral feedings.[10]
- EN is warranted if the GI tract is functioning and additional nutritional intake is needed.[11]
- Indications and contraindications for enteral nutrition (EN) are listed in Tables 10.7 and 10.8.
- A wide variety of dietary terms are used to describe nutrition plans for patients.
- Commonly prescribed diets are described in Table 10.9.

Enteral Nutrition Products

In general, EN products are selected after a thorough and complete assessment of the patient's digestive/absorptive state and fluid and electrolyte demands.

Table 10.7 INDICATIONS FOR ENTERAL NUTRITION

Acquired immunodeficiency syndrome
Anorexia nervosa
Carcinoma with severe weight loss
Correction of malnutrition secondary to chronic disease
Endotracheal intubation
Esophageal stricture
Handicapping conditions
Hypermetabolic state (i.e., severe burn or trauma)
Inborn errors of metabolism
Neurologic disorders
Oral or esophageal injury
Severely impaired growth and development
Swallowing difficulties/dysphagia

From Davis AM. Pediatrics. In: Matarese LE, Gottschlich MM, eds. *Contemporary Nutrition Support Practice: A Clinical Guide.* Philadelphia, PA: WB Saunders; 1998:347–364; Marian M, McGinnis C. Overview of enteral nutrition. In: Gottschlich MM, ed. *The ASPEN Nutrition Support Core Curriculum: A Case-Based Approach-The Adult Patient.* Silver Springs, MD: American Society for Parenteral and Enteral Nutrition; 2007:187–208; and Kumpf VJ, Chessman KH. Enteral nutrition. In: DiPiro JT, Talbert RL, Yee GC, et al., eds. *Pharmacotherapy: A Pathophysiologic Approach.* 6th ed. New York, NY: McGraw-Hill; 2005:2615–2634, with permission.

- Commonly available EN products are described in Table 10.10.[12,13,14]
- Starting EN within 24 to 48 hours after severe injury has positive effects, whereas postponing it for 4 to 5 days may be too late to achieve reduced infectious complications.[15]
- EN may be delivered via numerous routes depending on the patient's clinical condition: (Table 10.11).[13]
  - Nasogastric (placed from the nose into the stomach).
  - Gastrostomy (stoma created from the abdominal wall into the stomach).
  - Jejunostomy (stoma created from the abdominal wall into the jejunum)[11].
- Complications of EN are gastrointestinal, metabolic, and mechanical (Table 10.12).[2,16,17]

Table 10.8 CONTRAINDICATIONS FOR ENTERAL NUTRITION

Gastrointestinal hemorrhage
Gastrointestinal obstruction
High-output enterocutaneous fistula (i.e., >500 mL/d)
Intestinal ischemia
Intractable diarrhea or vomiting despite medical therapy
Nutritional intervention not warranted
Paralytic ileus
Peritonitis
Severe malabsorption
Short bowel syndrome with <100 cm small bowel remaining with malabsorption

Reprinted with permission from Marian M, McGinnis C. Overview of enteral nutrition. In: Gottschlich MM, ed. *The A.S.P.E.N. Nutrition Support Core Curriculum: A Case-Based Approach—The Adult Patient.* Silver Springs, MD: A.S.P.E.N. 2007:187–208, with permission from the American Society for Parenteral and Enteral Nutrition (A.S.P.E.N.). A.S.P.E.N. does not endorse the use of this material in any form other than its entirety.

 Administration of Enteral Nutrition

The proper administration of EN products is important to achieve and enhance patient tolerance. The following points should be considered when administering a particular product.

- Continuous drip given over a 24-hour period is the preferred method for administration of tube feedings in the hospital setting.
- Potential complications associated with tube feedings (e.g., hyperglycemia, pulmonary aspiration, and diarrhea) can be reduced by continuous feedings.
- Bolus feedings are an option if the feeding tube is in the stomach and previous feedings have been well tolerated.

Initiation of Enteral Feedings

To initiate a continuous tube feeding (Table 10.13):

1. Perform an abdominal examination. Presence of abdominal distention, nausea, bloating, and bowel sounds should be evaluated.

Table 10.9 TYPES OF ORAL DIETS

Type	Description	Indication	Example
Clear liquid	Provides fluid and calories; low in irritants, and contains foods that require minimal digestion	Prior to diagnostic tests or bowel surgery; recovery phase after surgery; transition from nothing by mouth to more advanced diet	Fatfree clear broth, tea, coffee, plain flavored gelatin, carbonated beverages, hard candy, clear fruit juices, popsicles
Full liquid	Provides adequate calories and protein; requires minimal chewing and digestion	Difficulty swallowing, chewing, or digesting solid foods; transition to more advanced diet	Blenderized foods, such as soup; all liquids allowed
Pureed	Provides adequate nutrition; facilitates ingestion of food with no chewing	Very limited chewing ability; severe mouth sore; motor deficits; esophageal strictures; head and neck surgery; transition to more advanced diet	Solid foods moistened and blended to a mashed potato–like consistency; all liquids allowed
Soft mechanical	Provides adequate nutrition; facilitates ingestion of solid foods with minimal chewing	Difficulty chewing and/or swallowing whole foods	Solid foods softened or moistened; all liquids allowed
General	Meets nutritional needs for maintenance, repair, growth, and development	All patients not requiring restrictions, modifications, or special additions to their dietary regimen	All foods are allowed; milk products, meat, bread and cereal products, fruits and vegetables, saturated and unsaturated fats, and added sugar

Table 10.10 PROFILE OF ENTERAL NUTRITION PRODUCTS

Type	Description	Indication	Example
Adult			
Standard without fiber	Isotonic; 1–1.2 kcal/mL; may contain fiber; not sweetened	Most patient populations; generally for tube feeding only (not palatable for oral supplementation)	Isosource HN (No), Osmolite (MJ), FiberSource HN (No), Jevity (R)
High protein	NPC:N <125:1; may contain fiber	Critically ill (i.e., trauma, burn); pressure sores; surgical wounds; high fistula output	Isosource VHN (No), Replete (N), Promote with fiber (R)
Concentrated	Hypertonic; 1.5–2 kcal/mL; low electrolyte content	Fluid restriction (i.e., cardiac, renal, pulmonary, or hepatic failure)	Isosource 1.5 (No), Osmolite 1.5 (N), Resource 2.0 (No), TwoCal HN (R)
Peptide-based	Protein supplied in the form of dipeptides and tripeptides; higher fat content supplied as MCT	Intolerance to standard formulations due to malabsorption; chronic pancreatitis; cystic fibrosis; celiac disease	Peptinex DT (N), Perative (R), Peptamen (N), Subdue (MJ)
Diabetic	Isotonic; 1–1.2 kcal/mL; high fat, low carbohydrate	Hyperglycemia; limited evidence	Glucerna (R), Resource Diabetic (No), Glytrol (N)
Hepatic	Hypertonic; 1.2–1.5 kcal/mL; high BCAA:AAA	Grade II or greater encephalopathy; not for use in the absence of encephalopathy	Nutri-Hep (N)
Immune modulating	Contains glutamine, arginine, nucleotides, and/or omega-3 fatty acids	Critically ill (i.e., trauma, burn, sepsis), perioperative	Impact with Glutamine (No), Perative (R), Crucial (N), AlitraQ (R)
Pulmonary	1.5 kcal/mL; contains omega-3 fatty acids, gamma-linolenic acid, and antioxidants	Acute respiratory distress syndrome	Oxepa (R)
Renal	Hypertonic; caloric dense (2 kcal/mL); moderate protein; low electrolyte and mineral content	Renal failure with difficult-to-control electrolyte and mineral; for dialyzed patients	Nepro (R), NovaSource Renal (No); Renalcal (N)

(continued)

Table 10.10 PROFILE OF ENTERAL NUTRITION PRODUCTS (continued)

Type	Description	Indication	Example
Pediatric			
Standard	Isotonic; 0.8–1 kcal/mL; contains at least one source of cow's milk; may contain fiber	Children 1–10 y	Enfamil Kindercal (MJ), PediaSure (R), PediaSure with Fiber (MJ), Kindercal with Fiber (R), Kindercal with Fiber (R)
	0.8–1 kcal/mL	Children 1–10 y with malabsorption, cow's milk protein allergy	Neocate One+ (SHS), EleCare (R), Peptamen Jr (N), Vital Jr (R), Tolerex (No)
Cow's milk-based	Isotonic; 0.67–0.8 kcal/mL; carbohydrate source is lactose (lactosefree formulations are available); high milk content	Term infants	Enfamil LIPIL (MJ), Enfamil Lactofree LIPIL (MJ), Similac Advance (R), Similac Lactose Free Advance (R)
Soy-based lactose free	Hypotonic; 0.67 kcal/mL; cow's milk protein free and lactosefree	Term infants who have allergies, lactose intolerance, or galactosemia	Enfamil ProSobee LIPIL (MJ), Similac Isomil Advance (R)
Preterm	Isotonic; 0.67–0.8 kcal/mL; easily digested	Preterm infants <2–3 kg	Enfamil Premature LIPIL (MJ) Similac Care Advance 20 Advance (R), Similac Care Advance 24 Advance (R)

NPC:N, nonprotein calorie:nitrogen ratio; MCT, medium-chain triglyceride; BCAA:AAA, branched-chain amino acids:aromatic amino acids; No, Novartis; MJ, Mead Johnson Nutritionals; R, Ross Products; N, Nestle Clinical Nutrition; SHS, SHS International Ltd.

Adapted with permission from Kumpf VJ, Chessman KH. Enteral nutrition. In: DiPiro JT, Talbert RL, Yee GC, Matzke GR, Wells BG, Posey LM, eds. *Pharmacotherapy: A Pathophysiologic Approach*. 6th ed. New York, NY: McGraw-Hill; 2005:2615–2634; and Carlson SJ. Enteral formulations. In: Merritt R, ed. *The ASPEN Nutrition Support Practice Manual*. 2nded. Silver Spring, MD: American Society for Parenteral and Enteral Nutrition; 2005:63–75, with permission.

Table 10.11 TYPES OF FEEDING TUBES

Type	Location	Indications	Advantages	Disadvantages
Nasogastric	Stomach	Normal gastric emptying Short term (<30 d)	Easily placed at bedside Allows intermittent and bolus feeding	Aspiration risk Discomfort to patient
Nasoduodenal/nasojejunal	Small bowel	Impaired gastric emptying Short term (<30 d)	Easily placed at bedside Reduced aspiration risk	
Percutaneous gastrostomy/ open gastrostomy	Stomach	Normal gastric emptying Long term	Allows intermittent and bolus feeding	Surgical risk Aspiration risk Requires stoma site care
Percutaneous jejunostomy/ open jejunostomy	Small bowel	Postoperative feeding Impaired gastric emptying Long term	Reduced aspiration risk	Continuous and cyclic feeding only Requires stoma site care

Reprinted with permission from Kumpf VJ, Chessman KH. Enteral nutrition. In: DiPiro JT, Talbert RL, Yee GC, et al., eds. *Pharmacotherapy: A Pathophysiologic Approach.* 6th ed. New York, NY: McGraw-Hill; 2005:2615–2634.

Table 10.12 TUBE FEEDING COMPLICATIONS

Complication	Causes	Management
Gastrointestinal		
Diarrhea (most common)	Bacterial contamination of formula; improper administration; use of antibiotics; lactose intolerance; impaction; malnutrition; liquid drug formulations containing sorbitol; bowel infection from C. difficile and pseudomembranous colitis	Discard tubing after 24 h; use only 8–12 h of feeding; use isotonic formula at tolerable rate by continuous delivery; avoid or recognize drugs causing diarrhea; avoid lactose-containing formulas; rule out impaction before treating diarrhea; use elemental formula; add fiber to formula
Constipation	Low-residue formula used in long-term, tube-fed patients; dehydration	Provide additional fluids by mouth or tube feeding; increase ambulation or use a high-fiber, high-residue formula; administer bulking agents (psyllium); administer laxatives
Bloating	Presence of a mild ileus; intolerance to lipids in formula; swallowing excessive amounts of air (e.g., head and neck surgery)	Use formulas with no fiber; increase ambulation; administer laxative; start promotility agents; check gastric residuals
Inadequate gastric emptying	Gastric atony, prepyloric ulcers, bowel ileus; drugs such as theophylline, dopamine, anticholinergics calcium channel blockers, and narcotics that relax the lower esophageal sphincter	Verify tube placement; monitor stomach content residuals before bolus feedings or every 2–6 h during continuous feedings
Vomiting	Psychological association with the illness; unpleasant odor of formulas containing free amino acids or the reinstilling of large amounts of aspirated gastric residuals	Reduce anxiety; use intact protein-containing formulas or antiemetic when indicated; reduce the rate of delivery; feed beyond the pylorus; slowly advance feeding rate
Nausea	Delayed gastric emptying; gastric distention; formula too hot or too cold, or given too rapidly	Stop feedings and determine cause; check gastric residual to determine the progress of gastric emptying after 1–2 h; restart feedings at lower rate and slowly advance

Metabolic		
Hyperglycemia	Common in patients who are diabetic, hypermetabolic, or receiving corticosteroids	Check blood glucose frequently with advancing enteral feedings; administer insulin as needed; hydrate patient or change to a lower carbohydrate content formula
Electrolyte disturbance	Fluid imbalance; medication use; renal insufficiency; feeding formulation	Monitor fluid intake and output and serum chemistries; replace electrolytes as necessary
Mechanical		
Tube obstruction	Formula with a caloric density of 1.5–2.0 kcal/mL; inadequate crushing of medications or inadequate dilution/flushing of psyllium or antacids	Use feeding pumps for dense formulas and/or larger-bore feeding tubes; give medications as elixirs; flush tube with 30 mL of water after medications; use pancreatic enzymes
Displacement	Vomiting; cough; incorrect tube placement; detached tape holding tube to nose	Check tube placement by radiograph; listen for air being injected through the tube into the stomach with a stethoscope, followed by aspiration of a small amount of gastric contents
Irritation	Esophageal reflux, peptic esophagitis; pressure necrosis of esophageal and tracheal wall at cuff inflation site	Provide nose and mouth care; change tape; increase salivation in the mouth by allowing chewing gum, hard candy, or ice chips
Aspiration	Gastric contents refluxing into bronchus secondary to delayed gastric emptying; improper placement of tube in tracheal or bronchus; incompetent lower esophageal sphincter	Place feeding tube beyond the pylorus; use small, soft feeding tube; keep maximum gastric content residuals to <250 mL; raise head of bead to 45 degrees

From ASPEN Board of Directors and the Clinical Guidelines Task Force. Guidelines for the use of parenteral and enteral nutrition in adult and pediatric patients. *JPEN J Parenter Enteral Nutr.* 2002;26(1 Suppl):1SA–138SA; Malone AM, Seres DS, Lord L. Complications of enteral nutrition. In: Gottschlich MM, ed. *The ASPEN Nutrition Support Core Curriculum: A Case-Based Approach–The Adult Patient.* Silver Springs, MD: American Society for Parenteral and Enteral Nutrition; 2007:246–263; and Haddad RY, Thomas DR. Enteral nutrition and enteral tube feeding: review of the evidence. *Clin Geriatr Med.* 2002;18(4):867–881, with permission.

Table 10.13 INITIATION OF CONTINUOUS ENTERAL NUTRITION

Age	Initial Rate	Advance, if Tolerated	Goal Rate
0–12 mo	1–2 mL/kg/h	Every 2–8 h	6 mL/kg/h
1–6 y	1 mL/kg/h	Every 2–8 h	4–5 mL/kg/h
>6 y	25 mL/h	Every 2–8 h	100–150 mL/h
Adult—gastric	25 mL/h	Every 4–6 h	Variable
Adult—jejunal	25 mL/h	Every 24 h	Variable

Adapted with permission from Davis AM. Pediatrics. In: Matarese LE, Gottschlich MM, eds. *Contemporary Nutrition Support Practice: A Clinical Guide*. Philadelphia, PA: WB Saunders; 1998:347–364.

2. Placement of the tube should be confirmed by irrigation with air or aspiration of stomach or small bowel contents. Radiologic verification of the tube may also be used.
3. After determination of the final goal rate based on energy requirements, continuous feeding may be initiated. If the patient has a gastric tube, start enteral feeding at 25 mL/hour. If the tube is in the small bowel, start feeding at 25 mL/hour.
4. If the tube is in the stomach, perform an abdominal examination and check gastric residuals every 4 hours. Feedings may be increased by 25 mL/hour every 4 to 6 hours, if the feeding is tolerated, until the goal rate is achieved. If the tube is in the small bowel, feedings may be increased by 25 mL/hour each day until the goal rate is achieved.
5. If diarrhea or abdominal discomfort is present after the advancement of the feeding, the previous rate may used for another 24-hour period.

Monitoring Enteral Nutrition

Once tube feedings are initiated, the patient must be monitored to ascertain efficacy of the nutritional support regimen and to identify and correct intolerance problems, metabolic complications, or other adverse effects (Table 10.14).[12]

Drug–Nutrient Compatibility

Drug–nutrient interactions may occur when medications and EN are given via a tube.

Table 10.14 MONITORING PARAMETERS FOR ENTERAL NUTRITION

Accurate records of input and output

Evidence of intolerance (abdominal distention/pain, nausea, emesis)

Frequency and consistency of stool output

Laboratory parameters, including serum electrolytes, complete blood count, serum glucose, inflammatory markers (i.e., C-reactive protein [CRP])

Markers for nutrition status (prealbumin, nitrogen balance)

Physical examination for hydration or nutrient deficiency or excess

Review of medications

Weight trends

- To avoid potential drug–nutrient incompatibilities, tube feedings should be discontinued and ≥30 mL of water instilled through the tube before and after drug administration.[18,19]
- The most frequent compatibility problems involve strongly acidic or buffered syrups with pH values <4 (Table 10.15).[20]
- Incompatibilities between formulas and drugs can cause immediate dumping, and the increased viscosity and particle size can clog feeding tubes.[20]
- At pH values <5, in vitro clotting has occurred with Pulmocare, Ensure Plus, Osmolite, Enrich, Ensure, and Resource.[21]

▣ Medication Administration[18,19]

Medication dosage forms possess different characteristics that can affect how they are tolerated when administered through enteral feeding tubes.

- Immediate-release tablets may be crushed and mixed with water to form a slurry and administered through a feeding tube. Similarly, capsules may be opened and the contents made into a slurry for administration.
- Sublingual, buccal, time-released, or enteric coated tablets may have an altered therapeutic effect or increased side effects and toxicity when crushed.

Table 10.15 DRUG–NUTRIENT COMPATIBILITY

Product	Ensure	Osmolite	Vivonex
Acetaminophen elixir	C	C	C
Amphojel	NA	I	C
Bentyl liquid	NA	I	C
Benadryl elixir	C	C	C
Cibalith-S syrup	I	I	C
Dimetapp elixir	I	I	I
Feosol elixir	I	I	C
Guaifenesin liquid	I	I	C
Imodium	NA	C	C
KCl liquid	I	I	I
Lanoxin elixir	C	C	C
Morphine liquid	C	C	C
Phenytoin suspension	I	I	NA
Phenytoin injection	C	C	NA
Sudafed syrup	I	I	C
Thorazine concentrate	I	I	C

C, compatible; NA, no data available; I, incompatible.
Adapted with permission from Sacks GS. Drug–nutrient considerations in patients receiving parenteral and enteral nutrition. *Pract Gastroenterol.* 2004:39–48.

- Some medications may be administered as a liquid dosage form. However, liquid dosage forms may have higher osmolality and a significant amount of sorbitol, which increase the possibility of diarrhea.
- See Table 10.16 for examples of medications that should not be given through a tube.

■ Pediatric Enteral Nutrition

In general, children are at an earlier risk for nutrient deficiencies than adults due to lower energy and protein stores. Therefore, earlier intervention may be required.

Table 10.16 SELECTED MEDICATIONS THAT SHOULD NOT BE GIVEN VIA FEEDING TUBE

Medication	Dosage Form	Mechanism
Bisacodyl (Dulcolax)	Tablet	Enteric coated
Bupropion (Wellbutrin XL)	Tablet	Sustained release
Carbamazepine (Tegretol XR)	Tablet	Sustained release
Carbidopa/levodopa (Sinemet CR)	Tablet	Sustained release
Clarithromycin (Biaxin-XL)	Tablet	Sustained release
Diclofenac (Voltaren)	Tablet	Delayed release
Diltiazem (Cardizem CD*a*, Cardizem SR*a*, Tiazac)	Capsule	Sustained release
Felodipine (Plendil)	Tablet	Extended release
Fluoxetine (Prozac Weekly)	Capsule	Sustained release
Lansoprazole (Prevacid*a*)	Capsule	Delayed release
Mesalamine (Asacol, Pentasa)	Tablet, capsule	Sustained release
Mycophenolate (CellCept)	Tablet, capsule	Teratogenic
Omeprazole (Prilosec)	Capsule	Delayed release
Pancreatic enzymes (Creon 10, Creon 20, Pancrease, Ultrase, Zymase)	Capsule	Enteric coated spheres
Pantoprazole (Protonix)	Tablet	Sustained release
Verapamil (Verelan*a*, Calan SR)	Capsule, tablet	Sustained release

*a*Capsule may be opened and contents administered by tube with fluid.
Adapted with permission from Sacks GS. Drug–nutrient considerations in patients receiving parenteral and enteral nutrition. *Pract Gastroenterol.* July 2005:39–48.

- Table 10.5 shows the growth targets of infants and children. Children who are unable to meet these targets may be candidates for nutrition support.[5,6]
- EN is the preferred method of nutrition support if oral access is not available. Indications for EN in pediatrics are listed in Table 10.7.[6,12,13]

Table 10.17 COMPARISON OF COW'S MILK TO HUMAN MILK

Nutrient	Cow's Milk	Human Milk
Fat (% of total calories)	50	50–55
Triglycerides	Long-chain saturated fatty acids	Long-chain polyunsaturated and monounsaturated fatty acids
Protein (% of total calories)	22%	6%
Whey casein[a]		55:45
Taurine and cystine[b]	Low levels	Abundant
Carbohydrate (% of total calories)	31%	42%
Carbohydrate source[c]	Lactose	Lactose
Renal solute load	228 mOsm/L	75 mOsm/L
Sodium	2.2 mmol/100 mL	0.7 mmol/100 mL
Ca/PO$_4$ ratio	1.3:1	2:1

[a]Whey is a soluble, noncurdling protein that remains in solution throughout the digestive process. Casein is relatively insoluble.
[b]Taurine is an essential amino acid involved with the development of the central nervous system. Cysteine is an essential amino acid in infants.
[c]Lactose enhances the absorption of calcium and magnesium.

- Table 10.13 provides continuous infusion recommendations based on age and weight.[6]
- In infants, EN is intended to provide adequate replacement for human breast milk.
- For those infants allergic or intolerant to various components of human breast milk or standard infant formulas, enteral nutrition should provide adequate substitute feeding.
- Table 10.17 compares the content of cow to human milk.[6,22,23]
- Formulas may be modified to meet the protein, vitamin, and mineral requirements of the child, although this results in a concentrated formulation.[22]
- Caution must be used to not exceed the kidney's ability to concentrate and excrete renal solute when concentrated EN formulations are used.[6,22]

References

1. Hammond K. History and physical examination. In: Matarese LE, Gottschlich MM, eds. *Contemporary Nutrition Support Practice: A Clinical Guide*. Philadelphia, PA: WB Saunders; 1998:17–32.

2. ASPEN Board of Directors and the Clinical Guidelines Task Force. Guidelines for the use of parenteral and enteral nutrition in adult and pediatric patients. *JPEN J Parenter Enteral Nutr*. 2002;26(1 Suppl):1SA–138SA.

3. World Health Organization Technical Report Series; 894. Obesity: Preventing and Managing the Global Evidence: Report of a WHO Consultation. Geneva, Switzerland: World Health Organization; 2004 (reprint).

4. Blackburn GL, Bistrian BR, Maini BS, et al. Nutritional and metabolic assessment of the hospitalized patient. *JPEN J Parenter Enteral Nutr*. 1977;1(1):11–22.

5. Chessman KH, Kumpf VJ. Assessment of nutrition status and nutrition requirements. In: DiPiro JT, Talbert RL, Yee GC, et al., eds. *Pharmacotherapy: A Pathophysiologic Approach*. 6th ed. New York, NY: McGraw-Hill; 2005:2559–2578.

6. Davis AM. Pediatrics. In: Matarese LE, Gottschlich MM, eds. *Contemporary Nutrition Support Practice: A Clinical Guide*. Philadelphia, PA: WB Saunders; 1998:347–364.

7. Russell MK, Mueller C. Nutrition screening and assessment. In: Gottschlich MM, ed. *The ASPEN Nutrition Support Core Curriculum: A Case-Based Approach-The Adult Patient*. Silver Springs, MD: American Society for Parenteral and Enteral Nutrition; 2007:163–186.

8. Russell MK, McAdams PM. Laboratory monitoring of nutritional status. In: Matarese LE, Gottschlich MM, eds. *Contemporary Nutrition Support Practice: A Clinical Guide*. Philadelphia, PA: WB Saunders; 1998:47–64.

9. Dickerson RN. Using nitrogen balance in clinical practice. *Hosp Pharm*. 2005;40(12):1081–1085.

10. DeChicco RS, Matarese LE. Determining the nutrition support regimen. In: Matarese LE, Gottschlich MM, eds. *Contemporary Nutrition Support Practice: A Clinical Guide*. Philadelphia, PA: WB Saunders; 1998:185–191.

11. Kirby DF, Delegge MH, Fleming CR. American Gastroenterological Association technical review on tube feeding for enteral nutrition. *Gastroenterology*. 1995;108(4):1282–1301.

12. Marian M, McGinnis C. Overview of enteral nutrition. In: Gottschlich MM, ed. *The ASPEN Nutrition Support Core Curriculum: A Case-Based Approach-The Adult Patient*. Silver Springs, MD: American Society for Parenteral and Enteral Nutrition; 2007:187–208.

13. Kumpf VJ, Chessman KH. Enteral nutrition. In: DiPiro JT, Talbert RL, Yee GC, et al., eds. *Pharmacotherapy: A Pathophysiologic Approach*. 6th ed. New York, NY: McGraw-Hill; 2005:2615–2634.

14. Carlson SJ. Enteral formulations. In: Merritt R, ed. *The ASPEN Nutrition Support Practice Manual*. 2nd ed. Silver Spring, MD: American Society for Parenteral and Enteral Nutrition; 2005:63–75.

15. Minard G, Kudsk KA. Is early feeding beneficial? How early is early? *New Horiz*. 1994;2(2):156–163.

16. Malone AM, Seres DS, Lord L. Complications of enteral nutrition. In: Gottschlich MM, ed. *The ASPEN Nutrition Support Core Curriculum: A Case-Based*

Approach-The Adult Patient. Silver Springs, MD: American Society for Parenteral and Enteral Nutrition; 2007:246–263.

17. Haddad RY, Thomas DR. Enteral nutrition and enteral tube feeding. review of the evidence. *Clin Geriatr Med.* 2002;18(4):867–881.

18. Sacks GS. Drug-nutrient considerations in patients receiving parenteral and enteral nutrition. *Pract Gastroenterol.* 2004:39–48.

19. Beckwith CM, Feddema SS, Barton RG, et al. A guide to drug therapy in patients with enteral feeding tubes: dosage form selection and administration methods. *Hosp Pharm.* 2004;39(3):225–237.

20. Cutie AJ, Altman E, Lenkel L. Compatibility of enteral products with commonly employed drug additives. *JPEN J Parenter Enteral Nutr.* 1983;7(2):186–191.

21. Marcuard SP, Perkins AM. Clogging of feeding tubes. *JPEN J Parenter Enteral Nutr.* 1988;12(4):403–405.

22. Bechard LJ, Duggan C. Modifying enteral formulas. In: Corkins MR, Shulman RJ, eds. *Pediatric Nutrition in Your Pocket.* Silver Springs, MD: American Society for Parenteral and Enteral Nutrition; 2002:110–115.

23. Magelli MA, Grinder CP. Meeting the special enteral nutrition needs of infants and children. *J Pediatr Pharm Prac.* 1996;1(2):113–129.

11 Parenteral Nutrition

Gordon Sacks and Amy Hodgin

Parenteral Nutrition

Parenteral Nutrition (PN) provides carbohydrate, protein, lipid, electrolytes, vitamins, and minerals intravenously to patients who are unable to assimilate nutrients via the gastrointestinal (GI) tract. It can maintain weight and metabolic integrity, replete malnourished patients with deficits in lean body mass, and restore hematologic and immune function integrity.

- PN may be started and given in a hospital, a skilled nursing facility, or a patient's home.
- PN should be used only when the gut is unavailable or dysfunctional.
- Indications and contraindications for PN are listed in Tables 11.1 and 11.2.

Central versus Peripheral Administration

PN may be given via a peripheral or a central intravenous line.

- Providing nutrition through a central line is the preferred method.
- Peripheral PN (PPN) is used when a patient requires intravenous nutritional support but does not have a central access device.
- Guidelines for administering peripheral PN are listed in Table 11.3.
- Central PN (CPN) refers to PN infused through central veins, including the subclavian, internal jugular, and femoral veins.
  - PN via a central vein requires a central venous access device due to its hyperosmolarity (>1,000 mOsm/L).[1]

Table 11.1 INDICATIONS FOR PARENTERAL NUTRITION

Anticipated nonfunctioning gastrointestinal (GI) tract for at least 5–7 d

Enterocutaneous fistula (high output >500 mL/d)

Short bowel syndrome

Intestinal obstruction

Radiation enteritis

Motility disorders (ileus, intestinal pseudo-obstruction)

Severe malnutrition with a dysfunctional or inaccessible GI tract

Severe pancreatitis

Hyperemesis of pregnancy with intolerance to enteral nutrition

Severe hypermetabolic states in which enteral feeding is contraindicated or inadequate

Inborn errors of metabolism (pediatrics)

Intractable diarrhea of infancy (pediatrics)

Extreme prematurity (pediatrics)

From Mirtallo J, Canada T, Johnson D, et al. Safe practices for parenteral nutrition. *JPEN J Parenter Enter Nutr.* 2004;28:S39–S70; and American Society of Parenteral and Enteral Nutrition (ASPEN) Board of Directors and the Clinical Task Force. Guidelines for the use of parenteral and enteral nutrition in adult and pediatric patients. *JPEN J Parenter Enter Nutr.* 2002;26(Suppl):1SA–138SA; Errata: 2002;26:114,.with permission.

- Total nutrient admixture, also known as 3-in-1, refers to a solution containing dextrose, amino acids, and intravenous lipid emulsion (Table 11.4).
- Table 11.5 lists common access devices for CPN.

Table 11.2 CONTRAINDICATIONS FOR PN

Adequate nutrition stores and expected gastrointestinal (GI) function returning within 5–7 d

GI function is not impaired

Nutritional intervention not warranted

Table 11.3 GUIDELINES FOR PERIPHERAL PARENTERAL NUTRITION (PPN)

Used for <7 d
Hypo-osmolar solution (600–900 mOsm/L)
Final dextrose concentration: <10% (adults), 12.5% (children)
Final amino acid concentration: <5% (adults), 3.5% (children)
Large volume is required for compatibility; limit PPN to patients with no fluid restriction
Monitor for vein irritation
Consider addition of hydrocortisone, 5 mg/d, and heparin, 100–1,000 units/d, to decrease risk of vein irritation

From Isaacs JW, Millikan WJ, Stackhouse J, Hersh T, Rudman D. Parenteral nutrition of adults with 900-milliosmolar solution via peripheral vein. *Am J Clin Nut.* 1977;30:552–559; and Payne-James JJ, Khawaja HT. First choice for total parenteral nutrition: the peripheral route. *JPEN J Parenter Enter Nutr.* 1993;17:468–478, with permission.

Safe Prescribing Practices

Guidelines published by the American Society of Parenteral and Enteral Nutrition (ASPEN) are considered the gold standard for PN.[1,2]

- PN order sheets commonly contain abbreviated guidelines and information enabling physicians to devise patient-specific PN.
- Each institution should create guidelines for the uniform prescribing of PN to decrease the risk for errors (Table 11.6).
- Components that should be considered for inclusion on the PN order form are listed in Table 11.7.

Table 11.4 COMPONENTS OF 2-IN-1 VS. 3-IN-1 SOLUTIONS

Component	2-in-1	3-in-1/Total Nutrient Admixture
Dextrose	Yes	Yes
Amino acids	Yes	Yes
Lipid	No	Yes

Table 11.5 TYPES OF CENTRAL VENOUS ACCESS DEVICES

Type	Description	Advantages	Disadvantages
Peripheral catheter	Short-term access; may be placed at the bedside	Easily placed	Increased infection risk
Peripherally inserted central catheter (PICC)	Short- or long-term access; may be placed at the bedside; enters the antecubital vein and threaded into the subclavian vein; placement verified radiographically	Easily placed; decreased infection risk; less expensive than other long-term options	
Tunneled	Long-term access; placed surgically through the vein on the upper chest; useful for home total parenteral nutrition (PN) patients	Decreased infection risk; increased patient comfort	Surgical risks; requires proper care
Implanted port	Long-term access; placed surgically underneath the skin near the clavicle; useful for home PN patients	Decreased infection risk; increased patient comfort; aesthetically pleasing	Surgical risks; requires proper care; requires needle changes to gain access to port

Reprinted with permission from Mirtallo J, Canada T, Johnson D, et al. Task Force for the Revision of Safe Practices for Parenteral Nutrition. Safe Practices for Parenteral Nutrition. *JPEN J Parenter Enteral Nutr.* 2004;28(suppl):S39–S70 with permission from the American Society for Parenteral and Enteral Nutrition (A.S.P.E.N.). A.S.P.E.N. does not endorse the use of this material in any form other than its entirety.

Table 11.6 COMMON PRESCRIBING ERRORS

Prescribing practices
Formulation compatibilities
Prescribing nomenclature
Calculation of dosages

Source: From Mirtallo J, Canada T, Johnson D, et al. Safe practices for parenteral nutrition. *JPEN J Parenter Enter Nutr.* 2004;28:S39–S70, with permission.

Table 11.7 COMPONENTS OF ORDER FORM
Organized and clearly written for prescribers and anyone else who may use the form
Ingredients listed in the same format and order as the parenteral nutrition (PN) label
Components ordered in units per day (i.e., mg/d, μg/d) or kg per d
Specify central or peripheral access device
Infusion rate guidelines
Dosing guidelines
Recommended laboratory tests

Reprinted with permission from Mirtallo J, Canada T, Johnson D, et al. Task Force for the Revision of Safe Practices for Parenteral Nutrition. Safe Practices for Parenteral Nutrition. *JPEN J Parenter Enteral Nutr.* 2004;28(suppl):S39–S70 with permission from the American Society for Parenteral and Enteral Nutrition (A.S.P.E.N.). A.S.P.E.N. does not endorse the use of this material in any form other than its entirety.

Fluid Requirements

Fluid requirements should be considered in PN to prevent overhydration or dehydration.

- In healthy adult individuals, a fluid intake of 30 to 40 mL/kg maintains normal fluid balance.[1,2]
- Fluid requirements can be increased by fever, losses from vomiting, diarrhea, nasogastric suction, and fistula drainage, underlying disease.
- Most adults require 35 mL/kg actual body weight to maintain fluid balance.
- A method for calculating fluid requirements in children is displayed in Table 11.8.
  - In infants, use of radiant warmers and treatment with phototherapy increases fluid requirements by 10% to 20%.

Minimizing Fluid in PN

Under certain clinical conditions when a patient is fluid overloaded (e.g., congestive heart failure, chronic renal failure, hypoproteinemia, pulmonary edema), the fluid in PN must be minimized.

- Commercial amino acids are available as dilute (8.5%, 10%) and concentrated (15%, 20%) solutions.
- Because of the low concentrations, amino acid stock solutions add considerable fluid to PN.

Table 11.8 CALCULATION OF FLUID
REQUIREMENTS

	Daily Baseline Fluid Requirements
Adult	35 mL/kg
Children:	
0–10 kg	100 mL/kg
11–20 kg	1,000 mL—50 mL/kg for each kg >10 kg
>20 kg	1,500 mL—20 mL/kg for each kg >20 kg

Reprinted with permission from Mirtallo J, Canada T, Johnson D, et al. Task Force for the Revision of Safe Practices for Parenteral Nutrition. Safe Practices for Parenteral Nutrition. *JPEN J Parenter Enteral Nutr.* 2004;28(suppl):S39–S70 with permission from the American Society for Parenteral and Enteral Nutrition (A.S.P.E.N.). A.S.P.E.N. does not endorse the use of this material in any form other than its entirety.

- In patients who require less fluid, a more concentrated amino acid solution should be used.

Nutritional Requirements

Energy Requirements

The kilocalories a patient needs daily are determined by the basal metabolic rate, level of activity, and increased metabolism caused by the stress of trauma or disease. The basal metabolic rate varies with age, weight, height, gender, and disease state.

- True basal energy expenditure (BEE) can be measured only in a contained metabolic chamber.
- Resting energy expenditure (REE) can be determined by using formulas based on population studies or at a patient's bedside using indirect calorimetry with a metabolic measurement cart.[3]
- Indirect calorimetry is a useful tool but is expensive, and reproducible results require a skilled and experienced technician.
- Underlying disease and trauma influence indirect calorimetry results.
- Indirect calorimetry cannot be used in patients on continuous positive oxygen airway pressure with chest tubes or when the fraction of inspired is ≥50%.
- Indirect calorimetry has limited validity in infants and small children in whom a large amount of physiologic "dead space" is present.

Calculating Energy Requirements

It has been estimated that almost 200 different published formulas derived from population studies are available to calculate REE. Because these

Table 11.9 ACTIVITY AND STRESS FACTORS FOR HARRIS-BENEDICT EQUATION[15]

Activity Factors	Use	Stress Factors	Use
Confined to bed	1.2	Minor operation	1.2
Ambulatory	1.3	Skeletal trauma	1.3
Sepsis	1.6	Major burn	1.5–2.1

Reprinted with permission from Long CL, Schaffel N, Geiger JW, et al. Metabolic response to injury and illness: Estimation of energy and protein needs from indirect calorimetry and nitrogen balance. *JPEN J Parenter Enteral Nutr.* 1979;3:452–456, with permission from the American Society for Parenteral and Enteral Nutrition (A.S.P.E.N.). A.S.P.E.N. does not endorse the use of this material in any form other than its entirety.

formulas are derived from population studies, they are approximations, and the clinical response of the patient should be monitored to determine if the correct kilocalories are being supplied. When energy requirements are calculated, the patient's actual body weight (ABW) is customarily used.

Method 1:
Harris-Benedict equation[3]

$$\text{Male: } 66.5 + (13.75 \times wt) + (5 \times ht) - (6.8 \times age)$$
$$\text{Female: } 655 + (9.6 \times wt) + (1.7 \times ht) - (4.7 \times age)$$

where wt (weight) is in kg, ht (height) is in cm, and age is in years.

Multiplying REE by activity and stress factors in Table 11.9 gives the approximate kilocalories needed. In practice, multiplying REE by 1.2 to 1.4 should supply sufficient kilocalories to account for activity and the stress of trauma and/or disease for most patients.

Method 2:
Kcal/kg per day
The kcal/kg per day method is often used because most patients will require 25 to 35 kcal/kg per day.[2,4]

- Current practice advocates estimating 25 total kcal/kg per day in most adult patients.
- Table 11.10 lists estimated energy requirements for different stress situations.

Method 3:
Hypocaloric feeding for obese patients

Table 11.10 ENERGY REQUIREMENTS USING KCAL/KG/D METHOD

Stress	Energy (kcal/kg/d)
Maintenance/routine surgery	25–30
Minor infection	30
Major surgery/sepsis	30–35
Thermal/head injury	40

Patients with excess body stores of fat (body mass index [BMI] >30 kg/m^2) may be hypocalorically fed.

- Table 11.11 summarizes energy requirements.
- Clinical outcomes to support this strategy include improved wound healing, decreased insulin requirements, and decreased number of intensive care unit days.[5,6]

Protein Requirement

The protein requirement is closely related to the patient's clinical situation.

- Protein requirements vary with degree of metabolic stress (Table 11.12).
- For healthy adults, 0.8 g/kg per day has proven enough to maintain positive nitrogen balance.[2,7]
- Critically ill or hypermetabolic patients generally require 1.5 g/kg per day.[2]
- Patients with chronic renal failure may require slightly less protein, whereas patients with acute renal failure probably do not need protein restriction.
- Daily protein requirements are based on the ABW.
- If a patient is obese (BMI >30 kg/m^2), ideal body weight (IBW) should be used.
- If a patient is edematous, estimated dry weight should be used.

Table 11.11 HYPOCALORIC REGIMEN STRATEGIES

22–25 kcal/kg IBW/d
11–14 kcal/kg ABW/d

IBW, ideal body weight; ABW, actual body weight.
Source: From Choban PS, Dickerson RN. Morbid obesity and nutrition support: is bigger different? *Nutr Clin Pract.* 2005;20:480–487; and Dickerson RN. Hypocaloric feeding of obese patients in the intensive care unit. *Curr Opin Clin Nutr Metab Care.* 2005;8:189–196, with permission.

Table 11.12 PROTEIN REQUIREMENTS

Clinical Situation	Protein (g/kg/d)
Maintenance	0.8–1.0
Moderately stressed	1.1–1.5
Severely stressed	1.5–2.0
Chronic renal failure, no dialysis	0.8–1.2
Renal failure, hemodialysis	1.0–1.2
Renal failure, continuous renal replacement	1.5–2.5
Obese, hypocaloric feeding	2.0 (based on IBW)

Reprinted with permission from Mirtallo J, Canada T, Johnson D, et al. Task Force for the Revision of Safe Practices for Parenteral Nutrition. Safe Practices for Parenteral Nutrition. *JPEN J Parenter Enteral Nutr.* 2004;28(suppl):S39–S70 with permission from the American Society for Parenteral and Enteral Nutrition (A.S.P.E.N.). A.S.P.E.N. does not endorse the use of this material in any form other than its entirety.

Lipid Emulsion
Lipid emulsion is used to deliver calories and to prevent and treat essential fatty acid deficiency (EFAD).[2]

- To prevent EFAD, ≥8% of the total kcal/day must be given as lipid emulsions.
- The usual proportion of fat kilocalories is 15% to 30% of total kcal/day.
- In adults who tolerate lipid emulsion (i.e., those whose serum triglycerides do not rise above 500 mg/dL), a greater proportion of fat calories (≤40%) may provide a balanced nutrient solution.
- The percentage of total kcal/day contributed by lipid should not exceed 60% or an infusion rate >0.11 g/kg per hour).[1]

Electrolytes[1,2]
Standard concentrations of electrolytes in PN solutions vary with institutional guidelines.

- The concentrations shown in Table 11.13 are derived from healthy populations and are general guidelines.
- The electrolyte concentration of a PN solution should be based on the patient's chemistry and clinical condition. Patients may have significant deficits or excesses of serum electrolytes.
- Baseline laboratories and the patient's clinical situation should be considered when determining electrolyte requirements.
- In the institutionalized setting, PN formulations are infused over 24 hours, and electrolyte imbalances should be taken care of immediately.

Table 11.13 GUIDELINES FOR AMOUNT OF ELECTROLYTES TO BE ADDED TO PARENTERAL NUTRITION SOLUTIONS

Electrolyte	Adults	Children
Sodium	0–140 mEq/L	2–4 mEq/kg (max: 100–120 mEq/d)
Potassium	40–60 mEq/L (max: 100 mEq/L)	2–3 mEq/kg (max: 100–120 mEq/d)
Chloride	0–140 mEq/L	3–5 mEq/kg
Phosphate	0–20 mmol/L	0.3–1 mmol/kg
Calcium	4.5–9.0 mEq/L	0.5–1.0 mEq/kg
Magnesium	8–12 mEq/L	0.2–1 mEq/kg
Acetate	Varies	Varies

- Oral or intravenous supplementation of electrolytes may be used in addition to the PN.
- Early after nutrition support is instituted in the malnourished patient, potassium, magnesium, and phosphate shift intracellularly because of increased synthesis of cells.
- As a result, serum concentrations of potassium, magnesium, and phosphate fall. This is known as the refeeding syndrome. It should be anticipated in malnourished patients and serum electrolytes monitored carefully during this period.[8]
- Commercially available stock solutions of the salts used to provide electrolytes in PN solutions are listed in Table 11.14.
- Under conditions of metabolic acidosis, it is common to increase or maximize the concentration of acetate salts because acetate is converted metabolically to bicarbonate by the liver, which raises pH. The concentration of chloride salts, which lower pH, is minimized.[9]
- It is not always possible to entirely remove chloride because amino acid solutions contain intrinsic amounts of chloride counterions.
- Under conditions of metabolic alkalosis, acetate is minimized to avoid raising pH and chloride maximized to lower pH. Eliminating acetate completely is not possible because there are acetate salts intrinsically in amino acid solutions.[9]
- Severe cases of metabolic acidosis or alkalosis should be resolved by fluids and electrolyte solutions and not by PN.

Table 11.14	ELECTROLYTE SALTS OF COMMERCIALLY AVAILABLE SOLUTIONS
Sodium chloride	
Sodium acetate	
Sodium phosphate	
Potassium chloride	
Potassium acetate	
Potassium phosphate	
Calcium gluconate	
Magnesium sulfate	

Vitamins[1,2]

Vitamin requirements for adults and children are based on the recommended daily allowances. The compositions of the most used adult and pediatric preparations are shown in Table 11.15.

Trace Elements[1,2]

Concentrations of trace elements in commonly used commercial preparations are listed in Table 11.16.

- Copper and manganese are eliminated primarily via the bile. For adult patients with cholestasis, copper and manganese are withheld and appropriate amounts of zinc, selenium, and copper are added to the PN separately.
- Patients receiving PN for long periods may develop deficiencies in trace elements due to inadequate intake or underlying diseases.[10]

Additions to PN Formulations

Many compounds can be added safely to PN and total nutrient admixtures (TNAs) although it is usually best to keep the formulation as simple as possible.

- Additions to TNAs should be very limited because of the risk of "cracking" the emulsion. To determine whether a compound is compatible, major references of intravenous stability and compatibility should be consulted such as Trissel's work on compatibility for PN.[11]
- If no data can be found, any requested addition should be considered incompatible.
- Table 11.17 lists commonly added components to PN formulations.

Table 11.15 COMPOSITION OF ADULT AND PEDIATRIC MULTIVITAMIN SOLUTIONS

Vitamins	Adult Multivitamins/ 10 mL	Pediatric Multivitamins/5 mL
A	3,300 IU	2,300 IU
D	200 IU	400 IU
C	200 mg	80 mg
Thiamine (B1)	6 mg	1.2 mg
Pyridoxine (B6)	6 mg	1.0 mg
Riboflavin (B2)	3.6 mg	1.4 mg
Niacin (B3)	40 mg	17 mg
Pantothenic acid	15 mg	5 mg
E	10 IU	7 IU
Folic acid	600 mcg	140 mcg
Cyanocobalamin (B12)	5 mcg	1.0 mcg
K	150 mcg	200 mcg
Biotin	60 mcg	20 mcg

Reprinted with permission from Mirtallo J, Canada T, Johnson D, et al. Task Force for the Revision of Safe Practices for Parenteral Nutrition. Safe Practices for Parenteral Nutrition. *JPEN J Parenter Enteral Nutr.* 2004;28(suppl):S39–S70 with permission from the American Society for Parenteral and Enteral Nutrition (A.S.P.E.N.). A.S.P.E.N. does not endorse the use of this material in any form other than its entirety.

Characteristics of PN Components

The major components of PN (dextrose, amino acids, lipid emulsions) are typically prescribed in terms of grams. Therefore, the amount of calories must be considered when determining energy requirements. Table 11.18 lists common components of PN and the amount of energy provided per gram. Certain clinical situations may exclude the use of lipid emulsions. Contraindications to the use of lipid emulsions are listed in Table 11.19.

Compatibility Issues with PN

Although TNAs must be compounded carefully because precipitates cannot be seen by the unaided eye, any PN formulation can form precipitates

Table 11.16 COMPOSITION OF ADULT AND PEDIATRIC TRACE ELEMENT SOLUTIONS

Trace Element	Adult Solution	Pediatric Solution
Zinc	5 mg	100 μg
Manganese	0.5 mg	6 μg
Copper	2 mg	20 μg
Chromium	20 μg	0.2 μg
Selenium	100 μg	—

Reprinted with permission from Mirtallo J, Canada T, Johnson D, et al. Task Force for the Revision of Safe Practices for Parenteral Nutrition. Safe Practices for Parenteral Nutrition. *JPEN J Parenter Enteral Nutr.* 2004;28(suppl):S39–S70 with permission from the American Society for Parenteral and Enteral Nutrition (A.S.P.E.N.). A.S.P.E.N. does not endorse the use of this material in any form other than its entirety.

Table 11.17 COMMON ADDITIONS TO PARENTERAL NUTRITION SOLUTIONS

Component	Usual Dose	Indication
Regular insulin	0.1 units/g of dextrose; adjust for blood glucose	Hyperglycemia
H_2 antagonists	Ranitidine: 150 mg; adjust for renal dysfunction	Stress ulcer prophylaxis if has risk factors; gastroesophageal reflux disease

Table 11.18 TYPICAL COMPONENTS OF PARENTERAL NUTRITION SOLUTIONS

Component	Kcal/g	Comments
Dextrose 70%	3.4	Maximum infusion rate: 5mg/kg/min (adult), 20 mg/kg/min (pediatric)
Amino acid 10%	4.0	—
Amino acid 15%	4.0	Concentrated form of amino acid
Lipid, intravenous 10%	10	Should not be used for nutrition support
Lipid, intravenous 20%, 30%	10	—

Table 11.19 LIPID EMULSIONS CONTRAINDICATIONS

Triglyceride levels >400–500 mg/dL
Acute pancreatitis with hyperlipidemia
Lipoid nephrosis when accompanied by hyperlipidemia
Neonates with hyperbilirubinemia since lipids displace bilirubin from albumin. If bilirubin is <10 mg/dL (direct <2 mg/dL) and free fatty acid to albumin ratio is 4, lipid may be given because displacement is unlikely
Egg allergy because egg yolk phospholipids are used as emulsifiers

either during compounding, storage, or administration. See Table 11.20 for ways to prevent incompatibility when compounding a PN formulation.

Administration of PN

PN should be initiated slowly to prevent intolerance. Because of the risk of hyperglycemia with large doses of dextrose, the initial day of nutrition support should not contain >200 g/day.

To initiate continuous PN:

1. Calculate the final goal fluid, energy and protein requirements. Protein and a maximum of dextrose (200 g) may be initiated on the first day.

Table 11.20 PREVENTION OF PRECIPITATION

Use calcium gluconate for compounding, rather than calcium chloride
Phosphate should be added near the beginning and calcium near the end of compounding
Do not add ascorbic acid to solution due to its degradation of calcium
The sum of calcium and magnesium should be <20 mEq/L
Add iron with caution secondary to higher cation valence and increased destabilizing potential
Keep solution away from high temperatures

From Trissel LA. *Calcium and Phosphate Compatibility in Parenteral Nutrition.* 1st ed. Houston, TX: Tri Pharma Communications; 2001, with permission.

If lipid emulsion is included in the PN formulation, it may be withheld until the next day.

2. Start at a rate of 25 mL/hour.
3. Check blood glucose via finger sticks every 6 hours. If blood glucose remains <150 mg/dL, the rate may be increased by 25 mL/hour until the goal rate is reached.
4. On day 2, if the patient has tolerated PN, it may be adjusted to include the goal amount of dextrose, protein, and lipid. If the lipid emulsion is to be hung separately, it may be ordered on this day.
5. If the patient does not tolerate the dextrose load, do not advance to goal calories on day 2. Adjust insulin and reassess the next day.
6. If PN must be discontinued, the rate of administration is gradually tapered to prevent rebound hypoglycemia. A typical approach is to reduce the hourly rate by 50% per hour until the final rate is ≤25 mL/hour. If the solution is discontinued abruptly, infuse 10% dextrose until nutrition is able to be restarted.

Monitoring PN

PN is an invasive therapy, and patients should be monitored carefully for metabolic abnormalities throughout the course of the therapy. The suggested regimen in Table 11.21 provides some guidelines for monitoring patients who require PN. Monitoring of patients receiving PN should be individualized according to clinical status, chemical abnormalities, and severity of illness.

Table 11.21 MONITORING PARAMETERS FOR PARENTERAL NUTRITION

Weight trends
Accurate records of input and output
Evidence of intolerance
Laboratory parameters, including serum electrolytes, complete blood count, glucose, inflammatory markers
Markers for nutrition status (prealbumin, nitrogen balance)
Physical examination for hydration or nutrient deficiency or excess
Review of medications

Table 11.22 PARENTERAL NUTRITION (PN) COMPLICATIONS

Complication	Causes	Management
Mechanical		
Pneumothorax	Placement by inexperienced personnel	Possible chest tube placement; minimize number of catheter insertions; placement by experienced personnel
Air embolism	Air inspiration during line placement	Placement by experienced personnel
Catheter occlusion	Formation of fibrin sheath outside of catheter	Anticoagulation locally with urokinase or streptokinase; routine line flushing
Venous thrombosis	Trauma to vein, hypercoagulopathy, sepsis	Anticoagulation; catheter removal
Metabolic		
Hyperglycemia	Common in patients who are diabetic, hypermetabolic, or receiving corticosteroids	Slowly initiate PN; check blood glucose frequently prior to advancing nutrition; administer insulin if needed
Hypoglycemia	Overuse of insulin in PN; abrupt discontinuation of PN	Decrease amount of insulin administered; avoid abrupt discontinuation of PN by tapering rate of infusion; administer 10% dextrose if PN is abruptly discontinued
Hypertriglyceridemia	Inadequate clearing of lipids from bloodstream; pathologic hyperlipidemia	Decrease lipid volume administered; increase length of infusion time; avoid lipid administration >60% of total calories; assess risk factors for hypertriglyceridemia

Electrolyte disturbance	Fluid imbalance; refeeding syndrome; medication use; renal insufficiency	Monitor fluid intake and output and serum chemistries; replace electrolytes as necessary
Essential fatty acid deficiency	Inadequate lipid intake	Provide 8%–10% of total calories as lipids
Prerenal azotemia	Excessive protein administration; dehydration; insufficient nonprotein calories	Increase fluid intake; decrease protein administered; increase nonprotein calories; analyze nitrogen balance
Gastrointestinal (GI)		
Cholestasis	Exact cause unknown; possible excess glucose, protein, amino acid; impaired bile flow; absence of intraluminal nutrients needed to stimulate hepatic bile secretion	Avoid overfeeding; use GI tract as soon as clinically able
Gastrointestinal atrophy	Atrophy of villi; colonic hypoplasia	Use GI tract as soon as clinically able
Infectious		
Catheter-related sepsis	Inappropriate line placement technique; inadequate catheter care; type, location, and duration of catheter	Remove catheter and place at alternate site; adequately care for catheter site; possible treatment with intravenous antibiotics

From Btaiche IF, Khalidi N. Metabolic complications of parenteral nutrition in adults, Part 1. *Am J Health-Syst Pharm.* 2004;61:1938–1949; Btaiche IF, Khalidi N. Metabolic complications of parenteral nutrition in adults, Part 2. *Am J Health-Syst Pharm.* 2004;61:2050–2059, with permission.

Table 11.23	INDICATIONS FOR PARENTERAL NUTRITION—PEDIATRICS
Omphalocele	
Short bowel syndrome	
Congenital malformation	
Gastroschisis	
Malrotation/volvulus	
Intestinal pseudo-obstruction	
Hirschsprung disease	

Source: From American Society of Parenteral and Enteral Nutrition (A.S.P.E.N.). Board of Directors and the Clinical Task Force. Guidelines for the use of parenteral and enteral nutrition in adult and pediatric patients. *JPEN J Parenter Enter Nutr.* 2002;26(Suppl):1SA–138SA; Errata: 2002;26:114, with permission.

Complications of PN

Complications of PN can be categorized as mechanical, metabolic, hepatobiliary, and infectious. The complications associated with PN, as well as possible causes and suggested management, are given in Table 11.22. Health care professionals caring for patients receiving PN should be experienced in the detection and resolution of these complications.

Pediatric Considerations

Enteral nutrition (EN) is the preferred method of nutrition support. However, when this route is contraindicated or inaccessible, PN may be instituted. Typical indications for PN in pediatrics are shown in Table 11.23.

Nutrient requirements for infants and children vary with gender, age, growth rate, and disease state.

- Numerous equations and methods exist to estimate nutrient needs.
- Premature infants may require a greater amount of calories for the "catch up" growth period.
- Table 11.24 summarizes estimated energy and protein requirements dependent on age.
- Electrolyte requirements are similar to those of adults.
- Table 11.25 gives dose ranges for electrolyte goals according to age and weight.
- Children are at risk for essential fatty acid deficiency; therefore most regimens should include lipid emulsion.

Table 11.24 ENERGY AND PROTEIN REQUIREMENTS—PEDIATRICS

Age	Calories (kcal/kg/d)	Protein (g/kg/d)
Preterm	120–150	2.5–3
<6 mo	90–120	2.5–3
6–12 mo	80–100	2–2.5
Toddler	80–12	1.5–2
Child	60–90	1.5–2
Adolescent	30–75	0.8–2

Reprinted with permission from Mirtallo J, Canada T, Johnson D, et al. Task Force for the Revision of Safe Practices for Parenteral Nutrition. Safe Practices for Parenteral Nutrition. *JPEN J Parenter Enteral Nutr.* 2004;28(suppl):S39–S70 with permission from the American Society for Parenteral and Enteral Nutrition (A.S.P.E.N.). A.S.P.E.N. does not endorse the use of this material in any form other than its entirety.

- Stability of 3-in-1 formulations has not been verified in this population. Intravenous lipid emulsions should be infused separately from the dextrose/amino acid formulation.
- Pediatric PN formulations contain significant amounts of cysteine, histidine, and tyrosine, amino acids that are considered semiessential for

Table 11.25 INTRAVENOUS ELECTROLYTE REQUIREMENTS—PEDIATRICS

Electrolyte	Neonates	Infants/Children	Adolescents
Sodium	2–5 mEq/kg/d	2–6 mEq/kg/d	60–150 mEq/d
Potassium	1–4 mEq/kg/d	2–3 mEq/kg/d	70–180 mEq/d
Chloride	1–5 mEq/kg/d	2–5 mEq/kg/d	60–150 mEq/d
Magnesium	0.3–0.5 mEq/kg/d	0.3–0.5 mEq/kg/da	10–30 mEq/d
Calcium	3–4 mEq/kg/d	1–2.5 mEq/kg/d	10–20 mEq/d
Phosphorus	1–2 mmol/kg/d	0.5–1 mmol/kg/d	10–40 mmol/d

Reprinted with permission from Mirtallo J, Canada T, Johnson D, et al. Task Force for the Revision of Safe Practices for Parenteral Nutrition. Safe Practices for Parenteral Nutrition. *JPEN J Parenter Enteral Nutr.* 2004;28(suppl):S39–S70 with permission from the American Society for Parenteral and Enteral Nutrition (A.S.P.E.N.). A.S.P.E.N. does not endorse the use of this material in any form other than its entirety.

infants. In addition, taurine is included because it has been reported to prevent cholestasis associated with PN in children.

References

1. Mirtallo J, Canada T, Johnson D, et al. Safe practices for parenteral nutrition. *JPEN J Parenter Enter Nutr.* 2004;28:S39–S70.
2. American Society of Parenteral and Enteral Nutrition (ASPEN) Board of Directors and the Clinical Task Force. Guidelines for the use of parenteral and enteral nutrition in adult and pediatric patients. *JPEN J Parenter Enter Nutr.* 2002;26(Suppl):1SA–138SA; Errata: 2002;26:114.
3. Harris JA, Benedict FG. A Biometric Study of Basal Metabolism in Man. Publication No.279. Washington, DC: Carnegie Institute; 1919.
4. Cerra FB, Benitez MR, Blackburn GL, et al. Applied nutrition in ICU patients. A consensus statement of the American College of Chest Physicians. *Chest.* 1997;111:769–778.
5. Choban PS, Dickerson RN. Morbid obesity and nutrition support: is bigger different? *Nutr Clin Pract.* 2005;20:480–487.
6. Dickerson RN. Hypocaloric feeding of obese patients in the intensive care unit. *Curr Opin Clin Nutr Metab Care.* 2005;8:189–196.
7. Miles JM. Yes, protein should be included in calorie calculations for a TPN prescription. *Nutr Clin Pract.* 1996;11:204–205.
8. Kraft MD, Btaiche IF, Sacks GS. Review of refeeding syndrome. *Nutr Clin Pract.* 2005;20:625–633.
9. Sacks GS. The ABC's of acid-base balance. *J Pediatr Pharmacol Ther.* 2004;9:235–242.
10. Triplett WC. Clinical aspects of zinc, copper, manganese, chromium and selenium metabolism. *Nutr Int.* 1985;1(2):60.
11. Trissel LA. *Calcium and Phosphate Compatibility in Parenteral Nutrition.* 1st ed. Houston, TX: Tri Pharma Communications; 2001.
12. Isaacs JW, Millikan WJ, Stackhouse J, Hersh T, Rudman D. Parenteral nutrition of adults with 900-milliosmolar solution via peripheral vein. *Am J Clin Nut.* 1977;30:552–559.
13. Payne-James JJ, Khawaja HT. First choice for total parenteral nutrition: the peripheral route. *JPEN J Parenter Enter Nutr.* 1993;17:468–478.
14. Krzywda EA, Andris DA, Edmiston CE, et al. Parenteral access devices. In: Gottschlich MM, DeLegge MH, Mattox T, et al., eds. The A.S.P.E.N. Nutrition Support Core Curriculum: A Case-Based Approach—The Adult Patient. 1st ed. Silver Spring, MD: A.S.P.E.N.; 2007:300–322.
15. Long C. Metabolic response to injury and illness: estimation of energy and protein needs from indirect calorimetry and nitrogen balance. *JPEN J Parenter Enteral Nutr.* 1979;3:452.
16. Btaiche IF, Khalidi N. Metabolic complications of parenteral nutrition in adults, Part 1. *Am J Health-Syst Pharm.* 2004;61:1938–1949.
17. Btaiche IF, Khalidi N. Metabolic complications of parenteral nutrition in adults, Part 2. *Am J Health-Syst Pharm.* 2004;61:2050–2059.

12

A Pharmacy Calculations Anthology

Shelley L. Chambers-Fox and Teresa A. O'Sullivan

The practice of pharmacy requires proficiency in calculations, so during both early and advanced practice experiences students should take every opportunity to practice and perfect their ability to accurately perform calculations. This chapter is an anthology of both common and rare (but complex) calculations encountered in pharmacy practice.

General Principles for Solving Pharmacy Calculations

- Calculation accuracy is greatly improved by independent double checks (i.e., two trained practitioners independently calculate then compare answers). The calculation error rate for a single individual is around 10% (based on results from comprehensive exams). Independent double checks catch 95% of errors,[1] so double checks will catch all but 5% of an individual's errors, reducing the likelihood that a calculation error will reach the patient from 10% to 0.5% ($0.1 \times 0.05 \times 100 = 0.5\%$).
- Published[2] strategies for increasing accuracy in pharmacy calculations include the following:
  - Using references to identify unknown definitions or equations.
  - Writing equations on paper rather than trying to solve mentally.
  - Identifying substance and units for each number in the equation.
  - Using proportional/ratio analysis for calculations involving two different but related expressions of drug amounts.
  - Using dimensional analysis for calculations involving more than two different expressions of drug amounts.

 ‣ Consciously double-checking accuracy by ensuring that all numbers, units, and substances are correctly transcribed/identified, and that all substances and their units on either side of an equation's equal sign (after crossing out matching numerator-denominator substances and their units on either side of the equal sign) are the same.

- Medications are manufactured in forms allowing most recipients to receive small but measurable drug amounts. In general, doses of oral solid medications will be one or two tablets or capsules; doses of liquid medications will be anywhere from 1 mL to 2 teaspoonfuls. If a calculation results in a drug amount that is unreasonably high (e.g., 75 tablets of a manufactured dosage form) or low (e.g., 0.0005 mL of a manufactured liquid dosage form), then the calculation is probably incorrect.

- Many medication dosing recommendations are expressed as a range. Dose calculations for individual patients must identify a single dose, not a dosing range.

- Tablets can be cut in half, but cutting exact half-tablets is difficult even when tablets are scored. Avoid recommending doses that require a patient to cut tablets in half unless there is a clear benefit to the patient. *Capsules cannot be cut in half.*

- Calculated doses should be rounded to a measurable number, requiring familiarity with the precision of the measurement device used for medication dosing.

- Many widely used methods of communicating information about medications have been identified as potentially dangerous.[3] Health care professionals need to avoid using abbreviations in general. See Table 12.1 for a list of abbreviations to avoid.

Conversion Factors and Definitions

A list of conversion factors between the systems commonly used in the United States and the metric system is presented in Table 12.2. Three approaches for converting between Celsius and Fahrenheit systems are shown in Table 12.3, and the equations and definitions commonly used in pharmacy calculations are presented in Table 12.4.

Examples of Calculations Used for Compounding

Percent Volume/Volume (v/v) Concentration Example

A pharmacist needs 38% alcohol in a vehicle to dissolve a drug at the required concentration. The prescription requires 120 mL of an oral liquid

Table 12.1 ABBREVIATIONS TO AVOID

Do Not Use	To Mean	Because	Instead
Trailing zero[a]	e.g., "2.0 mg"	Decimal point is missed: interpreted number higher than actual number by factor of 10	Use 2 mg rather than 2.0 mg
Lack of leading zero	e.g., ".2 mg"	Decimal point is missed: interpreted number higher than actual number by factor of 10	Use a leading zero e.g., 0.2 mg
U	unit	Mistaken for "0," the number "4," or "cc"	Write out "unit"
IU	international unit	Mistaken for "IV" or the number "10"	Write out "international unit"
μ	micro	Mistaken for either u (unit) or m (milli)	Write micro or use mc (e.g., mcg = microgram)
QD, qd	every day	Mistaken for QOD or qod	Write "daily"
QOD, qod	every other day	Mistaken for QD or qd	Write "every other day"
DC	"discharged" or "discontinue"	Confused for one another	Write out full word
Abbreviations for drug names e.g., NTG, HCTZ	Full drug names e.g., nitroglycerin, hydrochlorothiazide	Abbreviations can be misunderstood and misinterpreted	Write out full name of drug
Chemical-like abbreviations MS, MSO$_4$, and MgSO$_4$	Morphine sulfate or magnesium sulfate	Confused for one another	Write "morphine sulfate" and "magnesium sulfate"

[a] A trailing 0 can be used when needed to identify the level of measurement precision, such as for compounding and reporting of laboratory values and imaging studies.

Table 12.2 CONVERSION FACTORS

Unit of Measure	Exact Equivalent	Approximate Equivalent
1 meter (m)	39.4 in.	—
1 inch (in.)	2.54 cm	—
1 kilogram (kg)	2.2 pounds (lb avoir)	—
1 gram (g)	15.4 grain (gr)	—
1 grain (gr avoir)	64.8 mg	60 mg or 65 mg
1 ounce (oz avoir)	28.35 g	30 g
1 pound (lb avoir)	454 g	—
1 teaspoon (tsp)	5 mL	—
1 tablespoon (tbs or Tbsp)	15 mL	—
1 fluid dram (f℥)	3.69 mL	5 mL (1 tsp)
1 fluid ounce (f℥)	29.57 mL	30 mL
1 pint (pt; 16 f℥)	473 mL	480 mL
1 quart (32 f℥; 2 pt)	946 mL	1 liter (1 L)
1 gallon (gal; 4 qt)	3,785 mL	

solution (soln). How much alcohol is needed to make 120 mL 38% (v/v) alcohl?

$$38\% = \frac{38 \text{ mL alcohol}}{100 \text{ mL soln}} = \frac{x \text{ mL alcohol}}{120 \text{ mL soln}} \qquad x = 45.6 \text{ mL alcohol}$$

The alcohol the pharmacist will use to make this is Alcohol USP, which is 95% ethanol:

$$95\% = \frac{95 \text{ mL ethanol}}{100 \text{ mL alcohol USP}} = \frac{45.6 \text{ mL ethanol}}{y \text{ mL alcohol USP}} \qquad y = 48 \text{ mL alcohol USP}$$

Table 12.3 THERMOMETRY CONVERSIONS

$$^\circ F = \frac{(^\circ C)(9)}{5} + 32 \quad or \quad ^\circ F = (^\circ C \times 1.8) + 32 \quad or \quad (5)(^\circ F) = (9)(^\circ C) + 160$$

$$^\circ C = \left(\frac{^\circ F - 32}{9}\right)(5) \quad or \quad ^\circ C = (^\circ F - 32) \times 0.556 \quad or \quad (9)(^\circ C) = (5)(^\circ F) - 160$$

Table 12.4 FORMULAS AND DEFINITIONS USED IN PHARMACY PRACTICE

Term	Definition	Formula
Actual body weight (ABW) or total body weight (TBW) in kg	An individual's actual weight, measured in kg	(ABW in lb)(1 kg/2.2 lb) = ABW in kg
Adjusted body weight in kg	An adjustment made to lean body weight (LBW) to account for drug distribution	AdjBW = 0.4 (TBW − LBW) + LBW
Body surface area (BSA) in meters squared	Size of body surface that provides a better relationship to drug clearance than weight	$BSA = \sqrt{\dfrac{Height\ (in\ cm) \times Weight\ (in\ kg)}{3600}}$
Creatinine clearance (CrCl) in mL/min	Rate at which creatinine is cleared by the kidneys; approximates how well kidneys are functioning	(Cockcroft-Gault equation) $\dfrac{(140 - age) \times (actual\ BW\ in\ kg)}{(GF)(S_{cr})}$ GF (glomerular filtration) = 72 for males, 85 for females S_{cr}: serum creatinine
Lean body weight (LBW) or ideal body weight (IBW) in males	Total body weight of nonfat tissue/fluids in males	50 kg + (2.3 × inches over 5 ft)
Lean body weight (LBW) or ideal body weight (IBW) in females in kg	Total body weight of nonfat tissue/fluids in females	45.5 kg + (2.3 × inches over 5 ft)
Milliequivalent (mEq)	1 mEq = weight of a substance that can replace or combine with 1 millimole (1 mg) of H^+	$1\ mEq = \dfrac{mg\ FW\ weight}{(ions \times valence)}$
Milliosmole (mOsm)	a millimole (6.022 × 10^{20}) of dissolved particles	$= \dfrac{weight\ in\ g \times no.\ species \times 1{,}000}{MW\ in\ g}$ where MW is molecular weight

(continued)

Table 12.4 FORMULAS AND DEFINITIONS USED IN PHARMACY PRACTICE *(continued)*

Term	Definition	Formula
Minimum weighable quantity (MWQ)	The smallest weight of substance that can be measured with ≤5% error	$\dfrac{\text{Balance sensitivity requirement}}{\text{Acceptable error rate (5\%)}}$
Osmolarity (mOsm/L)	Number of milliosmoles in a liter of solution	$= \dfrac{\text{concentration in g/L} \times \text{no. species} \times 1000}{\text{MW in g}}$
Parts per million; ppm (weight/volume)	g per 1,000,000 mL solution	g/mL × 1,000,000
Parts per million; ppm (weight/weight)	g per 1,000,000 g mixture	g/g × 1,000,000
Parts per billion; ppb (volume/volume)	mL per 1,000,000,000 mL solution	mL/mL × 1,000,000,000
Percent (% weight/volume)	grams per 100 or in 100 mL	g/mL × 100
Percent (% volume/volume)	mL per 100 or in 100 mL	mL/mL × 100
Percent (% weight/weight)	grams per 100 or in 100 g	g/g × 100
Ratio strength (1:1000 weight/volume)	grams in 1,000 mL solution	g/mL × 1,000
Ratio strength (1:2 500 volume/volume)	mL in 2,500 mL solution	mL/mL × 2500
Ratio strength (1:500 weight/weight)	grams in 500 g mixture	g/g × 500
Sodium chloride equivalent (E value)	Weight of sodium chloride equivalent to 1 g of drug	E g NaCl = 1 g drug
Specific gravity	Ratio of the weight of a substance to the weight of an equal volume of water	$\text{Sp G} = \dfrac{\text{g/mL substance}}{\text{g/mL water}}$
USP Volume	Volume of isotonic solution that can be made from 1 g of drug and water.	USP mL isotonic solution = 1 g drug

Percent of Concentrated and Dilute Acids

Remember that the chemists use the convention of % weight/weight (w/w) for concentrated acids and % weight/volume (w/v) for dilute acids. If a pharmacist uses 50 mL concentrated phosphoric acid (85%, sp gr 1.71) to make 500 mL of diluted phosphoric acid, what is the percent concentration of the dilution (w/v)?

What weight of phosphoric acid does 50 mL of the concentrated acid contain?

$$\frac{85 \text{ g PA}(1.71 \text{ g soln})}{100 \text{ g solution } (1 \text{ mL soln})} = \frac{145 \text{ g PA}}{100 \text{ mL soln}}$$

$$\frac{145 \text{ g PA}}{100 \text{ mL soln}} = \frac{x \text{ g PA}}{50 \text{ mL soln}} \qquad x = 72.7 \text{ g PA}$$

What is the new concentration w/v?

$$\frac{72.7 \text{ g}}{500 \text{ mL}} = \frac{x \text{ g}}{100 \text{ mL}} \qquad x = 14.5 \text{ g and as a percent } 14.5\%$$

Ratio Strength Calculations

The dose of epinephrine required for a child is 0.022 mg. Can this volume be more conveniently drawn from epinephrine 1:1,000 or 1:10,000?

$$\frac{1 \text{ g epi}}{1,000 \text{ mL}} = \frac{1,000 \text{ mg epi}}{1,000 \text{ mL}} = 1 \text{ mg epi/mL} \quad 0.022 \text{ mg}\frac{(1 \text{ mL})}{1 \text{ mg}} = 0.022 \text{ mL}$$

$$\frac{1 \text{ g epi}}{10,000 \text{ mL}} = \frac{1,000 \text{ mg epi}}{10,000 \text{ mL}} = 0.1 \text{ mg/mL} \quad 0.022 \text{ mg}\frac{(1 \text{ mL})}{0.1 \text{ mg}} = 0.22 \text{ mL}$$

Parts per Million Calculation

A patient reads that the fluoride concentration of her drinking water is 0.8 ppm. How much fluoride does she consume from drinking three 8-oz glasses of water per day?

$$\frac{8 \text{ oz}}{\text{glass}} \frac{(3 \text{ glasses})}{(\text{day})} \frac{(30 \text{ mL})}{(\text{oz})} \frac{(0.8 \text{ g})}{10^6 \text{ mL}} \frac{(1,000 \text{ mg})}{(1 \text{g})} = \text{weight/day}$$

$$= \frac{0.576 \text{ mg fluoride}}{\text{day}}$$

Aliquot Dilutions

- If the available balance or volumetric equipment cannot accurately measure the quantity required, the pharmacist can weigh out a multiple of the quantity and dilute it such that the desired amount is contained in a measurable quantity. This is called an aliquot dilution and can be done as follows:

Example: The pharmacist will compound 30 mg Klonopin (clonazepam) capsules for a child with seizures. She has a typical torsion balance with a sensitivity of 5 mg and

$$\text{Minimum weighable quantity (MWQ)} = \frac{\text{sensitivity or linear accuracy}}{\text{fraction error}}$$

$$\text{Minimum weighable quantity} = \frac{5 \text{ mg}}{0.05} = 100 \text{ mg}$$

1. Select a multiple of the amount that will equal or exceed the MWQ for the balance:

$$30 \text{ mg} \times 4 = 120 \text{ mg clonazepam to weigh out}$$

2. Select the weight of the dilution that will contain the amount of active ingredient that is needed (the aliquot weight). This number must also equal or exceed the MWQ.

    The pharmacist decides that 1/4 of the dilution will weigh 200 mg: Multiply it by the same factor:

$$200 \times 4 = 800 \text{ mg total dilution}$$

$$- \frac{120 \text{ mg drug}}{680 \text{ mg lactose}}$$

Mix these two well.

3. Take 1/4 or 200 mg of the dilution, and it will contain 30 mg clonazepam.

Simple Dilutions

What volume of adult strength acetazolamide injection, 100 mg/mL, should be used to make 10 mL of the neonatal concentration, 5 mg/mL?

$$\frac{\text{Original concentration}}{\text{Diluted concentration}} = \frac{\text{Diluted volume}}{\text{Original volume}}$$

$$\frac{100 \text{ mg/mL}}{5 \text{mg/mL}} = \frac{10 \text{ mL}}{y \text{ mL}}$$

Rearranging for y:

$$(100 \text{ mg/mL}) \, (y \text{ mL}) = (5 \text{ mg/mL}) \, (10 \text{ mL})$$

$$C_1 V_1 = C_2 V_2$$

$$V_1 = \frac{(5 \text{ mg/mL}) \, (10 \text{ mL})}{(100 \text{ mg/mL})} = 0.5 \text{ mL adult strength acetazolamide}$$

Blending Two Concentrations

   Rx   Tobramycin 1% eye drops
           Disp 10 mL
           Sig: 1 gtt od tid

The pharmacist will make these drops from the commercially available eye drops, which have a strength of 0.3 %, and the injectable tobramycin, 40 mg/mL. What volume of each strength should be used to make the 10 mL eye drops?

$$40 \text{ mg/mL} \times 100 = 4{,}000 \text{ mg/100 mL} = 4 \text{ g/100 mL} = 4\%$$

Set

$$x = \text{fraction of tobramycin injection}$$

$$1 - x = \text{fraction of tobramycin eye drops}$$

The equation is

$$1\% = 4\% \, x + (1 - x) 0.3\%$$

Multiplying by 0.3,

$$1 = 4x + 0.3 - 0.3x$$

Combine the like terms:

$$1 - 0.3 = 4x + 0.3 - 0.3 - 0.3x$$

$$0.7 = 3.7x$$

Solving for x

$$\frac{0.7}{3.7} = \frac{3.7x}{3.7}$$

$x = 0.19$ = fraction of injectable tobramycin

$1 - x = 0.81$ = fraction of tobramycin eyedrops

To make 10 mL:

$0.19 \times 10\,\text{mL} = 1.9\,\text{mL}$ injectable tobramycin

$0.81 \times 10\,\text{mL} = 8.1\,\text{mL}$ tobramycin eye drops

Tonicity Calculations

- E value calculates the weight of sodium chloride equivalent to 1 g of drug or other solute.
- In some cases the E value of the drug has been tabulated,[4] and the amounts of water and isotonic vehicle to be added to prepare an isotonic product can be calculated using proportions.

E Value Calculation

Rx   Cromolyn sodium 40 mg/mL
benzalkonium chloride 0.01%
Dispense 10 mL

How much sodium chloride is required to make the solution isotonic if the E for cromolyn sodium = 0.11?

1. Amount of NaCl equivalent to drug: For cromolyn:

$40\,\text{mg/mL} \times 10\,\text{mL} = 400\,\text{mg} = 0.4\,\text{g}$ cromolyn   E value $= 0.11$

$$\frac{0.4\,\text{g drug}}{1\,\text{g drug}} = \frac{x\,\text{g NaCl}}{0.11\,\text{g NaCl}}$$

$x = 0.044\,\text{g NaCl}$

For benzalkonium chloride:
$0.01/100 \times 10\,\text{mL} = 0.001\,\text{g}$ benzalkonium chloride E value $= 0.16$

$$\frac{0.001\,\text{g drug}}{1\,\text{g drug}} = \frac{x\,\text{g NaCl}}{0.16\,\text{g NaCl}}$$

$x = 0.00016\,\text{g NaCl}$

2. How much NaCl to make the solution isotonic?

$$\frac{0.9\,\text{g NaCl}}{100\,\text{mL}} = \frac{y\,\text{g NaCl}}{10\,\text{mL}} \qquad y = 0.09\,\text{g NaCl}$$

3. How much NaCl to add?

0.09 g	NaCl
− 0.044 g	contributed by the cromolyn
−0.00016 g	contributed by the benzalkonium chloride
0.04584	= 0.046 g NaCl to add

Oral Suspensions for Reconstitution:

Rx   Zithromax 250 mg/5 mL
     Sig: 2 tsp today and 1 tsp qd × 4 additional days.

The patient is an 87-year-old man with pneumonia. The pharmacist has a 30-mL size bottle of azithromycin (Zithromax) powder for reconstitution that if reconstituted with 18 mL water will have a concentration of 200 mg/5 mL. How many milliliters of water should be added to prepare it in the prescribed concentration?

What volume is the powder?

30 mL
−18 mL
12 mL represented by the powder

How much total drug is in the bottle?

$$\frac{(200\,\text{mg})}{(5\,\text{mL})}(30\,\text{mL}) = 1{,}200\,\text{mg drug total}$$

What total volume should be used to make the concentration equal 250 mg/5 mL?

$$\frac{(5\,\text{mL})}{250\,\text{mg}}(1{,}200\,\text{mg}) = 24\,\text{mL total volume}$$

How much water should be added?

24 mL total volume
− 12 mL represented by the powder
12 mL water to add

Proportionate Parts

A convenient method for recording formulae that are made in widely varying amounts is proportionate parts. For example, the formula of a popular suppository base consists of

PEG 1000   3 parts
PEG 4000   1 part

A prescription requires 22 g of the suppository base. How much of each component does the pharmacist need?

PEG 1000   3 parts
PEG 4000   1 part
Total   4 parts

$$\frac{3 \text{ parts PEG 1000}}{4 \text{ parts total}} = \frac{x \text{ g PEG 1000}}{22 \text{ g total}} \qquad x = 16.5 \text{ g PEG 1000}$$

$$\frac{1 \text{ part PEG 4000}}{4 \text{ parts total}} = \frac{x \text{ g PEG 4000}}{22 \text{ g total}} \qquad x = 5.5 \text{ g PEG 4000}$$

Compounding with Commercially Available Dosage Forms

- Pharmacists will often use commercially available dosage forms in compounding rather than drug powders.
- For example, an ointment may be prepared from so many milliliters of an injection and an ointment base that absorbs solutions or a suspension may be compounded by crushing tablets or opening capsules.
- When using an injectable product, the volume of the solution that contains a specified amount of drug can be easily calculated *because the weight per unit volume is on the label.*
- With solid dosage forms the concentration of drug in solid mixture is specified per tablet or per capsule rather than per gram or milligram.
- Tablets and capsules will always have ingredients other than drug in the dosage form.
  ‣ One hydralazine tablet contains 50 mg drug, 10 tablets are required to provide 500 mg.
  ‣ But what if a prescription requires 480 mg?
- It will be necessary to know the weight of the tablet or in the case of capsules *of the capsule contents*, to determine what weight of hydralazine tablets contains 480 mg.

Rx Lamotrigine 4 mg capsules
    Make capsules
    Dispense 28
    Sig: Open 1 capsule on soft food twice daily

Lamotrigine is an anticonvulsant drug available as 25-, 100-, 150-, and 200-mg tablets.

How much drug is required to make the 28 capsules?

$$4 \text{ mg/cap} \times 28 \text{ caps} = 112 \text{ mg is needed}$$

If the pharmacist uses 25-mg tablets and they weigh 80 mg each, how much crushed tablet powder is required to make the 28 capsules?

$$(112 \text{ mg drug}) \frac{(80 \text{ mg tab powder})}{25 \text{ mg drug}} = 358.4 \text{ mg tab powder}$$

And what weight of tablet powder will contain the dose?

$$\frac{358.4 \text{ mg tab powder}}{28 \text{ doses}} = 12.8 \text{ mg tab powder/dose}$$

Test Capsules, Test Suppositories

- When making capsules or suppositories, the pharmacist is faced with determining what weight of the drug mixture will fit in the volume dictated by a capsule shell or suppository mold.
- This is done by preparing a test capsule or suppository using diluent and drug.
- The weight of the test capsule or suppository can be used to determine how much diluent or suppository base to use for a given batch.

Consider the lamotrigine capsules above. The pharmacist plans to pack them into a no. 4 capsule. If the test capsule weighs 135 mg, how much lactose should be used to make the 28 lamotrigine capsules?

$$135 \text{ mg/capsule} \times 28 \text{ capsules} = 3780 \text{ mg total mixture}$$
$$\frac{-358.4 \text{ mg tab powder}}{} \text{ containing our drug}$$
$$3421.6 \text{ mg lactose to add}$$

Rx Avandia 8-mg suppositories
    Dispense 7
    Sig: 1 rectally q AM.

These suppositories can be made from Avandia tablets. A batch of five Avandia 8-mg tablets weighs 1,570 mg. If the test suppository weighs 2.4 g, how many grams PEG 1000 and PEG 4000 should be used to make the seven suppositories?

1,570 mg/5 tab = 314 mg/tab = 0.314 g
2.4 g × 7 = 16.8 g suppository mixture
tablets weigh 0.314 g × 7 = 2.198
16.8 − 2.198 = 14.602 g base needed

$$\frac{3 \text{ parts PEG 1000}}{4 \text{ parts total}} = \frac{x \text{ g PEG 1000}}{14.602 \text{ g total}} \qquad x = 10.95 \text{ g PEG 1000}$$

$$\frac{1 \text{ parts PEG 4000}}{4 \text{ parts total}} = \frac{x \text{ g PEG 4000}}{14.602 \text{ g total}} \qquad x = 3.65 \text{ g PEG 4000}$$

Examples of Calculations Used for Dosing

Doses Based on Age and Weight

A 3-year-old, 36 lb patient with otitis media is to receive cephalexin. The recommended dose is 75–100 mg/kg per day in four divided doses. If 90 mg/kg is used, what volume in teaspoonsful of Keflex suspension, 250 mg/5 mL, should the child receive in each dose?

$$(36 \text{ lb}) \frac{(1 \text{ kg})}{(2.2 \text{ lb})} \frac{(90 \text{ mg})}{(\text{kg/day})} \frac{(\text{day})(1 \text{ tsp})}{(4 \text{ doses})(250 \text{ mg})} = 1.47 \text{ tsp} = 1.5 \text{ tsp/dose}$$

Doses Based on Lean Body Weight

Because some drugs partition largely into body water or lean tissue and to a much lesser extent into adipose, an obese patient could receive more drug than required to produce therapeutic levels in the lean tissues if the dose were based on actual body weight. It is preferable, then, to calculate the patient's ideal or lean body weight and use this as the basis for calculating the dose of such drugs. The following equations can be used to calculate lean body weight (LBW):[5]

$$\text{LBW (males)} = 50 \text{ kg} + (2.3 \times \text{ in. over 5 ft})$$
$$\text{LBW (females)} = 45.5 \text{ kg} + (2.3 \times \text{ in. over 5 ft})$$

The digitalizing or loading dose of digoxin tablets is 10–15 μg/kg. What is the appropriate dose for a 62-year-old woman who is 5 ft 1 in. and weighs 188 pounds (85.5 kg)?

Calculate lean body weight:

$$\text{LBW (females)} = 45.5 \, \text{kg} + (2.3 \times 1)$$
$$= 47.8 \, \text{kg}$$

Calculate the digitalizing dose:

$$(47.8 \, \text{kg}) \frac{(12.5 \mu\text{g})}{(1 \, \text{kg})} = 597.5 \, \mu\text{g}$$

The patient should receive one 250-μg tablet immediately and a second 250-μg tablet in 6 to 8 hours.

Doses Based on Surface Area

Because body surface area has a stronger relationship to renal clearance and to metabolic capacity than does body weight, BSA is preferred for calculating doses of drugs with narrower margins of safety. Body surface area may be calculated from the following equation:

$$\text{BSA} = \sqrt{\frac{\text{Height(in cm)} \times \text{Weight(in kg)}}{3600}}$$

BSA is body surface area in m^2. An adult patient is to receive cytarabine, 25 mg/m^2 for one dose, followed by cytarabine, 100 mg/m^2 every 24 hours for seven doses. The patient is 6 ft 1 inch and 163 pounds. How many milligrams of cytarabine should the patient receive in the first dose and how many in each subsequent dose?

Convert his weight:

$$(163 \, \text{lb}) \frac{(1 \, \text{kg})}{(2.2 \, \text{lb})} = 74 \, \text{kg}$$

Convert his height:

$$(73 \, \text{in.}) \frac{(2.54 \, \text{cm})}{(1 \, \text{in.})} = 185 \, \text{cm}$$

Calculate his body surface area:

$$BSA = \sqrt{\frac{\text{Height (in cm)} \times \text{Weight (in kg)}}{3600}}$$

$$BSA = \sqrt{\frac{(185 \text{ cm}) \times (74 \text{ kg})}{3600}}$$

$$BSA = 1.95 \text{ m}^2$$

Calculate the initial dose:

$$(1.95 \text{ m}^2)\frac{(25 \text{ mg})}{(\text{m}^2)} = 49 \text{ mg}$$

Calculate each subsequent dose:

$$(1.95 \text{ m}^2)\frac{(100 \text{ mg})}{(\text{m}^2)} = 195 \text{ mg}$$

Doses Based on Creatinine Clearance

Drugs that are primarily cleared from the body by the kidneys may accumulate to toxic levels in patients with renal dysfunction if either the dose or the frequency of administration is not modified. The literature on a number of drugs provides dosing tables for adjusting drug regimens based on the extent of renal dysfunction. A useful estimate of the degree of renal dysfunction is the creatinine clearance (normal range, 100–140 mL/minute; CrCl). Creatinine is an endogenous substance that is filtered by the kidneys but not significantly reabsorbed or secreted. Thus its clearance is an estimate of glomerular filtration rate. Serum creatinine levels can be easily measured and used to calculate creatinine clearance using the following formula:

The method of Cockcroft and Gault is adjusted for lean body weight:[6]

$$\text{CrCl (males)} = \frac{(140 - \text{age}) \times \text{LBW}}{72 \times S_{cr}}$$

$$\text{CrCl (females)} = \frac{(140 - \text{age}) \times \text{LBW}}{85 \times S_{cr}}$$

- CrCl is creatinine clearance in mL/minute, age in years.
- LBW is lean body weight in kg.

- S_{cr} is serum creatinine in mg/dL.
- Use total body weight (TBW) if TBW <LBW.
- Use adjusted body weight (AdjBW) if obese >125% of LBW.
- AdjBW = 0.4 (TBW − LBW) + LBW.

>> A 79-year-old male patient has a urinary tract infection. He is 69 in. tall, 155 lb, and his S_{cr} = 1.7 mg/dL. Calculate this patient's estimated CrCl.

$$LBW = 50 + (2.3 \times 9) = 70.7 \text{ kg} \quad 155 \text{ lb}/2.2 \text{ lb/kg} = 70.5 \text{ kg}$$

$$CrCl = \frac{(140 - 79) \times 70.5}{72 \times 1.7} = \frac{4300.5}{122.4} = 35.1 \text{ mL/min}$$

The labeling of cefixime makes the following recommendations for patients with renal dysfunction:

CrCl >60 mL/min	No dosage adjustment needed
CrCl 20–60 mL/min:	300 mg daily
CrCl <20 mL/min:	200 mg daily

How many 100 mL bottles of cefixime suspension, 100 mg/5mL, should be dispensed to provide the patient above with 14 days' therapy?

$$\frac{(300 \text{ mg})}{(\text{day})} \frac{(5 \text{ mL})}{(100 \text{ mg})} \frac{(1 \text{ bottle})}{(100 \text{ mL})} (14 \text{ d}) = 2.1 \text{ bottles} \ (3 \text{ bottles})$$

Calculation of Injectable Volumes

The pharmacy has an order for a 120-lb patient for amikacin sulfate, 7.5 mg/kg loading dose, in 100 mL D5W. Amikacin is available in vials containing 100 mg/2 mL, 500 mg/2 mL, and 1 g/4 mL.

$$120 \text{ lb} \frac{(1 \text{ kg})}{(2.2 \text{ lb})} \frac{(7.5 \text{ mg})}{(\text{kg})} = 409 \text{ mg amikacin}$$

$$\text{Use the 500 mg vial:} \ \frac{500 \text{ mg}}{2 \text{ mL}} = \frac{409 \text{ mg}}{y \text{ mL}} \quad y = 1.64 \text{ mL}$$

- Note: This volume, 1.64 mL, would be added to a 100-mL bag of D5W, which means that the resulting volume would be 101.64 mL.

- This is typically how IV additives are made *rather* than first withdrawing 1.64 mL of D5W and then adding the drug solution so that the final volume is 100 mL.
- Although small volumes of overfill are sometimes ignored in subsequent calculations, this example will include them.
- This practice may vary from hospital to hospital.

Administration Rate Calculations

Large-volume parenterals (LVPs) are administered in two ways:

1. Drip set: an apparatus that is attached to the LVP bag with tubing that runs to the patient and has a drip chamber that can be used to observe and count the number of drops flowing through over a specified time. Flow rate is expressed in *drops per minute*.
   a. Drip sets deliver from 10 drops/mL to 60 drops/mL.
   b. Typical rates are between 0.7 and 2.5 mL/minute (25–80 drops/minute).
2. Infusion pump: a programmable device that allows the nurse/pharmacist to set the number of *milliliters per hour or milligrams per hour* that it will deliver through the tubing to the patient.
   a. Typical rates are between 42 and 150 mL/hour.
3. Overfill: In addition to the overfill created by additives, most parenteral products contain some planned overfill. Manufacturers provide a slight excess volume since it is impossible to transfer 100% of the volume from a container into a syringe.
   a. Some pharmacies ignore overfill in their calculations of volume and flow rate and others do not.

Consider the patient who is receiving amikacin. The first dose is usually infused over 30 minutes. What drip rate should be set with a drip set that delivers 20 drops/mL?

The order includes $100 + 1.64 = 101.64$ mL drug solution.

$$\frac{(101.64 \text{ mL})}{30 \text{ min}} \frac{(20 \text{ drops})}{(\text{mL})} = \frac{67.8 \text{ drops}}{\text{min}} \text{ or } \frac{68 \text{ drops}}{\text{min}} \text{ drug solution}$$

Administration Rate Using Infusion Pumps

Here is an infusion pump example: A doctor wants to dose a patient at $2 \mu g/kg/minute$ with dopamine in the intensive care unit (ICU). The patient weighs 70 kg. The concentration of drug in the bag is 80 mg/100 mL.

What flow rate in mL per hour should be set to infuse the dopamine solution?

$$(70\,\text{kg}) \frac{(2\,\mu\text{g})}{(\text{kg/min})} \frac{(1\,\text{mg})}{(1{,}000\,\mu\text{g})} \frac{(100\,\text{mL})}{(80\,\text{mg})} \frac{(60\,\text{min})}{(1\,\text{hr})} = \frac{10.5\,\text{mL}}{\text{hr}}$$

The 2004 Joint Commission on Accreditation of Healthcare Organizations (JCAHO) medication error reduction program recommended programming pumps in mg/hour instead of mL/hour. What is the infusion rate in mg/hour?

$$(70\,\text{kg}) \frac{(2\,\mu\text{g})}{(\text{kg/min})} \frac{(1\,\text{mg})}{(1{,}000\,\mu\text{g})} \frac{(60\,\text{min})}{(1\,\text{hr})} = \frac{8.4\,\text{mg}}{\text{hr}}$$

Calculating Osmolarity

In clinical practice the pharmacist may want to know the concentration of particles exerting osmotic pressure in an injection or ophthalmic product so that it may be adjusted if it differs substantially from that of serum or tears. The osmolarity or moles of solute particles per liter of serum or tears is between 275 and 295 mOsm/L. This parameter can be estimated from the following equation.

$$\text{mOsm/L} = \frac{\text{wgt of substance in g/L}}{\text{molecular weight (MW) in g}} \times \text{number of species} \times 1{,}000$$

For example, the calculated osmolarity of 1 g of ampicillin sodium (FW 371.4) in 10 mL of SWI would be

$$\text{mOsm/L} = \frac{1\,\text{g}/0.01\,\text{L}}{371\,\text{g}} \times 2 \times 1{,}000 = 539\,\text{mOsm/L}$$

Bulky Powders for Reconstitution

Many drugs are not stable in solution.

- Manufactured as powders for reconstitution, the pharmacy adds diluent before they can be administered.
- Some of these powders represent a very large volume; they may include buffers or with oral products, flavors, sweeteners, and dyes, which increase the volume of the powders to be dissolved.
- It cannot be assumed that the volume of the powder to be reconstituted is negligible; that is, dissolving 1 g of ampicillin in 10 mL water produces a concentration of 100 mg per mL.

- The manufacturer will give specific instructions on how much diluent to use to produce a specified concentration.

A pharmacist needs to make cefazolin injection for ophthalmic use at a concentration of 25 mg/0.1 mL. He has cefazolin powder for reconstitution: to 1 g, add 2.5 mL of diluent, for a resulting concentration of 333.3 mg/mL. How many milliliters of normal saline should be added to make the 25 mg/0.1 mL for ophthalmic use?

$$\frac{1\,g}{x\,mL} = \frac{0.3333\,g}{1\,mL} \quad x = 3\,mL \quad 3\,mL - 2\text{-}5\,mL = 0.5\,mL$$

represented by the powder

$$\frac{1,000\,mg}{x\,mL} = \frac{25\,mg}{0.1\,mL} \quad x = 4\,mL \quad 4\,mL - 0.5\,mL = 3.5\,mL$$

saline to add

Milliequivalents

One milliequivalent is the weight of a substance that can replace or combine with 1 millimole (1 mg) of H^+.

How many milliequivalents of Ca are there per milliliter of a 10% calcium gluconate injection?

Formula: $C_{12}H_{22}CaO_{14}$
FW   430
Valence 2×1 Ca ion

So there are

$$\frac{2\,mEq\ Ca\ ion}{430\,mg\ Ca\ gluc}$$

$$10\%\,Ca\ gluc = \frac{10\,g\ Ca\ gluc}{100\,mL} \frac{(2\,mEq\ Ca)}{(0.43\,g\ Ca\ gluc)} = 0.465\ mEq\ Ca/mL$$

References

1. The virtues of independent double checks—they really are worth your time? In: Institute for Safe Medication Practices Medication Safety Alert [Internet] Institute for Safe Medication Practices, 2003 Mar 6. Available at: www.ismp.org. Accessed July 23, 2007.

2. Brown MC. Introduction to pharmaceutical calculations, *Am J Pharm Educ.* 2003;67(2): Article 67.

3. Anon. ISMP's List of Error-Prone Abbreviations, Symbols and Dose Designations, Institute for Safe Medication Practices, Available at www.ismp.org, Accessed January 30, 2008.

4. Stoklosa MJ, Ansel HC. *Pharmaceutical Calculations*, 12th ed. Philadelphia, PA: Lippincott, Williams & Wilkins; 2006:161–162.

5. Shargel L, Wu-Pong S, Yu ABC. Applied Biopharmaceutics and Pharmacokinetics. 5th ed. New York, NY: McGraw-Hill; 2005.

6. Cockcroft DW, Gault MH. Prediction of creatinine clearance from serum creatinine. *Nephron.* 1976;16:31–41.

13 Clinical Pharmacokinetics

Molly E. Gates and Sandra B. Earle

USE OF PHARMACOKINETIC PRINCIPLES TO ENHANCE DRUG THERAPY

Pharmacists are uniquely qualified in their understanding and application of pharmacokinetic (PK) principles as tools to optimize the use of drugs in patients. Using PK, the pharmacist can properly evaluate measured drug concentrations and design dosage regimens. In addition, by understanding what determines pharmacokinetic parameters, drug and disease interactions can be predicted. This chapter provides a table of equations, a glossary, and some general concepts of clinical therapeutic drug monitoring and dosage regimen design. This is not an all-encompassing review of clinical pharmacokinetics but can serve as a refresher of basic ideas and important caveats. Please see more detailed texts and literature references for further details.

Evaluation of Measured Drug Concentrations: Therapeutic Drug Monitoring (TDM)

Indications for Therapeutic Drug Monitoring

Most drugs do not require determination of drug concentrations for optimization of drug therapy. If you can give a standard dosage regimen and get the wanted effect in all/most patients, there is no reason to measure drug concentrations. TDM may be useful only if the following criteria are in place:

- Absence of a well-defined dose–response relationship.
- A well-defined concentration–response relationship (pharmacodyamics).

- A relatively narrow therapeutic range.
- Interpatient variability in dose regimen–concentration relationship (pharmacokinetics).
- Accurate drug assays available.

In addition to serving as a guide for dosage adjustment, drug concentrations may be used to assess patient adherence.

For appropriate interpretation of the measured drug concentrations, the following information should be either known or obtained:

- What condition is being treated?
- Is the patient suffering from any dose-related toxicities and/or signs of lack of efficacy?
- Is the patient at steady state (SS)?
- Were all doses given at the appropriate time, and if not, when were they given?
- When was (were) the sample(s) drawn in relation to the dose given?
- Are there any patient-specific factors that can influence pharmacokinetic parameters (i.e., volume status, albumin concentrations, etc.)?

Unbound Free versus Total Concentrations

Total concentrations of drugs are made up of the sum of both drug bound to plasma proteins as well as drug that is free from the binding proteins. Only free or unbound drug molecules can interact at the pharmacologic sites. Therefore, free concentrations correlate more closely with drug effect. It is much easier (and cheaper) for the lab to measure total drug rather than just the free drug concentration. Thus, most drug concentrations are reported as total concentrations, and most therapeutic ranges are in terms of total drug concentrations. As long as the free fraction of drug in the plasma (fraction unbound in plasma [fup]) remains constant, the total concentration will be proportional to the free concentration. As soon as the fup changes, this will no longer be true. It is almost always acceptable to look at total concentrations and feel confident that they are proportional to the free concentration, except when fup is thought to be altered by drugs or disease or is changing with concentration.

Sampling Times

As a general rule, the trough concentration (Cmin) is usually monitored. If the Cmin (trough) is within the therapeutic range (TR), the patient is likely not suffering from lack of efficacy due to inadequate serum concentrations. This does not ensure, however, that the patient's average concentration at steady state (Css,avg) and maximum concentration at steady state (Css,max) are appropriate. Since the time to Cmax can vary significantly for orally administerd drugs, it is hard to determine when to draw a concentration to capture the Cmax. If any two concentrations are drawn during the elimination phase, an elimination rate constant (k), half-life ($t^{1}/_{2}$), volume of distribution (V), and drug out (CL) can be determined along with Cmax, Cmin, and any other concentration. There are drugs for which both the trough and the peak concentrations may be monitored (e.g., aminoglycosides). If trying to determine k when giving a short infusion, be sure to allow sufficient time after giving a drug for initial distribution. A good rule of thumb is to wait 1 hour after giving a $^{1}/_{2}$-hour infusion and wait $^{1}/_{2}$ hour if giving an infusion over an hour.

It is important to be sure that the blood sample drawn will have a concentration that will be above the minimum detection limit of your lab. The pharmacist should predict what the concentration will be before it is drawn, to ensure it is within the detectable range. A Cmin measurement may be too low to detect. If a concentration-related toxicity is suspected, a serum concentration sample should be drawn as soon as possible to determine the toxicity range for that patient.

Dosage Regimen Design

Initial Dosing

Depending on the therapeutic concentration goals, a loading dose (LD) may or may not be needed. A LD is needed when it will take too long to achieve therapeutic concentrations when using a maintenance dosing regimen. This includes drugs with a long $t^{1}/_{2}$. A LD is based on the target concentration and the Vc. Giving a LD does not change the time to steady state (SS); only $t^{1}/_{2}$ determines when SS will be achieved.

$$LD = V_C \times C_{target}$$

Intial maintenance dosage regimens are determined by choosing a target Css,avg and target peak-to-trough ratio (P:T). The dosage regimen is made up of the dose rate (DR) and the dose interval (τ). The DR is a determinant of the Css,avg achieved, and the τ determines what P:T will be seen. When a drug is given to a patient for the first time, population averages are used as the patient's PK parameters. Target Css,avg along with population CL and bioavailability (F) estimates determine the initial DR:

$$Css,avg = \frac{F \times DR}{CL}$$

Dosing once every $t^1/_2$ is a good rule of thumb, but P:T ratio can be targeted with a population k.

$$P : T = \frac{1}{e^{-k\tau}}$$

Modification of Dosing Regimen

After starting a patient on a dosage regimen based on population information, optimization of the indiviual patient's drug therapy must be verified. This includes evaluating the patient clinically. The drug concentrations are only one tool in evaluating therapy. Evaluating the patient's clinical status in light of his or her drug concentrations will help to determine if a change in dosing regimen is necessary. To evaluate Css,avg, you must be at SS. It is often appropriate to measure concentrations before reaching SS to avoid toxicity or lack of efficacy.

If the patient is at SS, the pharmacist should determine if the Css,avg is appropriate for the patient. If the Css,avg is too high, the patient's drug exposure may be too high, putting him or her at risk for concentration-related toxicity; therefore the DR should be decreased. If the Css,avg is too low, the opposite would be true and the DR should be increased. What would cause a change in Css,avg? The determinants of Css,avg are drug in ($F \times DR$) and drug out (CL).

$$Css,avg = \frac{F \times DR}{CL} = \frac{Drug\ In}{Drug\ Out}$$

If CL or F is altered, there will be a resulting change in Css,avg, possibly necessitating a change in DR. If there is a possible change in plasma protein binding, it will be important to consider the Css,avg, free rather than just the Css,avg. If a change in DR is deemed necessary and the patient is at SS, as long as there is no reason to think there might be a change in CL or F, Css,avg becomes proportional to DR. Therefore the adjustment in DR can be made using a simple proportion:

$$\frac{DR_1}{Css,avg_1} = \frac{DR_2}{Css,avg_2}$$

It is often important to consider the variability in the Cmax and Cmin concentrations (P:T). If the Cmax is too high and the Cmin is too low (large P:T) the dosing interval may be too long, so the dosing interval should be shortened, giving the drug more often during the day. It is rare (with the exception of aminoglycosides) that a Cmax would be too low and the Cmin too high (too small P:T). In this case, the τ should be increased. This would allow for greater change between the Cmax and Cmin. What would cause a change in this variability (P:T)? Changes in V or CL will cause a change in $t^{1/2}$ therefore change the P:T.

Determination of Concentrations Other than Those Measured

If a drug follows a first-order, one-compartment elimination model, concentrations at any time during the dosing interval can be determined if one concentration and a k is known. Therefore Css,max, Css,min, and any other concentration can be quantified using the one-compartment decay equation. k can be determined if two concentration time points are known. Css,avg can be determined by calculating the area under the concentration curve ($AUC_{0-\tau}$) at SS.

$$C_t = C_0 e^{-kt}$$

$$k = \frac{lnC_2 - lnC_1}{t_2 - t_1}$$

$$C_{ss,avg} = \frac{AUC_{ss\,0-\tau}}{\tau}$$

Predicting Drug and Disease Interactions

Drugs administered concurrently and diseases that patients have can alter PK parameters. This may result in changes in Css,avg or P:T ratios that could cause concentration-related toxicity or lack of efficacy. To predict these changes, the determinants of Css,avg and P:T must be understood.

Altered Css,avg can come about from a change in F and/or a change in CL. A change in F can occur due to a change in fraction absorbed (fa), fraction that escapes gut metabolism (fg), or fraction that escapes first-pass effect (ffp). A change in formulation or addition of drug that adsorbs the first drug, for example, could decrease fa causing a decrease in F and therefore a decrease in Css,avg. The DR should be increased to maintain a given Css,avg. The determinants of CL are complex as many organs may be involved. To simplify, consider a drug cleared only by the liver. Hepatic clearance is also complex, depending on blood flow to an organ (Q), enzyme activity (CLint), and free fraction (fup) for clearance. To make predictions possible, it is helpful to consider two extremes: drugs with high extraction efficiencies (and therefore high first-pass effects) and drugs with low extraction efficiencies (no or little first-pass effect). Low first-pass drugs are dependent on enzyme activity and fup to determine CL_H. If the object (first) drug was a CYP P450 2D6 substrate and a new drug is added that is a CYP P450 2D6 inhibitor, a decrease in the CL of the object drug would be expected. This would cause an increase in Css,avg, possibly resulting in concentration-dependent toxicity. The DR should be decreased before the patient would possibly suffer from a toxicity. A good resource for updated CYP P450 data is medicine.iupui.edu/flockhart/table.htm. Many variations of drug and disease interactions can alter Css,avg.

$$Css,avg = \frac{F \times DR}{CL} = \frac{Drug\ In}{Drug\ Out}$$

Changes in P:T are rarely as clinically significant as changes in Css,avg but still should not be ignored. For example, if there is a decrease in V, the $t^{1/2}$ would decrease and k would increase. This will make for more variation between the Css,max and Css,min (increase P:T). This may result in Cmax causing toxicity and/or Cmin causing lack of efficacy. Decreasing the τ (giving the drug more often) should allieviate the problem. A change in CL or V resulting in a smaller P:T (less variance between Css,max and Css,min) probably does not require a change in τ, but τ could be extended allowing the patient to take a drug less often.

GLOSSARY

Bioavailability (F): units—none (fraction). The fraction of the administered dose that is available to the systemic circulation. Determined by fa, fg and ffp. It is important in determining the dose rate needed to achieve a certain targeted Css,avg if given by other than intravenous route.

Fraction absorbed (fa): fraction of drug given that is able to be absorbed into the circulation.

Fraction that escapes gut metabolism (fg): fraction of drug absorbed that is able to escape metabolism in the gut wall and escape efflux pumps that are in the gut wall (like P-glycoprotein).

Fraction that escapes first pass effect (ffp): fraction of drug that escapes metabolism in the liver as the blood passes through the liver before reaching the systemic circulation. Ffp is related to the hepatic extraction ratio of a drug (E): ffp = 1− E.

Clearance (CL): units—vol/time. The volume of serum, plasma or blood that has all of the drug removed per unit of time by the eliminating organ. Total body clearance is the sum of the clearances of all the eliminating organs. It is also the rate of elimination with respect to the given plasma concentration ($CL = k/C$). Clearance of any organ is determined by the blood flow to that organ (Q) and the extraction efficiency of that organ (E). $CL = Q \times E$.

First order or linear elimination: the rate of elimination is directly proportional to the conentration of drug in the serum. It is independent of concentration.

Michaelis-Menten or nonlinear elimination: the rate of elimination does not change in proportion to the concentration of drug in the serum. As serum drug concentrations rise, the rate of elimination increases less than proportionally. This occurs when there is a capacity-limited elimination process. Examples are the hepatic enzymes and the transport sites for renal tubular secretion. When all available or nearly all available receptors are in use, the process reaches a saturation point, which results in the rate of elimination becoming fixed: $CL = \dfrac{Vmax}{Km + C}$

Hepatic extraction ratio (E): units—none. The fraction of the absorbed dose metabolized during each pass through the liver. It is determined by Q_H, $CLint_H$, and fup and is an important determinant of CL_H.

Dose regimen (DR): units—amt/time. The amount of drug administered per time. May be thought of as daily dose. Important in determining the Css,avg. One of the factors that pharmacists can control.

Dose interval (τ): units—time. the frequency of intermittent drug administration. Important in determining the variance between the Css,max and Cmin,ss or P:T. One of the factors that pharmacists can control. As a rule of thumb, drugs can be given once every half-life.

Peak-to-trough ratio (P:T): comparison of Cmax to Cmin. Important for understanding how much variation there is between the Cmax and Cmin concentrations within a dosing interval.

Half-life ($t^1/_2$): units—time. Time it takes for one half of the drug to be removed from the body if eliminated by first-order elimination.

Important for determining how often to dose a drug and how long it will take to get to steady state (ss). Determined by total body clearance (CL) and volume of distribution (V). Inversely related to elimination rate constant (k).

Elimination rate constant (k): units/time. The fraction of drug removed in a given time. Determined by measuring the slope of the terminal portion of the slope of the line formed by log serum concentrations versus time. Important for determining how often to dose a drug and how long it will take to get to steady state. Determined by total body clearance (CL) and volume of distribution (V). Inversely realted to half-life ($t^1/_2$).

Area under the concentration time curve (AUC): units— $\frac{amt \times time}{vol}$. The area measured under the concentration time curve that reults after administration of the drug. It relates patient exposure to a drug better than just a concentration at a point in time. In some cases it may be helpful in determining efficacy and/or toxicity of a given drug. It is determined by the dose given, F if given other than intravenously (IV) and CL.

Steady state (ss): the point in therapy when the amount of drug administered exactly replaces the amount of drug removed. SS is never techically achieved, but for clinical purposes 5 $t^1/_2$s (97% of SS) is considered to be at SS.

> Maximum concentration at steady state (Cmax,ss): units— amt/vol. The highest concentration achieved after intermittent dosage adminstiration at SS. Cmax,ss will remain constant from dose to dose. May correlate to possible dose-related toxicity problems.
>
> Minimum concentration at steady state (Cmin,ss): units— amt/vol. The lowest concentration within a SS dosing interval. Cmin,ss will remain constant from dose to dose. May correlate to possible dose-related lack of efficiacy.
>
> Average concentration at steady state (Css,avg): units— amt/vol. The drug concentration representing the average concentration achieved during a SS dosing interval. It is similar to but not determined by the average of the Css,max and Css,min. It is often the target concentration when determining what dose rate to administer.

Therapeutic range (TR): a statistical a range of desirable drug concentrations, for which *most* patients show effective therapeutic response with minimal drug-related side effects. Is *not* an absolute for every patient. Individual patients can have good therapeutic response with "subtherapeutic" drug concentrations or can experience toxicity with "therapeutic" drug concentrations. Therapeutic ranges are indication specific.

Volume of distribution (V): units—volume. Where the drug distributes in the body. Important for determining how long the drug stays in the body (determinant of $t\frac{1}{2}$) and whether a drug will be removed by hemodialysis (larger volumes will not be removed significantly). Is primarily determined by binding of the drug to plasma and tissue binding sites as well as lipophilicity.

> Central volume of distribution (Vc): hypothetical volume into which a drug initally distributes. It includes blood and highly perfused tissues. It is important for determining loading doses.
>
> Apparent volume of distribution (Vd): Calculated volume that would be necessary to account for all the drug or the concentration of drug in the body. It is calcuated by $Vd = \frac{Dose}{C}$ or by relating clearance and k $Vd = \frac{CL}{k}$.
>
> Volume of distribution at steady state (Vss): actual blood and tissue volumes into which the drug distributes. Can estimate the amount of drug in the body. Amount of drug in body $=$ Vss $\times$ Css,avg.

▨ DRUGS COMMONLY USING TDM

AMINOGLYCOSIDES (GENTAMICIN AND TOBRAMYCIN)

Use: parenteral antibiotics, Gram-negative infections

TR: extended interval dosing: peak 20 mg/L, trough too low to measure (<0.5 mg/L)

> Traditional dosing: peak 5–10 mg/L, trough <2 mg/L

CL: renal

> Approximated by glomerular filtration rate (GFR)

Vd: 0.25 L/kg

> Adjust for obesity and/or alterations in extracellular fluid status

$t\frac{1}{2}$: 2–3 hours

Concentration-related side effects: Nephro and ototoxicity[1-4]

Aminoglycoside dose regimens are determined in an unusual way because it targets peak and trough levels rather than targeting a Css,avg.

The dosing goals go on to be unconventional because a high peak concentration is the best predicter of efficacy and low troughs are necessary to avoid toxicity. Because of these goals, a relatively new dosing method has been used called extended interval or once daily dosing.[5] To improve the chance for a high peak and low trough, a longer dose interval is desirable. So rather than a conventional every 8 hours or every 12 hours dosing schedule, longer schedules of every 24 hours have been used targeting higher pea and lower trough drug in a dosing interval. This method has been tested in many patient groups with good success.

CLINICAL INSIGHTS

1. Serum concentrations should be monitored if aminoglycoside therapy is expected to be continued for more than a few days. Determination of two serum concentrations would enable the patient's pharmacokinetic parameters to be determined and the dosage regimen to be optimized for the treatment, but nomograms for extended interval dosing allow for only one midpoint concentration to be drawn.[5]

2. Although the disposition of aminoglycosides is better described by a two- or three-compartment model, no clinically significant difference is seen in predicted trough concentration using a one-compartment model versus a two-compartment model.[6] Be sure to wait for $1/2$ to 1 hour after the end of infusion to ensure the distribution phase has ended before drawing a peak.

3. Serum creatinine lags changes in renal function by ≥ 24 hours. Therefore, urine output, if available, should be used in conjunction with the serum creatinine to monitor aminoglycoside therapy.

4. Nephrotoxicity induced by aminoglycosides is usually reversible on discontinuance of the drug. Although high trough concentrations have been associated with renal toxicity, the high trough concentrations may also be the result, and not the cause, of renal dysfunction. In fact, elevated trough concentrations are an early indicator renal damage.[3,7]

Carbamazepine

Use: antiepileptic, generalized seizures
TR: 4-12 mg/L
CL: Hepatic 3A4
    Epoxide active metabolite
    Autoinduction
Vd: 1.4 L/kg
$t^1/_2$: initial 15 hours; after induction 10 hours

Concentration-related side effects: central nervous system (CNS) (nystagmus, ataxia, blurred vision, and drowsiness). *Not* concentration-related dermatologic and hematologic, the most serious of which is the rare but potentially fatal aplastic anemia.[8-10]

Carbamazepine undergoes autoinduction. It induces the enzymes responsible for its own clearance and the clearance of other drugs. Clearance increases with time of exposure. It takes 3 to 4 weeks for full induction. Therfore as clearance increases, concentrations and $t^1/_2$ decrease. Therefore dose rate should increase and τ decrease over the first month of administration. Also carbamazepine can induce the metabolism of other drugs, specifically other antiepileptics.

CLINICAL INSIGHTS

1. A baseline complete blood cell count (CBC) with differential, platelet count, serum sodium, and liver function tests should be obtained before the initiation of therapy. If possible, a baseline evaluation of gait and nystagmus should be obtained for future comparisons.
2. Rare but potentially fatal blood dyscrasias (aplastic anemia, agranulocytosis, thrombocytopenia, and leukopenia) have been reported. Signs of bone marrow toxicity (e.g., fever, sore throat, easy bruising) should be monitored. On the other hand, frequent monitoring of the CBC after the patient's condition is stabilized with carbamazepine is unnecessary and unlikely to detect toxicity.
3. Most of the CNS side effects can be minimized by a slow titration of dose increases.

Cyclosporine

Use: immunosuppression
TR: depends on assay
CL: Hepatic
    P-gp substrate
    3A4 substrate
Vd: 4 to 5 L/kg
$t^1/_2$: 6 to 12 hours
fu: <0.1 bound to lipoproteins
Concentration-related side effects: renal vasoconstriction (renal impairment), neurotoxicity (headache, tremor, parasthesias, seizures), and hypertension.

Cyclosporine is at risk for many interactions. Being a CYP 3A4 and P-glycoprotein substrate, many drugs and diseases can alter these, causing changes in CL and F. Also, cyclosporine is highly plasma protein bound, making binding displacement situations significant. The result of subtheapeutic concentrations is very serious. There are many cases of organ rejection resulting from drug–drug or drug–disease interactions that alter CL, F, or V of cyclosporine.

Digoxin

Use: congestive heart failure (CHF) and atrial fibrillation (a fib)
TR: CHF 0.5–1 μg/L
   a fib 1.5–2.5 μg/L
CL: renal (primarily) + hepatic
   P-gp substrate
   CHF decreases CL_H
   CL_R approximated by GFR
Vd: 3.8 (weight kg) + (3.1 × creatinine clearance [CrCl])
   Dosed on ideal body weight (IBW)
   Decreased in renal failure
$t^1/_2$: 36 to 48 hours
Dose-related side effects: decreased heart rate, arrhythmias, vision changes

Digoxin has a relatively large volume of distribution and long half-life. Volume and clearance are affected by many diseaes and drugs.

CLINICAL INSIGHTS[11-13]

1. Interpretation of serum digoxin concentrations for optimal dosing design should ideally be made after steady state is attained.
2. Blood sampling for determination of any digoxin serum concentrations must take into account its prolonged distribution phase. The clinician should wait ≥6 hours after an intravenous dose and 8 hours after an oral dose to obtain the blood sample. Therefore, a standard collection time (preferably as a trough concentration before administration of the patient's daily dose) should be instituted.
3. For rapid control of ventricular rate in the acute management of atrial fibrillation, digoxin loading doses generally are divided into three or four doses (e.g., one-half, one-quarter, one-quarter given every 6 hours) to assess the clinical effect of each dose before administration of the next. In this clinical setting, determination of digoxin concentration between dosings is likely of minimal benefit and is not cost effective.

4. Determination of digoxin concentrations is appropriate for patients with significant renal impairment, for patients with clinical deterioration after initial good response, when toxicity or drug interaction (e.g., with quinidine) is suspected, and for evaluating noncompliance and/or the need for continued therapy.

5. Some medical conditions (e.g., hypokalemia, hyperthyroidism, and hypothyroidism) can change the sensitivity of the patient to pharmacologic effects of digoxin independent of any change in concentration. Therefore, in addition to renal function and concurrent therapy, electrolytes (especially potassium) and thyroid status should be assessed.

Ethosuximide

Use: antiepileptic
TR: 40–100 mg/L[14–17]
CL: hepatic
  3A4 (subject to induction and inhibition)
Vd: 0.7 L/kg
$t\frac{1}{2}$: 50 hours

CLINICAL INSIGHTS

1. The incidence of adverse effects associated with ethosuximide therapy is relatively low and does not correlate well with drug concentrations. Many patients with concentrations >100 mg/L experience no side effects.[18] Drug concentrations are, therefore, primarily used to evaluate a patient's potential for clinical response and compliance.

2. Ethosuximide may exhibit nonlinear kinetics in the higher concentrations.[19,20] Therefore, caution needs to be exercised with dosage increments at the upper end of the therapeutic range.

Lidocaine

Use: local anesthetic, antiarrhythmic
TR: 2–5 mg/L[21–25]
CL: hepatic
  High E; therefore high first-pass drug
  CHF, cirrhosis ($\downarrow$Q) decrease CL
  Active metabolites: MEGX and GX
V_1: 0.5 L/kg
V_2: 1.3 L/kg
$t\frac{1}{2}$: 100 minutes
fu: 0.3 (AAG; see the following)

Concentration-related side effects: CNS side effects (e.g., dizziness, mental confusion, and blurred vision). Seizures are usually associated with concentrations >9 mg/L.[21-25]

Lidocaine is highly extracted by the liver, which results in a very low oral bioavailability. Its pharmacokinetic profile follows a two-compartment model. To maintain lidocaine concentration within the therapeutic range, it is necessary to administer minibolus doses (one half of original loading dose) every 8 to 10 minutes.

CLINICAL INSIGHTS

1. Concurrent medical conditions such as congestive heart failure and liver disease can decrease the clearance of lidocaine and the expected therapeutic responses with the usual doses. Therefore, a reduction of dose by as much as 40% may be necessary for these patients.
2. MEGX is primarily eliminated by the liver, and GX is eliminated by both the liver and the kidney. Therefore, in patients with liver and/or renal disease, accumulation of the metabolites may contribute to CNS toxicity.
3. AAG is an acute-phase reactant; as such, its concentration can increase with stress or pathophysiologic conditions such as acute myocardial infarction (especially during the first week after infarction). An increase in the serum concentration of AAG decreases the free fraction of lidocaine temporarily due to enhanced protein binding. The increase and subsequent decrease in AAG concentration can further complicate interpretation of lidocaine kinetics and effects in patients. Careful concentration and clinical monitoring are required .
4. Because lidocaine is rapidly distributed to the brain and the heart, intravenous bolus doses should be administered at a rate not faster than 50 mg/minute so that the patient is not exposed to transient but toxic concentrations of lidocaine, especially in the brain. Seizures and arrhythmias may occur and may not always be preceded by other toxic signs (e.g., confusion, dizziness).
5. The clearance of lidocaine decreases with continuous dosing.[25,26] Therefore, infusions lasting longer than 24 hours require diligent monitoring of concentrations and of clinical responses. If necessary, doses should be reduced.

Lithium

Use: treat bipolar disease
TR: 0.6–0.8 mEq/L

CL: renal
　　Treated like Na
　　Actively reabsorbed
　　$0.25 \times CrCl$
V: 0.7 L/kg
$t^1/_2$: 20 hours
Concentration-related side effects: Gastrointestinal (i.e., nausea, vomiting, anorexia, epigastric bloating, abdominal pain) and CNS (i.e., lethargy, fatigue, muscle weakness, and tremor).[27-29]

CLINICAL INSIGHTS

1. Administering lithium preparations with meals will decrease both the rate of absorption and the achievable peak concentration. Meals, therefore, may help minimize the incidence of some of the adverse effects (e.g., tremor and polyuria). Side effects may also be minimized in some patients by use of the slow-release lithium dosage formulations.
2. The daily dose of lithium should be divided into two or more doses, and trough concentrations should be obtained 12 hours after the last dose.
3. Lithium reabsorption follows sodium reabsorption in the proximal tubule. Therefore, patients with precipitous changes in fluid balance or electrolytes due to drug therapy (e.g., thiazide diuretics) that result in increased sodium (and lithium) reabsorption are at increased risk of toxicity.

Phenobarbital

Use: antiepileptic
TR: 15–40 mg/L[30,31]
CL: hepatic (primary) + renal
　　Low E
　　Enzyme inducer
V: 0.7 L/kg
$t^1/_2$: 5 days
fu: 0.5
Concentration-related side effects: depression and ataxia.[31]

CLINICAL INSIGHTS

1. For treatment of status epilepticus, a loading dose of 15 mg/kg can be administered intravenously, usually in three divided doses of 5 mg/kg.
2. Because phenobarbital distributes to fatty tissue, loading doses for morbidly obese patients should be based on total body weight.[32]

Phenytoin

Use: antiepileptic

TR: 10–20 mg/L

    Free: 1–2 mg/L

CL: hepatic

    Nonlinear

    Enzyme inducer 3A4

    Subject to induction and inhibition

V: 0.65 L/kg

$t^1/_2$: nonlinear since nonlinear CL

fu: 0.1 (albumin)

Concentration-related side effects: nystagmus, ataxia, and diminished mental capacity.[33] Gingival hyperplasia, folate deficiency, and peripheral neuropathy are not related to concentration.

Phenytoin has nonlinear clearance in the TR and high plasma protein binding, making dosing very difficult. The metabolism of phenytoin is saturable. Therefore, modest changes in DR can result in disproportionate changes in steady-state plasma concentrations. The high binding provides a challenge in the interpretation of phenytoin concentration in patients with altered protein binding (e.g., patients with renal failure or hypoalbuminemia and patients with concurrent drugs that displace phenytoin from the binding sites).

CLINICAL INSIGHTS

1. Oral bioavailability of phenytoin can be reduced significantly by concomitant oral nutrition supplements (e.g., Osmolite) administered as nasogastric feedings. The most practical way of circumventing this problem is to administer phenytoin intravenously. If that is not possible, then stop nasogastric (NG) feeding 2 hours before dose administration, flush the NG tube with 60 mL of water after dose administration, then wait 2 hours before resuming NG feeding.

2. Only Dilantin capsules should be dosed once daily. As with other sustained-release formulations, the capsules should not be crushed.

3. Hypotension can occur with intravenous administration due to the propylene glycol diluent.[34] Therefore, the rate of phenytoin infusion should not be >50 mg/minute. Fosphenytoin, a prodrug of phenytoin, is available for parenteral use. The addition of a phosphate group to the chemical structure of phenytoin results in a more soluble chemical

entity; therefore, there is no need for the propylene glycol as a diluent for fosphenytoin.

4. Fosphenytoin dosing should be based on phenytoin equivalent (the molecular weight of fosphenytoin is 1.5 times that of phenytoin).

5. Protein binding displacement makes interpretation of a total concentration difficult.[35–37] In this case the total concentration of phenytoin would be lower once a new steady-state condition is established. However, the unbound (pharmacologically active) concentration remains the same. Dose regimen adjustment is again not necessary in patients with an altered degree of binding only.

6. Equations to equate the measured total phenytoin concentration to that which would be observed under normal binding conditions should be used so that inappropriate dosage adjustments can be avoided.[38,39]

Procainamide[40–45]

Use: antiarrhythmic

TR: 4–8 mg/L

May need much higher concentrations in some patients

CL: hepatic and renal

CLH by acetylation (acetylation phenotype: slow and fast acetylators)

Active metabolite: NAPA (renal clearance)

V: 2 L/kg

$t^{1}/_{2}$: 3 hours

Concentration-related side effects: gastrointestinal disturbances, weakness, mild hypotension, and electrocardiogram (ECG) changes (10%–30% prolongation of the PR, QT, or QRS intervals).

CLINICAL INSIGHTS

1. Hypotension may occur if intravenous procainamide is administered too quickly. The rate of infusion should not be faster than 25 mg/minute.

2. The short plasma half-life of procainamide requires the use of 3- to 4-hour dosing intervals for the rapid-release products and every-6-hours intervals for the sustained-release formulations. This is in contrast to the usual longer dosing intervals with sustained-release formulations of other drugs.

3. Wax matrix carcasses or "skeletons" of the sustained-release tablets may come through intact in the stool. This is not a concern because the drug is absorbed despite the recovery of the wax matrix.

4. Most clinical laboratories report the concentrations of both procainamide and NAPA. The electrophysiologic activity of NAPA is different from that of procainamide, and monitoring of NAPA concentration is not necessary to evaluate efficacy. However, assessment of NAPA concentrations may be appropriate in some patients[45] (e.g., those with diminished renal function), because NAPA is primarily eliminated by the kidneys and accumulates to a much greater extent than procainamide.

5. In addition to concentration monitoring, a baseline QT interval should be obtained, if possible, before initiation of therapy or before dosage increase. Prolongation of QT interval >25%–50% of the baseline value necessitates at least the consideration of dosage reduction.

Valproic Acid [46–51]

Use: antiepileptic
TR: 50–100 mg/L
   Nonlinear protein binding at upper ranges
CL: hepatic
   Nonlinear clearance due to nonlinear protein binding
   3A4 substrate
   Can induce and inhibit CLint of other drugs
V: 0.005 to 0.2 (albumin). Nonlinear in upper end of therapeutic range
$t^1/_2$: 10 to 12 hours
Concentration-related side effects: gastrointestinal disturbances, sedation, drowsiness, and hepatoxicity. *Not* concentration-related alopecia, a benign essential tremor, and thrombocytopenia.

CLINICAL INSIGHTS

1. Although the rate of absorption from the use of enteric-coated tablets may be slower, this formulation can be used to minimize gastrointestinal side effects.

2. Diurnal variation in valproic acid clearance has been reported, and the concentrations of valproic acid in the afternoon or evening are lower than in the morning. Therefore, it is important to standardize consistent blood sampling times (e.g., morning trough concentration) for therapeutic drug monitoring.

3. Valproic acid can inhibit the metabolism of several other drugs such as phenobarbital. In addition, valproic acid can displace highly protein-bound drugs such as phenytoin from their albumin binding sites. Therefore, similar to other antiepileptic drugs, the potential of

drug–drug interactions should be considered when adding or deleting drugs to a patient's regimen.

4. Although valproic acid–induced hepatotoxicity is rare, it is a serious complication of therapy and should be considered in any patient with elevated liver enzymes. Unfortunately, the predictive value of laboratory monitoring for occurrence of hepatotoxicity induced by valproic acid is low.

Vancomycin[52-63]

Use: antibiotic used for Gram-positive infections

TR: Peak <40 to 50 mg/L, trough ~10 mg/L

Nonlinear protein binding at upper ranges

CL: renal

Approximated by CrCl

V: 0.7 L/kg *or* $0.17 \times$ (age) + $(0.22 \times$ total body weight [TBW] in kg) + 15

Fu: 0.5

t $\frac{1}{2}$: 6–7 hr

Concentration-related side effects: nephrotoxicity when combined with other nephrotoxins or other assaults to kidney; rarely ototoxicity.

CLINICAL INSIGHTS

1. Red man syndrome (characterized by flushing, tachycardia, and hypotension) is associated with histamine release. Its incidence is higher with rapid infusion rates. To minimize its occurrence, vancomycin should be infused slowly (e.g., 1 g over ≥60 minutes). Even at this rate of infusion, some patients will experience flushing and tachycardia. The syndrome may also be managed by premedication with an antihistamine.

2. Efficacy is tied to having adequate concentrations of drug available. Therefore keeping a "therapeutic through" is very important.

References

1. Jackson GG, Arcieri G. Ototoxicity of gentamicin in man: a survey and controlled analysis of clinical experience in the United States. *J Infect Dis.* 1971;124(Suppl):130.

2. Schentag JJ, et al. Clinical and pharmacokinetic characteristics of aminoglycoside nephrotoxicity in 201 critically ill patients. *Antimicrob Agents Chemother.* 1982;5:721.

3. Wilfret JN, et al. Renal insufficiency associated with gentamicin therapy. *J Infect Dis.* 1971;124(Suppl):148.

4. Federspil P, et al. Pharmacokinetics and ototoxicity of gentamicin, tobramycin, and amikacin. *J Infect Dis*. 1976;134(Suppl):200.

5. Nicolau D, et al. Experience with a once-daily aminoglycoside dosing program administerd to 2,184 adult patients. *Antimicrob Agents Chemother*. 1995;39:650–655.

6. Hatton RC, Massey KL, Russell WL. Comparison of the predictions of one- and two-compartment microcomputer programs for long-term tobramycin therapy. *Ther Drug Monit*. 1984;6:432–437.

7. Goodman EL, et al. Prospective comparative study of variable dosage and variable frequency regimens for administrations of gentamicin. *Antimicrob Agents Chemother*. 1975;8:434.

8. So EL, et al. Seizure exacerbation and status epilepticus related to carbamazepine-10,11 epoxide. *Ann Neurol*. 1994;35:743–746.

9. Rane A, Hojer B, Wilson JT. Kinetics of carbamazepine and its 10.11-epoxide metabolite in children. *Clin Pharmacol Ther*. 1976;19:276–283.

10. Bertilsson L. Clinical pharmacokinetics of carbamazepine. *Clin Pharmacokinet*. 1978;3:128.

11. Smith TW. Digitalis toxicity: epidemiology and clinical use of serum concentration measurements. *Am J Med*. 1975;58:470.

12. Smith TW, Harber E. Digoxin intoxication: the relationship of clinical presentation to serum digoxin concentration. *J Clin Invest*. 1970;49:2377.

13. Aronson JK, Hardman M. ABC of monitoring drug therapy: digoxin. *Br J Med*. 1992;305:1149–1152.

14. Browne TR, et al. Ethosuximide in the treatment of absence seizures. *Neurology*. 1975;25:515.

15. Sherwin AL, et al. Improved control of epilepsy by monitoring plasma ethosuximide. *Arch Neurol*. 1973;27:178.

16. Penry JK, et al. Ethosuximide: relation of plasma levels to clinical control. In: Woodbury DM, Penry JK, Schmidt RP, eds. *Anti-epileptic Drugs*. New York, NY: Raven Press; 1972:431–441.

17. Sherwin AL, Robb JP. Ethosuximide: relation of plasma levels to clinical control. In: Woodbury DM, Penry JK, Schmidt RP, eds. *Anti-epileptic Drugs*. New York, NY: Raven Press; 1972:443–448.

18. Sherwin AL, et al. Plasma ethosuximide levels: a new aid in the management of epilepsy. *Ann Royal Coll Surg Can*. 1971;14:48.

19. Bauer LA, et al. Ethosuximide kinetics: possible interactions with valproic acid. *Clin Pharmacol Ther*. 1982;31:741–745.

20. Smith GA, et al. Factors influencing plasma concentrations of ethosuximide. *Clin Pharmacokinet*.1979;4:38–52.

21. Gianelly R, et al. Effect of lidocaine on ventricular arrhythmias in patients with coronary heart disease. *N Engl J Med*. 1967;277:1215.

22. Jewett DE, et al. Lidocaine in the management of arrhythmias after acute myocardial infarction. *Lancet*. 1968;1:266.

23. Seldon R, Sasahara AA. Central nervous system toxicity induced by lidocaine. *JAMA*. 1967;202:908.

24. Thompson PD. Lidocaine pharmacokinetics in advanced heart failure, liver disease, and renal failure in humans. *Ann Intern Med*. 1973;78:499.

25. LeLorier J, et al. Pharmacokinetics of lidocaine after prolonged intravenous administrations in uncomplicated myocardial infarction. *Ann Intern Med*. 1977;87:700–702.

26. Davidson R, Parker M, Atkinson A. Excessive serum lidocaine levels during maintenance infusions: mechanisms and prevention. *Am Heart J.* 1982;104:203–208.

27. Elizur A, et al. Intra:extracellular lithium ratios and clinical course in affective states. *Clin Pharmacol Ther.* 1972;13:947.

28. Salem RB. A pharmacist's guide to monitoring lithium drug-drug interactions. *Drug Intell Clin Pharm.* 1982;16:745.

29. Amdisen A. Lithium. In: Evans WE, Schentag JJ, Jusko WJ, eds. *Applied Pharmacokinetics: Principles of Therapeutic Drug Monitoring.* 2nd ed. Vancouver: Applied Therapeutics; 1986:978–1002.

30. Buchthal F, et al. Relation of EEG and seizures to phenobarbital in serum. *Arch Neurol.* 1968;19:567.

31. Plass GL, Hine CH. Hydantoin and barbiturate blood levels observed in epileptics. *Arch Int Pharmacodyn Ther.* 1960;128:375.

32. Wilkes L, Danziger LH, Rodvold KA. Phenobarbital pharmacokinetics in obesity: a case report. *Clin Pharmacokinet.* 1992;22:481–484.

33. Kutt H, et al. Diphenylhydantoin metabolism, blood levels and toxicity. *Arch Neurol.* 1964;11:642.

34. Louis S, et al. The cardiocirculatory changes caused by intravenous dilantin and its solvent. *Am Heart J.* 1967;74:523.

35. Lund L. Effects of phenytoin in patients with epilepsy in relation to its concentration in plasma. In: David DS, Prichard NBC, eds. *Biological Effects of Drugs in Relation to Their Concentration in Plasma.* Baltimore, MD: University Park Press; 1972; 227.

36. Lascelles PT, et al. The distribution of plasma phenytoin levels in epileptic patients. *J Neurol Neurosurg Psychiatry.* 1970;33:501.

37. Reidenberg MM. The binding of drugs to plasma proteins and the interpretation of measurements of plasma concentrations of drugs in patients with poor renal function. *Am J Med.* 1977;62:466.

38. Winter M. *Basic Clinical Pharmacokinetics.* 3rd ed. Vancouver: Applied Therapeutics; 1994:312–316.

39. Liponi DL, et al. Renal function and therapeutic concentrations of phenytoin. *Neurology.* 1984;34:395.

40. Koch-Weser J. Pharmacokinetics of procainamide in man. *Ann N Y Acad Sci.* 1971;169:370.

41. Koch-Weser J, Klein SW. Procainamide dosage schedules, plasma concentrations and clinical effects. *JAMA.* 1971;215:1454.

42. Engel TR, et al. Modification of ventricular tachycardia by procainamide in patients with coronary artery disease. *Am J Cardiol.* 1980;46:1033.

43. Giardina EV, et al. Efficacy, plasma concentrations and adverse effects of a new sustained release procainamide preparation. *Am J Cardiol.* 1980;46:855.

44. Greenspan AM, et al. Large dose procainamide therapy for ventricular tachyarrhythmia. *Am J Cardiol.* 1980;46:453.

45. Vlasses PH, et al. Lethal accumulations of procainamide metabolite in renal insufficiency [abstract]. *Drug Intell Clin Pharm.* 1984;18:493.

46. Kodama Y, et al. Binding parameters of valproic acid to serum protein in healthy adults at steady state. *Ther Drug Monit.* 1992;14:55–60.

47. Pinder RM, et al. Sodium valproate: a review of its pharmacological properties in therapeutic efficacy in epilepsy. *Drugs.* 1977;13:81.

48. Graham L, et al. Sodium valproate, serum level, and critical effect in epilepsy: a controlled study. *Epilepsia.* 1979;20:303.

49. Sherard ES, et al. Treatment of childhood epilepsy with valproic acid: result of the first 100 patients in a 6-month trial. *Neurology.* 1980:30:31.

50. Suchy FJ, et al. Acute hepatic failure associated with the use of sodium valproate. *N Engl J Med.* 1979;300:962.

51. Donalt JT, et al. Valproic acid and fatal hepatitis. *Neurology.* 1979;29:273.

52. Alexander MB. A review of vancomycin. *Drug Intell Clin Pharm.* 1974;8:520.

53. Kirby WMM, et al. Treatment of staphylococcal septicemia with vancomycin. *N Engl J Med.* 1960;262:49.

54. Vancomycin in perspective. *Am J Dis Child.* 1984;183:14.

55. Cunha BA, Ristuccia AM. Clinical usefulness of vancomycin. *Clin Pharm.* 1982;2:417.

56. Rotschafer JC, et al. Pharmacokinetics of vancomycin: observations in 28 patients and dosage recommendations. *Antimicrob Agents Chemother.* 1982;22:391.

57. Blouin RA, et al. Vancomycin pharmacokinetics in normal and morbidly obese subjects. *Antimicrob Agents Chemother.* 1982;21:575.

58. Mollering RC, et al. Vancomycin therapy in patients with impaired renal function; a nomogram for dosage. *Ann Intern Med.* 1981;94:343.

59. Farber BF, Mollering RC Jr. Retrospective study of the toxicity of preparations of vancomycin from 1974 to 1981. *Antimicrob Agents Chemother.* 1983;23:138.

60. Ryback MJ, et al. Nephrotoxicity of vancomycin, alone and with an aminoglycoside. *J Antimicrob Chemother.* 1990;25:679–687.

61. Newfield P, Roizen MF. Hazards of rapid administration of vancomycin. *Ann Intern Med.* 1979;91:581.

62. Cook FV, Farrar WE. Vancomycin revisited. *Ann Intern Med.* 1978;88:813.

63. Lanese DM, et al. Markedly increased clearance of vancomycin during hemodialysis using polysulfone dialyzers. *Kidney Int.* 1989;35:1409.

PHARMACOKINETIC EQUATIONS

	Equations	When to Use	When Not to Use
Area under the Concentration Time Curve (AUC) Units: (amt/vol) × time	$$AUC_{0-\infty} = \left[\frac{(C_1 + C_2)}{2} \times (t_2 - t_1)\right]\left[\frac{(C_2 + C_2)}{2} \times (t_1 - t_2)\right] + \cdots + \frac{C_{last}}{k}$$	To determine $AUC_{0-\infty}$ given concentration time data after administration of drug	If only want to measure to end of τ
	$$AUC_{0-\infty} = \frac{Dose_{IV}}{CL}$$	Determine AUC or CL from AUC if dose given IV	If given by other than IV
	$$AUC_{0-\infty} = \frac{F \times Dose_{PO}}{CL}$$	Determine AUC or CL from AUC if dose given other than IV	

462

Bioavailability (F) Units: no units (fraction)	$F = fa \times fg \times ffp$	Determine F, fa, fg, or ffp given the others	Assume parallel tube model
	$ffp = \dfrac{Q_H}{Q_H + (CLint \times fup)}$ Low hepatic extraction drugs: $ffp \sim 1$ High hepatic extraction drug: $ffp \sim \dfrac{Q}{CLint \times fup}$	Determine ffp Assume the well-stirred jar model	
	$F = \dfrac{AUC_{nonIV}}{AUC_{IV}}$	Used to determine F when same dose is given by IV and nonintravenous route	
	$F = \dfrac{AUC_{nonIV}}{AUC_{IV}} \times \dfrac{Dose_{IV}}{Dose_{nonIV}}$	To determine F when comparing differing doses	If different doses given
Total Body Clearance (CL) Units: vol/time	$CL = CL_H + CL_R + \cdots$	To determine total body clearance, all organ clearances must be summed	

(continued)

463

PHARMACOKINETIC EQUATIONS (continued)

	Equations	When to Use	When Not to Use
Hepatic Cl(Cl$_H$) Units: vol/time	$CL_H = Q_H \times E_H$ Low extraction: $CL_H \cong CLint \times fup$ High extraction: $CL_H \cong Q_H$	• To determine what will alter hepatic clearance. • Low extraction drugs the rate limitation to clearance is the enzyme activity (CLint) and fraction unbound in plasma (fup) • High extraction drugs rate limitation to clearance is liver blood flow (Q)	
Hepatic extraction efficiency [E$_H$] Units: none	$E_H = \dfrac{CLint \times fup}{Q_H + (CLint \times fup)}$	According to the well-stirred jar model	
Hepatic intrinsic clearance [enzyme activity] [CLint] Units: vol/time	$CLint = \dfrac{Vmax}{Km \times C}$	Michealis-Menten Vmax: max rate of metabolism, capacity of the system, or number of enzymes available Km: concentration at which 1/2 Vmax is reached, measure of affinity	

Renal clearance (CL_R) Units: vol/time	$CL_R = (CL_{gf} + CL_{TS})(1 - E_{TR})$	CL_{gf}, filtration clearance; CL_{TS}, tubular secretion clearance; E_{TR}, efficiency of tubular reabsorption
Elimination rate constant (k) Units: vol/time	$$k = \frac{\ln C_2 - \ln C_1}{t_2 - t_1}$$ $$k = \frac{CL}{V}$$	To determine k when given two concentration-time points during the decay phase of a drug considered to be linear, and gathered during a time that is considered to be reflecting only one compartment • To determine how changes in V and/or CL might alter k • To determine k if given CL and V • To determine CL if given k and V • To determine V if given K and CL	If the concentrations given are not gathered during the decay phase of a drug that is considered to be linear and within one compartment

(continued)

PHARMACOKINETIC EQUATIONS (continued)

	Equations	When to Use	When Not to Use
Half-life ($t^{1/2}$) Units: time	$$t^{1/2} = \frac{0.693}{k}$$	To determine $t^{1/2}$ from k or vice versa	
	$$t^{1/2} = \frac{0.693 \times V}{CL}$$	To determine how changes in V and/or CL might alter $t^{1/2}$	
Central volume of distribution (Vc) Units: vol	$$Vc = \frac{Dose\ (injected\ instanteneously)}{C_0}$$	Used to determine Vc or dose to achieve a target C_0	
Apparent volume of distribution (Vd) Units: vol	$$Vd = \frac{Dose}{C}$$ $$k = \frac{CL}{Vd}$$		
Volume of distribution at steady state (Vss) Units: vol	$$Vss = Vp + \left[V_T \times \frac{fup}{fut} \right]$$ Given: $Vp = 0.07$ L/kg $V_T = 0.53$ L/kg	Determine Vss, fut, or fup; given the other parameters	

Dosing Equations

Model of decay of one-compartment, first-order elimination			

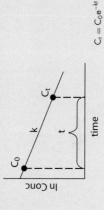

$C_t = C_0 e^{-kt}$

- To determine the concentration at any time (C_t) during the decay of a drug following one-compartment linear kinetics when given k, an earlier concentration (C_0) and the time between C_0 and C_t (t)
- To determine the concentration of an earlier concentration (C_0) when all the above conditions are met
- To determine the time (t) between two given concentrations (C_0 and C_t) when all the above conditions are met
- To determine elimination rate constant (k) when all the above conditions are met

- Multiple compartments
- Non linear clearance

(continued)

467

PHARMACOKINETIC EQUATIONS (continued)

	Equations	When to Use	When Not to Use
Model of decay, two compartments, linear	$C_t = C_1 e^{-k_1 t} + C_2 e^{-k_2 t}$	To determine the concentration at any time t during the decay of the drug if a two-compartment model	Nonlinear
Loading dose (LD) Units: amt	$LD = V_C \times (C_{target} - C_{observed})$	Determine LD when V_C, target concentration, and any drug already in body is known	
Concentration at steady state Units: amt/vol	$Css = \dfrac{DR}{CL}$	• To determine the plasma concentration at steady state (CSS) when a constant infusion is given at a certain dose rate (DR) and CL • To determine a DR if given a target Css and CL • To determine CL if given a DR and resulting CSS	If not at steady state If nonlinear CL

	$C_{ss,avg} = \dfrac{S \times F \times DR}{CL}$	• To determine the average concentration during a dosing interval at steady state • To determine how changes in DR, CL, and F will effect $C_{ss,avg}$ • S equals salt form
	$C_{ss,avg} = \dfrac{AUC_{ss,0-\tau}}{\tau}$	• To determine the $C_{ss,avg}$ given AUC_{ss} and τ
Concentration before steady state, constant infusion Units: amt/vol	$C_t = \dfrac{DR}{CL}(1 - e^{-kt})$	To determine the plasma concentration at time t prior to reaching steady state if given a constant infusion and the DR, CL, and k are known
Multiple dosing function (MDF) Units: none	$MDF = \dfrac{1 - e^{-nk\tau}}{1 - e^{-k\tau}}$ C_t at dose n = C_t at first dose $\times$ MDF	Use to multiply times any known concentration after first dose to any concentration at that same time on subsequent doses (n)

(continued)

PHARMACOKINETIC EQUATIONS (continued)

	Equations	When to Use	When Not to Use
Accumulation factor (Rac) Units: none	$$Rac = \frac{1}{1 - e^{-k\tau}}$$ Ct SS = Ct at first dose × Rac	Use to multiply times any known concentration after first dose to any concentration at that same time at SS	
Calculating new DR if known Css,avg at DR known	$$DR_{new} = \frac{DR_{given} \times C_{ss, target}}{C_{ss, observed}}$$	Determine new DR when measured concentration at SS and assumes CL and F remain constant	Nonlinear CL or Nonlinear F Cobserved not at SS
Calculating new dose regimen based on Css,avg	Determine DR $$DR = \frac{C_{target} \times CL}{F}$$	Determine DR if CL and F known at SS	Must be linear clearance and bioavailability
	Determine τ, dose q$t^{1/2}$ $$t\frac{1}{2} = \frac{0.693 \times V}{CL}$$ or base on known target peak and trough as below	Determine τ if can dose every $t^{1/2}$	
Calculating new dose regimen based on target Cmax and Cmin (i.e., aminoglycosides)	Determine optimal τ $$\tau = \left| -\frac{1}{k} \left[\ln \left(\frac{C_{min, target}}{C_{max, target}} \right) \right] \right| + t_i$$ t_i = time of infusion	Determine optimal dosing interval given target peak an troughs K must have been determined at SS	Multicompartmental Not at SS

	Determine optimal dose (using optimal τ from above) $R_o = V \times k \times C_{max,target}\left(\dfrac{1 - e^{-k\tau}}{1 - e^{-kt_i}}\right)$ DR is in terms of amt/time, *not dose*	• Determine optimal dose using optimal τ and target Cmax • V and k must have been determined at SS • Dose equals $R_o \times t_i$
	Determine what Css,max would be expected using a given dosing regimen $C_{max} = \dfrac{R_o}{V \times k}\left(\dfrac{1 - e^{-kt_i}}{1 - e^{-k\tau}}\right)$	Determine Css,max when given defined dosing regimen
	Determine what Css,min would be expected using a given dosing regimen $C_{min} = C_{max}\, e^{-k(\tau - t_i)}$	Determine Css,min when given defined dosing regimen
Adjustment of total phenytoin concentrations when protein binding displacement	In hypoalbuminemia: $C_{normal} = \dfrac{C_{observed}}{[(0.2)|A/b|] + (0.1)}$	Determine what would have been the observed concentration if normal binding Alb in gm/dl
	In renal failure: $C_{normal} = \dfrac{C_{observed}}{[(0.1)|A/b|] + (0.1)}$	Determine what would have been the observed concentration if normal binding Alb in gm/dl

14 Clinical Drug Monitoring

Teresa A. O'Sullivan and Ann K. Wittkowsky

Clinical drug monitoring is the most basic element of pharmaceutical care.[1] All the therapeutic knowledge the pharmacy student possesses is useless unless it can be applied in a structured and consistent manner to detect and solve patients' problems. This structured process is considered clinical drug monitoring. It includes each of the following activities:[2]

- Gathering objective and subjective patient information.
- Analyzing that information to determine medical and drug-related problems.
- Setting therapeutic goals for each medical and drug-related problem.
- Developing and enacting a treatment plan to reach the therapeutic goals.
- Developing and enacting a monitoring plan to see if the treatment works or causes any harm.
- Documenting all of the above (subjective and objective information, analysis, and plan) in a coherent and systematic manner so that the next care provider can continue the process.

Each of these activities is a necessary component of clinical drug monitoring. No single activity can be skipped, or good patient care will be sacrificed. The following steps provide a linear and methodic approach to these activities for the pharmacy student to follow when providing patient care.

Step 1. Gather Information: Prepare for the Interview

To effectively provide care, a pharmacist *must* talk to the patient. The discussion will be more comfortable and productive if the clinician first scans the patient's chart or profile to determine some discussion issues. The following should be considered:

- The current medication list (patient profile or most recent medication administration record [MAR]).
  - What medications has the patient been prescribed?
  - What likely disease states are present?
- Patient compliance/adherence (patient profile or most recent MAR).
  - How often does the patient get his or her medications for chronic conditions refilled? In an institutional setting, the pharmacist will want to check the MAR to see if the patient has been receiving or refusing medications.
- Disease state control (recent progress notes).
  - Monitoring notes written by other health care providers will be useful in an institutional or clinic ambulatory setting. Some community pharmacy practitioners are starting to document previous disease state control in their electronic profiles.
  - The pharmacist should look for disease state monitoring data obtained through interview, physical examination, and laboratory values. Well-written progress notes will include this information. In the absence of well-written progress notes, information from previous visits or admissions, an admission or discharge summary (for hospitals or long-term care settings), or current laboratory data can be reviewed to gain an idea of the patient's medical problems. In this situation, an interview with the patient or caregiver will provide invaluable information to determine disease state control.
- Cost (patient profile will contain costs; most recent MAR will not).
  - Are any chronic medications relatively expensive?
  - Is there any indication that lower-cost agents have not worked? Physicians distributing drug samples can facilitate the initiation of high-cost, brand name products without initial trials of low-cost agents.
  - Which agents are covered by the health insurance provider?
- Adverse drug effects (recent progress notes), including drug allergy information.
  - Are there any medications that may have been prescribed to treat side effects from other medications? When thinking about adverse drug reactions, the "as needed" or "prn" portion of the MAR is useful because prn medications are often given to combat side effects from routinely scheduled medications. For instance, if the patient begins asking for a laxative shortly after beginning opiate therapy for pain, opiate-induced constipation should be suspected.

The goal of this first step is to identify discussion questions quickly, *not* to read the patient's chart from beginning to end. The most important sources of information regarding patient problems are the patients themselves, not their charts. Only after the patient interview can the chart information be used efficiently.

To summarize, before interviewing the patient, the pharmacy student should look at the patient's medication list in the chart or profile in any setting, the MAR in an institutional setting, and any previous care notes that would indicate how well the patient's disease states are controlled.

Step 2. Gather Information: Interview the Patient

Obtaining subjective information from the patient is the most important step in the database-building process. The pharmacist must make it a priority to interview every patient to whom he or she provides care. If an interview with the patient is not possible (e.g., the patient is intubated) or unlikely to be informative (e.g., a patient has moderate to severe dementia), then the pharmacy student should interview the patient's caregiver.

- Before beginning the interview, the pharmacist should:
  - Introduce himself or herself and explain the role of the pharmacist on the health care team (which is to optimize the patient's drug therapy).
  - Ask if this is a good time to ask some questions about medication use. If it is not a good time for the interview (e.g., the patient is in a hurry, has visitors, or is going for a diagnostic test), another time should be scheduled.
- Many experienced clinicians use the standard organization for patient history and physical database (the "patient H&P database," Box 14.1) as a mental nudge for directing an interview. This helps to ensure that the proper information is gathered completely and consistently. The H&P database is also a standard format to use when presenting patient information at a formal case presentation.

Gathering Information about Prescription Medications

All prescription medications that the patient is currently taking should be reviewed. For each drug, the following should be noted:

- Drug, dose, route, frequency, indication (this is the *patient's* version of the indication).

> ### Box 14.1 Standard Organization of Patient History and Physical Data
>
> ID (identifying information): patient age, sex, race.
>
> CC (chief complaint): a one-phrase description of the patient's reason(s) for seeking medical and/or pharmaceutical care. Identification of the probable diagnosis is sometimes given as a chief complaint but is not strictly correct.
>
> HPI (history of the present illness): a summary of the events leading to the chief complaint. Organize chronologically if possible.
>
> PMH (past medical history): a brief summary of current diagnosed medical problems.
>
> - Organized by problem in order of most important (top) to the least important (bottom). Numbering or bulleting each medical problem will enhance organization. A pharmacist's PMH list should prioritize conditions based on the need for drug therapy monitoring.
> - Information about past health events can also be listed if they affect or explain current conditions.
> - Where possible, indicate time period since onset or duration of each problem.
>
> DH (drug history): some data may be obtained from the chart, but most will be obtained by interviewing the patient and, where possible, the patient's pharmacy. The drug history includes the following:
>
> - Name, dose, frequency, reason for use, duration of use, efficacy, toxicity, and indication of all prescription, OTC, and herbal medications that the patient has taken during the past month.
>   - All drug indications should be reflected in the past medical history.
>   - Note name and telephone number of pharmacy(ies) where patient obtains medications and medication-related information.
> - Medications previously (but not currently) used for a current medical condition; note why they were discontinued.
> - Recreational drug use, including current or past use of tobacco, ethanol, or illicit drugs.
>
> *(continued)*

Box 14.1 Standard Organization of Patient History and Physical Data (*continued*)

- Allergies or contraindications for drug use. The allergy history should include a detailed description of the allergic reaction, where possible.
- Compliance/adherence. Assess the patient's comprehension of drug therapy, knowledge of side effects/toxicity, compliance to drug regimen (including reliability), compliance aids, and needs for further intervention. Note any language or other barriers to compliance.

FH (family history): genetic predisposition or occurrence of relevant diseases in other family members. Only include if pertinent.

SH (social history): includes pertinent information regarding living situation, support systems, lifestyle, employment, and work environment (risks/chemical exposure) that may affect drug therapy.

ROS (review of systems): a subjective review of bodily systems as voiced by the patient during the interview.

PE (physical examination): an objective review of bodily systems obtained during the examination of the patient. At the very least, this should include vital signs (heart rate, blood pressure, respiratory rate, temperature), weight, and height.

- Both the ROS and the PE begin with general statements about the patient (subjective for ROS and objective for PE) and then move on to specific findings starting at the patient's head and moving down the body to the feet ("head to toe").

Labs (laboratory data): obtain all laboratory data pertinent to the problem list. At a minimum, report the baseline seven laboratory values (Na, K, CI, CO_2, glucose, BUN [blood urea nitrogen], and Cr), CBC (complete blood count) (WBC [white blood cell]/diff, Hct [hematocrit] and platelets), liver function tests (AST, ALT, alk phos, and total bili; albumin and PT/INR are reasonable indicators of metabolic capacity). If the patient is febrile and/or an infection is suspected, report Gram stain and C&S findings.

Dx (diagnosis): any diagnosis made by the physician regarding the chief complaint, particularly if the patient will require pharmacotherapy for the condition.

- Efficacy ("Tell me how you know that this medication is working for you.").
- Toxicity ("What problems do you think may be caused by this medication?"). If the patient says "None," the pharmacist can probe with a few of the most common side effects.
- Height and weight (if not otherwise available).
- Compliance ("How often do you actually take this medication?" or "Tell me what interferes with your ability to take the medication regularly." "What do you do if you miss a dose?"). The pharmacist should try to verify if cost, dosing frequency, adverse effects, or personal beliefs may be an obstacle to compliance.
- Medication management issues including the following:
  - How/where the patient stores medications.
  - Ease of administration for each dosage form.
  - The number and names of physicians the patient sees.
  - The name and telephone number of each pharmacy the patient uses.
  - How the patient remembers to order/pick up refills and transportation limitations (to the physician or pharmacy).
  - Technique and maintenance of devices used to facilitate drug delivery or monitor drug therapy.

Gathering Information about Nonprescription Medications

These include over-the-counter (OTC) medications, herbal and other natural remedies, vitamins and minerals, and nondrug therapy. The following "head to toe" review of systems approach should be used to inquire about nonprescription agents used by the patient. In addition to gaining valuable information about nonprescription agents the patient uses routinely or infrequently, it will also often identify disease states that may not have been identified through the prescription medication portion of the interview.

- Head, eyes, ears, nose, and throat (HEENT): nose, ear, or eye drops; nasal inhalers; analgesics used for headache or sinus pain; dental products.
- Respiratory tract: antihistamines, decongestants, OTC inhalers.
- Gastrointestinal: antacids, antiflatulents, antidiarrheals, laxatives, hemorrhoidal preparations.
- Genitourinary: urinary antibacterials; vaginal antiinfectives; usual amount of fluid consumed daily; what kind of fluid (e.g., soda versus water versus lite beer).

- Musculoskeletal: aspirin, antiinflammatory agents, acetaminophen, or combination pain medications.
- Hematologic: iron, B_{12}, folate.
- Dermatologic: psoriatic, seborrheic, antiinfective, or analgesic topical preparations; corn/callus pads or other foot care.
- Neurologic: medications for insomnia, motion sickness, anxiety, lethargy.
- Overall/systemwide: vitamins; naturopathic, homeopathic, or other alternative health care products. Tobacco and alcohol use, noting favored product, quantity, frequency, and duration of use. Nonprescribed (illicit) drugs for recreational purposes (patients are more likely to be honest if asked questions about illicit drug use in a matter-of-fact manner).

If the patient uses nonprescription products for a particular medical problem, the pharmacy student should establish how often the medical problem occurs, if the nonprescription therapy works, and if the therapy causes any side effects. Patients should be asked where they usually buy nonprescription products and how they obtain answers to questions about the products (i.e., if there is a pharmacist or other health care professional available to answer their questions).

Review of Disease States, Conditions, and Medications

These lists should be reviewed with the patient for confirmation. The pharmacy student should ask if there are other conditions that are not included on the list. Patients should be asked to describe their disease (e.g., "Just to give me an idea of your understanding of congestive heart failure, please describe what is happening."). The pharmacy student should probe for understanding of the effects of overtreatment, undertreatment, or sporadic treatment of the disease (e.g., "Tell me what long-term complications you may avoid if your blood pressure is lowered.") and any cultural and personal beliefs that might affect current or future drug therapy ("Tell me how you feel about medication use, in general." "How do you feel your medications affect your quality of life?"). Information about therapies used *previously* for each disease state may also be valuable.

Drug Allergies and Other Conditions

If a patient states that he or she is allergic to a certain drug or has had an adverse reaction to a certain drug, as much of the following information as possible should be obtained. This information should be obtained for every drug that the patient notes.

- Name of the drug to which the reaction occurred and information about similar reactions.
  - Occurrence of similar reaction when drugs in same class previously taken.
  - Number of times the drug was used previously without adverse sequelae.
- Reason the patient took the drug (and likelihood of viral infection within 2 weeks preceding drug use, if the reaction was a rash).
- Complete description of physical symptoms of the reaction. A physical assessment should be conducted if the adverse drug reaction is currently in progress.
- Timing of reaction versus administration of the drug ("How soon after you took the drug did this reaction happen?" "How many days or doses into therapy were you when this reaction occurred?"). Any information about other medications administered around the same time that the reaction occurred may also be useful.
- Other allergies or intolerances (e.g., food, nickel, latex). Drug vehicles or inert ingredients may contain something to which the patient will react.

If it is determined that a patient is incorrectly labeled as allergic to a drug or other substance, the primary care provider should be consulted about the possibility of removing the allergy label and flag from the patient's chart or profile.

▪ Step 3. Gather Information: Examine the Patient

Immediately after or during the interview, any physical examination necessary to test a hypothesis about drug-related problems should be conducted. Current and past laboratory data and diagnostic tests should be checked to determine changes that might indicate drug efficacy or toxicity. The patient's pharmacy should be contacted to confirm current prescription drugs and regimens. Questions about refill patterns will confirm compliance. A patient's family members, caregivers, or physician can be contacted if they can provide valuable information regarding the patient's response to therapy.

If a pharmacy student wishes to obtain information about an objective parameter that has not been previously measured, he or she must justify to the preceptor why the information would be helpful and cost justified. The student should also identify tests or procedures that must be done immediately versus those that can be delayed until the most emergent problem(s) is/are addressed.

■ Step 4. Determine and Prioritize Medical and Drug-Related Problems

A list of all the patient's current medical problems—conditions that the patient is experiencing or being treated for—should be identified. These medical problems should be numbered and placed in order of importance, starting with the medical problems needing the most immediate attention and ending with problems that can be addressed later. In a hospital setting, many of the patient's medical conditions will be identified by the physician in the patient chart. In the community pharmacy, medical problems may need to be inferred from the patient's drug therapy list and confirmed through patient interview.

Alongside each medical condition should be a corresponding list of drug-related problems (DRPs). Drug-related problems are issues pertaining specifically to drug therapy. Although eight DRPs were identified in the seminal publication[2] distinguishing the role of the pharmacist in the patient care team, these DRPs can be further consolidated into five easily remembered issues:

- Drug needed. (i.e., drug indicated but not prescribed, correct drug prescribed but not taken).
- Wrong drug. (i.e., inappropriate drug prescribed—no apparent current medical problem justifying use of drug, unneeded duplication of therapy, less expensive alternative available or drug not covered by formulary, drug not available; failure to account for pregnancy status, age of patient, or other contraindications; incorrect nonprescription agent self-prescribed by patient; harmful recreational drug use).
- Wrong dose. (i.e., prescribed dose too high—needs adjustments for kidney, liver function, age, or body size; correct prescribed dose but overuse by patient; prescribed dose too low—needs adjustment for age or body size; correct prescribed dose but underuse by patient; incorrect, inconvenient, or less than optimal dosing interval).

- Adverse drug reaction. (i.e., unwanted side effect, allergy, drug-induced medical problem or laboratory change).
- Drug interaction. (i.e., unwanted drug–drug, drug–disease, drug–nutrient, or drug–laboratory interaction).

Questions that a pharmacist should consider while examining a patient's list of medications to determine whether any of these issues are occuring are as follows:

- Are there any medical problems (diagnoses) identified by the prescriber or pharmacist for which no drug therapy has been prescribed? If so, does the condition probably need drug therapy?
- Are there any drugs prescribed for the patient with no apparent indication?
- Is the patient taking the medications as prescribed? If not, why not?
- Is the treatment working? If not, why not?
- Is the treatment causing intolerable side effects?
- Are the doses correct/optimal?
- Are any abnormal laboratory values drug induced?
- Could lower-cost medications produce a similar effect?

Step 5. Determine Therapeutic Goal for Each Medical Problem

The four primary goals for any drug therapy are to accomplish the following as needed:

- Cure a disease (e.g., infection).
- Eliminate or reduce a patient's symptoms (e.g., pain, congestive heart failure).
- Arrest or slow a disease process (e.g., kidney dysfunction, atherosclerosis).
- Prevent an unwanted condition (e.g., stroke, infection, pregnancy).

There are also general secondary goals that, if achieved, can aid in attaining the patient's primary goals. Secondary goals include the following:

- Avoiding unwanted adverse effects.
- Attaining medication regimen convenience.
- Achieving cost-effectiveness.
- Enhacing patient education.

Proxy or intermediate end points are most often monitored to determine therapeutic efficacy of a medication regimen.

- The best intermediate end points are predictive of the primary goals (which are essentially avoidance of adverse health-related events); for example, there is a reasonable correlation between a systolic blood pressure <130 mm Hg (an intermediate end point) and a lower risk of stroke (an unwanted condition).
- Many intermediate end points, however, are not strongly correlated with lower risk of adverse health events. For example, although it is true that the risk of stage 5 chronic kidney disease increases as blood pressure increases, it has not been shown definitively that lowering blood pressure lowers risk of progression to stage 5 chronic kidney disease.

Pharmacy students need to identify which intermediate end points most strongly predict achievement of the overall health goal.

Step 6. Identify Reasonable Therapeutic Alternatives for Each DRP

All reasonable therapeutic options (drug classes and nondrug therapies) used for a medical problem should be considered in the process of solving a DRP. For each therapeutic option, the following should be determined:

- The evidence for efficacy.
- The likelihood and severity of adverse medication effects.
- The number of daily doses.
- The effects (either positive or negative) of the option on the patient's other diseases.
- The cost relative to the other agents.

The pharmacy student should review this information during the practice experience for each treatment received by or considered for each assigned patient. The ability to clearly summarize the most recent evidence supporting (or disputing) each treatment option will facilitate providing the best possible care. The preceptor will query students extensively about therapeutic alternatives, so this important step should not be neglected.

Step 7. Choose and Individualize the Best Therapeutic Option

If a thorough job has been done collecting and evaluating the benefits and limitations of each therapeutic option, choosing the most reasonable therapeutic option should be easy. The option must then be individualized to fit the characteristics of the patient. This is where knowledge about height and weight (for pharmacokinetic dose considerations), concomitant diseases and medications (for drug–disease and drug–drug interactions), and adherence history (to determine frequency of doses) will be vital. If the plan includes drug therapy, then drug, dose, route, frequency, and duration of therapy need to be specified. All drug and nondrug plans should include some degree of patient education.

Step 8. Design a Monitoring Plan for Efficacy and Toxicity

After choosing a therapeutic regimen, a monitoring plan needs to be designed. The monitoring plan should include the following:

- Exactly what will be measured.
- Who will do the measuring.
- How often it will be done.
- When it may be time to change or discontinue the therapy.
- Why the backup plan is the next best option.

The student must be able to defend all of the above measures. This will be easy if the monitoring parameters are cheap, quick, and noninvasive but more difficult if they are expensive, lengthy, or invasive.

Step 9. Document the Decision-Making Process

It is professionally unacceptable and legally dangerous to provide care for a patient and not record both care decisions and the reasoning behind those decisions. Practice-based experiences are valuable because they allow students the necessary practice to eventually produce a brief yet informative note in a short amount of time.

All documentation notes should begin with the date and time that the information is recorded. Good notes will also include before the start of the note a brief one-phrase overview of the reason for the note. This one-phrase overview should identify the pharmacy origin of the note (making it easier for other health care providers to locate) and some indication of the problem (e.g., "Pharmacy note sub-optimally controlled blood pressure," "Pharmacy note regarding probable adverse drug reaction").

Format

There are several formats for documentation of medication regimen decision making, but all follow the same general flow of ideas:

- Patient data are presented first.
- Data analysis identifies an actual or potential DRP.
- A plan or recommendation is identified to address or prevent the identified DRP.

In the SOAP format (and its iterations), subjective information (the "S" in SOAP) is presented first.

- Subjective information is obtained verbally from the patient or caregiver and therefore is not directly observed or measured by the SOAP writer.
- Objective information (the "O" in SOAP) is presented next, and details data directly measured or observed by the SOAP writer.
- Information in the subjective and objective sections of a SOAP note do not use the subheadings of ID, CC, HPI, DH, SH, ROS, and PE used in the patient H&P database. See Box 14-1 for definitions of abbreviations.

The subjective and objective information in a SOAP note should be limited to only that information that pertains directly to the assessment or plan/ recommendation.

- The assessment section (the "A" in SOAP) of a SOAP note communicates the critical thinking of the writer. The assessment section should:
    › Identify a drug-related problem (DRP) and explain why the identified DRP needs correcting.
    › Contain a short list of reasonable therapeutic alternatives with a brief explanation of benefits and potential problems associated with each option, and treatment goals.
    › Reference evidence from the medical literature where appropriate. It is conventional to use a brief reference format of acceptable journal name/abbreviation, year of publication, volume, and first page number.

When written optimally, by the time the reader reaches the end of the assessment section, that reader will know exactly what is going to be recommended by the writer, and why.

- The plan section, which is the final step, (the "P" in SOAP; alternatively, pharmacists may choose to write "SOAR" notes, where the "R" stands for "recommendation") identifies the actions proposed by the writer. A pharmacist's recommendation or plan should include the following:
  - Drug, dose, route, frequency, and duration (when applicable).
  - What will be measured to determine if the therapy is working (i.e., effective), who will measure it, and how frequently this will be done.
  - What will be measured to determine if the recommended drug is causing a problem (i.e., toxicity), who will measure it, and what will be done if toxicity occurs. Toxicity monitoring will usually involve different monitoring parameters than the efficacy measures.
  - Specific counseling points about administration, dose, frequency of use, side effects or precautions if the writer's purpose is to document patient counseling.
  - When follow-up will occur (e.g., follow-up in 3 months for repeat blood pressure [BP] check).
  - The alternatives to treatment if efficacy is not achieved or if toxicity occurs.

SOAP notes in the ambulatory care setting are often used to document patient interactions for billing purposes. In such cases it is important to include in the note the number of minutes spent on the interaction/workup. This number is usually placed at the end of the note.

Other written formats for communicating information include preprinted check-off forms, such as care pathways or protocols, or dictation (i.e., transcription of taped information to written form). Because patient care activities such as unexpected DRPs cannot be recorded completely using a preprinted form, these activities should be documented by adding a written addendum to the progress notes.

Tips for Writing Patient Care Notes

- **Length.** As a general rule, care notes should not exceed one page. This can be most easily accomplished through careful use of phrases, rather than sentences, and by including *only* the information needed to support the assessment and plan and nothing more.
- **Number of problems.** Pharmacy students new to writing care notes should try to address only one DRP in each SOAP. With experience,

a student's will develop the skill to address more than one problem *succinctly* in a care note. To facilitate organization of such an assessment, each separate problem should be numbered. The recommendations for each separate problem should also be numbered with the numbered problem in the assessment (A) section having the same number in the plan/recommendation (P/R) section.

- Abbreviations. It may be safe to abbreviate common laboratory values (e.g., white blood cells [WBC], hemoglobin [Hgb]), the four main vital signs, and common diagnostic tests (e.g., chect x-ray study [CXR], radiograph [XRAY], computed tomography [CT], magnetic resonance imaging [MRI], forced expiratory volume [FEV_1], forced vital capacity [FVC]), but abbreviation of anything else may result in miscommunication among health care providers, increasing the risk of medication errors. Drug names should never be abbreviated. Many institutions have an approved abbreviations list; the pharmacy student should obtain a copy of this list on the first day at a new site. Pharmacy students should be well acquainted with potentially dangerous abbreviations and avoid their use.

- Common problems seen in care notes written by new or untrained writers include the following:

  ‣ Inclusion of extraneous information (example: identification of all medications a patient is receiving in the subjective or objective section when the assessment addresses only one or two of those medications).

  ‣ Exclusion of important information (example: identification of uncontrolled hypertension in the assessment with no or only one blood pressure reading in the objective section).

  ‣ Information in the wrong place (example: assessment information in the plan).

  ‣ Vague or unclear information. Avoid use of nonspecific words such as "decreased," "increased," "recent," "symptoms," "problems," "changes," "monitor," "review," and "follow."

  ‣ Lack of clear reasoning to support problem existence or choice of recommendation.

▨ Step 10. Meet with the Patient after Plan Implementation

It is important to meet with the patient after plan implementation to determine the success of the plan and the need for modification.

Example

An example of a complete patient workup will illustrate the patient care process. The scenario:

It is the first day of the clinical clerkship at a community pharmacy. Mr. Smith, a 68-year-old man who has been a patient at this pharmacy for several years, presents a prescription for "Coumadin 2 mg #30, 1 po daily" to the pharmacy student. The information sources available to the student are Mr. Smith, his pharmacy profile, and a log of his laboratory values, which the pharmacist has asked him to bring every time he comes to the pharmacy. The following information is the patient history and physical data, the student's assessment of Mr. Smith's situation, and the chart note.

Patient History and Physical Database

ID: A 68-year-old man.

CC: Needs an increase in warfarin dose due to decreased efficacy of past dose.

HPI: The patient takes warfarin daily for deep venous thrombosis (DVT) prevention. INR (international normalized ratio) today was 1.5, and the physician has decided to increase the warfarin dose from 5 mg by mouth daily to 7 mg by mouth daily. The patient has been instructed to take one 5-mg tablet and one 2-mg tablet daily and to return for reassessment in 2 weeks.

PMH:

- DVT, 2 months ago.
- Hip replacement surgery, 3 months ago.
- Atrial fibrillation, single episode 4 years ago; no symptoms are currently reported.
- Congestive heart failure (CHF), diagnosed 7 years ago.
- Chronic obstructive pulmonary disease (COPD), diagnosed 5 years ago.
- Anterior myocardial infarction (MI) 14 years ago indicating coronary artery disease (CAD); no current chest pain.

DH:

Prescription medications:

- Warfarin, 5 mg by mouth every day for 2 months (DVT; same dose since discharge from hospital 2 months ago).
- Digoxin, 0.25 mg by mouth every day for 7 years (CHF).
- Ipratropium, 2 puffs four times a day for 5 years (COPD).

- Albuterol, 2 puffs four times a day for 5 years (COPD).
  Nonprescription medications:
- Multivitamin with iron and minerals, one by mouth daily for 7 months.
- Psyllium, 1 scoop in a glass of water for constipation daily for 4 years.
- Bismuth salicylate, 4 tablespoonfuls as needed for diarrhea (took 1 dose twice in the past year for stomach flu).
- Alfalfa tablet 2 to 3 every day for health; friend recommended this to him about 1 month ago.
  Adherence information:
- Medication refill records indicate that the patient obtains refills on time.
- The patient obtains all prescription and OTC medications from this pharmacy.
- The patient bought alfalfa tablets at a health food store.
  Recreational drug use:
- 40-pack/year smoking history: quit 2 years ago.
- Occasional alcohol use: 1 to 2 drinks/week; no recent change in this amount.
  Allergies: denies history of medication or environmental allergies.

FH: Father died of acute MI at age 54.

SH: Retired; lives with spouse who assists with medication management at home; denies any changes in ingestion of vitamin K–containing foods

ROS: No current complaints

- Lungs: Clear sputum, no spells of coughing recently; denies shortness of breath (SOB), dyspnea on exertion (DOE), and paroxysmal nocturnal dyspnea (PND); sleeps with one pillow; is comfortable walking short distances (no change from 3 months ago).
- CV (cardiovascular): Denies chest pain.
- Skin: Denies bleeding or bruising.
- GI (gastrointestinal): Stools are dark brown.
- GU (genitourinary): Urine is clear, yellow; no blood.

PE: 5'10", 80 kg today (usual weight); HR (heart rate): 85, regular rhythm; BP: 135/82; RR respiratory rate): 20; temp 37.2°C; no bruising found on arms, legs, or face.

Pertinent Labs:

Today	2 weeks ago	4 weeks ago	6 weeks ago	8 weeks ago (at discharge)	8 weeks ago
INR: 1.5	INR: 1.9	INR: 2.4	INR: 2.6	INR: 2.3	Alb: 4.5

Current Medical Problems	Goal of Therapy	Measurable End Point
1. Recent DVT	Prevent recurrent thromboembolism	Therapeutic INR
2. CAD	Prevent angina and MI	No anginal episodes
3. CHF	Symptom control	No episodes SOB, edema, PND
4. COPD	Symptom control	No DOE, SOB, PND

Current Drug-Related Problems	Justification	Therapeutic Alternatives
1a. Underanticoagulation (wrong dose? drug interaction?)	Subtherapeutic INR Possible causes: • Diet (no recent change) • EtOH (patient denies) • Underlying disease state change (no evidence to support) • Drug interaction (recent addition of natural product that contains varying amounts of vitamin K) • Compliance (no evidence of noncompliance)	• Increase warfarin dose (problematic considering inconsistent amount of vitamin K in alfalfa tablets) • Discontinue (D/C) alfalfa • Heparin (prolonged heparin use would be more expensive than warfarin; short-term LMW heparin use might save cost of ultrasound to check for clot formation)
2a. Inadequate MI prophylaxis (needs drug?)	Current AHCPR guidelines recommend aspirin and beta-blocker for all patients post-MI unless contraindicated	• ASA, 81 mg PO daily (lower dose will minimize risk of bleeding) • ASA, 325 mg PO daily • beta-blocker (contraindicated secondary to CHF + COPD) *(continued)*

(Continued)

Current Drug-Related Problems	Justification	Therapeutic Alternatives
3a. Inadequate CHF and post-MI mortality benefit (needs drug?)	Current ACC/AHA guidelines recommend ACEI for all patients with CHF; SAVE, AIRE, and TRACE trials support use post-MI to reduce mortality	• ACE inhibitor • Angiotensin receptor antagonist
4a. COPD overmedicated (wrong drug?)	1995 Study conducted in the Netherlands showed increased costs and no additional benefit of two bronchodilators over one alone	• D/C albuterol (preferred due to CHF) • D/C ipratropium

EtOH, ethyl alcohol; LMW, low-molecular-weight; AHCPR, Agency for Health Care Policy Research; ACC/AHA, American College of Cardiology/American Heart Association.

Recommendation	Monitoring Plan
1. Anticoagulation • D/C alfalfa tablets • Start enoxaparin, 80 mg (1mg/kg) SQ q12hr. D/C when INR ≥2.0 • Continue warfarin at current dose. Instruct patient to self-administer SQ medication	• Return for INR check in 5 days • Patient to self-monitor for signs/symptoms (S/S) of DVT: calf warmth, tenderness or pain. Patient to call provider immediately if experiences chest pain or SOB • Patient to self-monitor for S/S minor, moderate, and major bleed: visual check for gum, urine, stool, skin bruising, epistaxis
2. MI prophylaxis • ASA, 81mg PO daily	• Patient to self-check for bleeding as noted above. Stool guaiac in 3 mo
3. CHF/post-MI mortality benefit • Lisinopril, 5 mg PO daily; first dose at bedtime; titrate dose upward weekly to maximal doses (20 mg PO q12hr) as tolerated per BP and serum creatinine (SCr)	• Check BP in 1 week (goal SBP 100–120) • Check SCr now for baseline and again in 1 week • Patient to self-monitor for and report dizziness/light-headedness and any increase in coughing frequency
4. COPD • D/C albuterol	• Patient to self-monitor for and report any increased incidence of SOB, DOE, PND

Today's date and time.

Pharmacy note regarding anticoagulation and other drug therapy for 68-year old white male.

S:

- Pertinent medical history: DVT, 2 months ago; CHF for 7 years; COPD for 5 years; anterior MI, 14 years ago.
- ROS: denies coughing, SOB, DOE, PND, chest pain, bleeding or bruising, blood in stool or urine.
- Occasional alcohol use: 1 to 2 drinks/week; no recent change in that amount.
- Denies any changes in ingestion of vitamin K–containing foods; has taken alfalfa tabs 2 or 3 daily for ~1 month per friend's advice (for general health).

O:

- 5′10″, 80 kg today (usual weight); HR: 85, regular rhythm; BP: 135/82; RR: 20.
- No bruising found on arms, legs, or face.
- INR: 1.5 today; 1.9 2 weeks ago; 2.4 4 weeks ago; 2.6 6 weeks ago; 2.3 at discharge 8 weeks ago.
- Pertinent prescription medications: warfarin, 5 mg PO daily (same dose for last 2 months); ipratropium, 2 puffs QID; albuterol, 2 puffs QID.

A:

1. INR ≤ 2.0 associated with $\uparrow$ risk of recurrent DVT. Addition of alfalfa coincides with $\downarrow$ INR control. Discontinuing alfalfa preferable to increasing warfarin dose since varying vitamin K tablet amount confounds dose titration. Since patient shows no signs/symptoms of acute DVT, addition of outpatient enoxaparin for a few days until INR in therapeutic range would be more cost-effective than admission to hospital to watch for recurrent DVT.

2. Suboptimal CHF and post-MI mortality benefit. Addition of aspirin for CAD and ACE inhibitor for CHF and post-MI associated with $\downarrow$ mortality. Beta-blocker use also associated with $\downarrow$ risk of subsequent MI but is relatively contraindicated in this patient because of CHF and COPD.

3. Dual-bronchodilator therapy not superior to single-bronchodilator therapy for COPD (*Am J Resp Crit Care Med* 1995;151:975). Ipratropium preferred over albuterol in this patient due to CHF.

P:

1. D/C alfalfa tabs. Start enoxaparin, 80 mg SQ (subcutaneous) q12hr. D/C when INR ≥2.0. Continue warfarin at current dose. Teach patient how to self-administer SQ medication. Return for INR check in 5 days. Instruct patient to self-monitor and report: calf warmth, tenderness or pain; chest pain or SOB; excessive blood in gums, urine, stool, nose, dermis.

2. Start: ASA (acetylsalicylic acid; aspirin), 81 mg PO daily; lisinopril 5 mg PO daily; first dose at bedtime; titrate dose up by 5 mg every week to max 20 mg PO daily as tolerated per BP ($\sqrt{}$ in 1 week; goal: SBP (systolic BP) 100–120) and SCr ($\sqrt{}$ today and in 1 week). Patient to report any dizziness or ↑ coughing.

3. D/C albuterol. Patient to report any ↑ in SOB, DOE, PND.

◼ SUMMARY

In summary, whether with a patient in the hospital, in the clinic, or at the pharmacy counter, the student should perform the following steps:

- Quickly scan the chart or profile to identify issues that need to be discussed with the patient.
- Obtain subjective data by interviewing the patient.
- Gather objective data by physical examination and review of pertinent laboratory parameters, MAR or patient fill records, and diagnostic tests and consultations.
- Summarize the patient's medical problems and drug-related problems and set goals for the therapy of those problems that need to be addressed immediately.
- Consider the potential benefits and hazards of all reasonable therapeutic alternatives. Select the alternative that has the highest likelihood of efficacy, a minimum of toxicity, and that seems the most cost-effective.
- Determine the optimal dose, route, frequency, and duration for the patient's pharmacokinetic, concomitant drug and disease state, economic, and compliance needs.
- Design and implement a monitoring plan to determine if the recommendation works or causes unreasonable toxicity.
- Document the decision-making process.

At first, this process will seem long and cumbersome, but with practice it will become quick and effortless. By taking the responsibility for clinical drug monitoring, the student will become a practitioner whom patients and health care colleagues will respect and trust.

References

1. Hepler CD, Strand LM. Opportunities and responsibilities in pharmaceutical care. *Am J Hosp Pharm*. 1990;47:533–543.
2. Strand LM, Cipolle RJ, Morley PC. Documenting the clinical pharmacist's activities: back to basics. *Drug Intell Clin Pharm*.. 1988;22:63–66.
3. Canaday BR, Yarborough PC. Documenting pharmaceutical care: creating a standard. *Ann Pharmacother*. 1994;28(11):1292–1296.

15

Antibiotics, Antivirals, and Infection

Jennifer M. Jordan, Devon Flynn, and David T. Bearden

Signs and Symptoms of Infection

Fever and an elevation in peripheral white blood cell count (WBC) are the classic nonspecific signs of infection. Fever is inexactly defined, but most clinicians consider temperatures >100.4°F (38°C) to be abnormal.[1] An increase in neutrophils, termed a "left shift" in white blood cells, is also frequently noted. It is important to note that some individuals may display neither sign of infection, due to a diminished host response. Reasons to lack a fever include advanced age, use of antipyretics, or sepsis. A low temperature in sepsis of <96.8°F (36°C) is actually a worse prognostic sign than a high temperature. Similarly, neutropenic patients may not have a WBC increase. Other signs and symptoms depend on the specific site of infection.

Cultures and Sensitivities Timeline

The treatment of infectious diseases is predicated on identifying and obtaining the pathogen causing the disease. This frequently occurs in several steps that may require several days (see Table 15.1) for completion. Each step reveals more data to aid in clinical decision making but also requires careful interpretation. It is important to note that the approximate times listed in Table 15.1 apply to most common bacterial cultures. Some more-difficult-to-grow organisms can take several days (fastidious organisms) to several weeks (*Mycobacterium tuberculosis*) to become positive.

Early Gram stain distinction of the organism shape and grouping provides important clues to the pathogen likely to be isolated (Table 15.2). In instances where only a single pathogen from a normally sterile site is likely, this information can be very helpful early in the treatment course.

Table 15.1 THE TYPICAL BACTERIAL CULTURE TIME LINE

Step	Time Frame	Antibiotic Choices	Example	Notes
1. Obtaining a specimen for culture	—	Broad empiric coverage for the likely pathogens at the suspected site of infection	Blood culture obtained; initially started empirically on vancomycin	—
2. Gram stain	Minutes	Add or alter therapy if empiric selection does not cover this group of organisms	No Gram stains are done on blood; no change in therapy	The presence of organisms does not always mean infection. Some sites are not sterile, and colonization cannot always be differentiated
3. Initial positive culture	12–48 h	Add or alter therapy if empiric selection does not cover this group of organisms; stop unnecessary additional coverage	Gram strain of growing organism reveals gram negative bacilli; stop vancomycin, start ceftazidime	The lack of a positive culture does not rule out infection. For most infections a positive culture may never be isolated due to technical issues, a difficult-to-grow organism, or transient bacterial appearance
4. Identification of species	24–48 hours	Add or alter therapy if empiric selection does not typically cover this organism	Organism identified as *Klebsiella pneumoniae*; continue ceftazidime	Using local susceptibility patterns at this step can give a better indication of the likelihood that initial therapy will be adequate
5. Anti-infective susceptibilities	48–72 hours	Narrow therapy to the specific organism's data	Susceptibilities reveal organism is resistant to ceftazidime but sensitive to ciprofloxacin; stop ceftazidime, start ciprofloxacin	Final antibiotic recommendations can now be made

Table 15.2 BACTERIAL SHAPES AND GRAM STAINS	
Gram Stain and Shape	**Likely Pathogen**
Gram Positive	
Cocci in clusters	*Staphylococcus* species
Cocci in chains	*Streptococcus* species (not *S. pneumoniae*)
Cocci in pairs and chains	*Enterococcus* species
Diplococci	*S. pneumoniae*
Gram Negative	
Bacilli (rods)	Many species
Diplococci	*Neisseria* species

From Koneman EW, Allen SD, Janda WM, et al. *Color Atlas and Textbook of Diagnostic Microbiology.* 5th Ed. Philadelphia, PA: Lippincott-Raven; 1997:2.

Not all positive cultures are clinically relevant. Attention to the type of organism isolated is also revealing. Normal flora is present at nonsterile sites and may contaminate samples (e.g., skin flora in blood samples or oral flora in sputum samples). Positive cultures of this sort that lack clinical symptoms (e.g., coagulase-negative staphylococci in a blood culture) are often considered contaminants. Similarly, not all negative cultures confirm a lack of infection. Even with documented infections, it is often difficult to isolate a specific bacterial cause. Finally, some types of organisms are notoriously difficult to culture. For example, anaerobes are often missed by typical cultures and need to be assumed present in some infections (e.g., diabetic foot, intra-abdominal infections).

Newer, rapid technology tests are currently being more widely used for the identification of important pathogens. For instance, polymerase chain reaction (PCR) testing can detect the gene responsible for methicillin-resistant *S. aureus* (*mec*A) within hours, cutting substantial time off selecting appropriate therapy.

■ Susceptibility Testing

The minimum inhibitory concentration (MIC) of an antibiotic against an organism is the concentration that inhibits growth in the laboratory. This concentration is determined and then compared to established guidelines that categorize the number into one of three groups—sensitive, intermediate, or resistant. Many laboratories will report only one of these three categories and not the exact concentration of the MIC. Clinically, the categories should generally guide antibiotic selection. An "intermediate" determination generally weighs against the use of that anti-infective.

There are times when a specific MIC may be important in decision making, and the laboratory can be asked to provide the actual concentration. Knowledge of the specific MIC is imperative for use in maximizing pharmacodynamic parameters in dosing regimens (see below). It is important to note that comparing a list of MIC values for various anti-infectives without knowing the concentrations required for a determination of sensitive, intermediate, or resistant is of little value. Lower does not always mean better. The typical concentration of the anti-infective in the blood and at the site of infection play an important role in setting the breakpoint values for determining susceptibility. An antibacterial with an MIC of 4 μg/mL can be preferable to one with an MIC of 2 μg/mL in the context of the tissue concentrations typically achieved.

 ## Choosing the Appropriate Antimicrobial Agent

The delay of appropriate antimicrobial therapy is related to higher rates of morbidity and mortality. This relationship creates a difficult challenge for clinicians who want to treat all the major pathogens until microbiologic laboratory data is available, while minimizing a patient's drug exposure to avoid toxicities, excessive costs, and the development of superinfections and resistance. The principles of treating infection can be simplified into the following steps:

1. Diagnosis of the infectious disease state (e.g., cellulitis).
2. Consideration of likely pathogens consistent with patient history, clinical presentation, and epidemiologic data (e.g., streptococcus or staphylococcus).
3. Choosing an antimicrobial regimen that has activity against the most likely pathogens and achieves adequate drug concentrations at the site of infection, and the patient is likely to tolerate (e.g., dicloxacillin).
4. Monitoring the patient for improvement and adjusting therapy based on clinical and microbiology data.

Pharmacists can play a key role in assisting prescribers with antimicrobial selection, dose optimization, and monitoring therapy for efficacy as well as toxicity.

Table 15.3 consists of the more common infectious diseases seen in clinical practice, likely pathogens, and possible empiric antibiotic

Table 15.3 COMMON INFECTIOUS DISEASES AND RECOMMENDED TREATMENT

Disease State	Typical Pathogens	Oral/IV Options	Comments
Cellulitis (uncomplicated, community-acquired)	S. pyogenes S. aureus	Dicloxacillin, Clindamycin, Nafcillin, Oxacillin, or Vancomycin	Emergence of CA-MRSA Bactrim, Doxycycline, Vancomycin, Linezolid
Cellulitis[a] (complicated, diabetic foot, decubitus ulcers)	S. aureus Streptococci Enteric GNB Pseudomonas	TMP/SMX or doxycycline plus a PCN or ceph TMP/SMX plus amoxicillin/clav Vancomycin plus piperacillin/tazo	Mild severity Moderate severity Severe infection
Bacterial meningitis (age ≥1 month, without head trauma or recent neurosurgery)	S. pneumoniae N. meningitidis	Vancomycin plus ceftriaxone or cefotaxime	Age >50 years, add ampicillin for Listeria
Acute otitis media	S. pneumoniae Viral H. influenzae M. catarrhalis	Amoxicillin	High-dose amoxicillin recommended
Acute rhinosinusitis	S. pneumoniae H. influenzae M. catarrhalis Viral	Amoxicillin	Observation with analgesics for mild cases
Acute pharyngitis	Viral streptococci	Penicillin	Document group A Streptococcus before treatment

Community-acquired pneumonia (previously healthy individual with no risk factors for DRSP)	*S. pneumoniae* *M. pneumoniae* *H. influenzae* *C. pneumoniae* Viral	Macrolide Doxycycline	Hospitalized patients should receive a respiratory quinolone or a β-lactam plus macrolide
Community-acquired pneumonia (comorbidities or antibiotics in previous 3 mo or high prevalence of macrolide resistance)	*S. pneumoniae* *M. pneumoniae* *H. influenzae* *C. pneumoniae* Viral	Respiratory FQ Macrolide *plus* amoxicillin or cefpodoxime or ceftriaxone or cefuroxime	If admitted to ICU, an IV β-lactam *plus* a macrolide or quinolone is recommended.
Health care–associated pneumonia (hospitalized <5 d, low risk for multidrug-resistant pathogen)	*S. pneumoniae* *H. influenzae* MSSA GNB	CRO Quinolone Ampicillin/sulbactam Ertapenem	Empiric regimens should cover > 90% of the local pathogens
Health care associated pneumonia (hospitalized ≥5 d and risk for multidrug-resistant pathogen)	Above pathogens *Pseudomonas* *Klebsiella* *Acinetobacter* MRSA	Anti-pseuodomonal β-lactam *plus* cipro or levofloxacin *plus* vanco or linezolid	Empiric regimens should cover > 90% of the local pathogens
Urinary tract infections (UTIs) (acute, female, uncomplicated)	*E. coli* Enteric GNB *S. saprophyticus*	TMP/SMX Nitrofurantoin Quinolone Fosfomycin	Moxifloxacin and gemifloxacin are not FDA approved for UTIs

(continued)

Table 15.3 COMMON INFECTIOUS DISEASES AND RECOMMENDED TREATMENT *(continued)*

Disease State	Typical Pathogens	Oral/IV Options	Comments
Intra-abdominal infections (community acquired)	E. coli Enteric GNB B. fragilis Streptococci Enterococci	β-lactam/β-lactamase inhibitor Third-generation cephalosporin plus metronidazole Quinolone plus metronidazole	Initial regimen should be based on local resistance patterns and severity of illness
Clostridium difficile diarrhea	C. difficile	Metronidazole Vancomycin oral	Vancomycin preferred for moderate to severe infections

CA-MRSA, community-acquired methicillin-resistant *Staphylococcus aureus*; GNB, Gram-negative bacilli; TMP/SMX, trimethoprim/sulfamethoxazole; PCN, penicillin nonsusceptibility; ICU, intensive care unit; MSSA, Methicillin-susceptible *Staphylococcus aureus*; CRO, ceftriaxone.

aInclude MRSA coverage.

From American Academy of Family Physicians and American Academy of Pediatrics. Diagnosis and Management of Acute Otitis Media 2004. Available at www.aafp.org/x26481.xml. Bisno AL, et al. Practice guidelines for the diagnosis and management of group A streptococcal pharyngitis. *Clin Infect Dis.* 2002;35:113–125; Guidelines for the management of aAdults with hospital-acquired, ventilator-associated, and healthcare-associated pneumonia. *Am J Respir Crit Care Med.* 2005;171:388–416; Lipsky BA, Berendt AR, Deery HG, et al. Diagnosis and treatment of diabetic foot infections. *Clini Infect Dis.* 2004;39:885–910; Mandell LA, Wunderink RG, Anzueto A, et al. Infectious Diseases Society of America/American Thoracic Society consensus guidelines on the management of community-acquired pneumonia in adults. *Clin Infect Dis.* 2007;44: S27–72; Rosenfeld RM. Clinical practice guideline on adult sinusitis. *Otolaryngol Head Neck Surg.* 2007;137:365–377; Solomkin JS, Mazuski JE, Baron EJ, et al. Guidelines for the selection of anti-infective agents for complicated intra-abdominal infections. *Clin Infect Dis.* 2003;37:997–1005; Stevens DL, Bisno AL, Chambers HF, et al. Practice guidelines for the diagnosis and management of skin and soft-tissue infections. *Clin Infect Dis.* 2005;41:1373–1406; Tunkel AR, Hartman BJ, Kaplan SL, et al. Practice guidelines for the management of bacterial meningitis. *Clin Infect Di.* 2004;39:1267–8124; and Warren JW, Abrutyn E, Hebel JR, et al. Guidelines for antimicrobial treatment of uncomplicated acute bacterial cystitis and acute pyelonephritis in women. *Clin Infect Dis.* 1999;29:745–758, with permission.

regimens. A detailed patient history, including history of present illness, allergy data, previous antibiotic therapy, health care exposure, presence of comorbidities, and laboratory data should be considered before recommending or starting any antimicrobial regimen. Complicated cases should be referred to an infectious disease specialist.

Unfortunately, the regimens as listed in Table 15.3 do not fit all patients. One must consider allergies, severity of disease, and local resistance patterns. Also, there are many drugs that would be effective, but listing every regimen is beyond the scope of this chapter. To assist in choosing alternative regimens, Table 15.4 lists most antimicrobials with their general spectrum of activity.

Special Bugs

Multidrug-resistant pathogens are becoming relatively common. The armamentarium to treat *Acinetobacter*, *Pseudomonas*, and *Enterobacter* species is becoming small with the increasing development of resistance.

SPECIAL CONSIDERATIONS

- *Acinetobacter*: There have been several outbreaks of multidrug-resistant *Acinetobacter* in the United States. Many of these strains are susceptible only to polymyxin B and tigecycline.
- *Enterobacter*: Inducible β-lactamases not seen with routine susceptibility tests may be present. Do not use third-generation cephalosporins. Drugs of choice for serious infections include carbapenems or cefepime.
- *Pseudomonas*: Fluoroquinolones or aminoglycosides should not be used as monotherapy for serious infections outside the urinary tract.
- Community-acquired methicillin-resistant *Staphylococcus aureus* (CA-MRSA): This staphylococcus is usually susceptible to several antibiotics. TMP/SMX and doxycycline are options for mild infections. CA-MRSA may cause necrosis and rapidly progressing life-threatening infections. Linezolid may be the drug of choice for pneumonia.
- Fungus and mold: See Table 15.5 for susceptibilities.

Pharmacokinetics-Pharmacodynamics of Antimicrobial Therapy: Optimizing Dosing

To optimize antimicrobial dosing, one must first understand pharmacokinetic/pharmacodynamic (PK/PD) principles that relate to the

Table 15.4 SPECTRUM OF ANTIMICROBIAL ACTIVITY TO COMMON PATHOGENS

| | Gram Positive | | | Gram Negative | | | | Anaerobes | | Comments |
	Strepto-cocci	MSSA	MRSA	Entero-coccus	E. coli	Kleb-siella	H. influ-enzae	Pseudo-monas	Oral An-aerobes	B. fra-gilis	
Penicillins											
Penicillin	+	–	–	–	–	–	–	–	+	–	Drug of choice for susceptible streptococci
Ampicillin Amoxicillin	+	–	–	+	+/–	–	+/–	–	+	–	Drug of choice for susceptible enterococci
Amp/sulbactam	+	+	–	+	+	+	+	–	+	+	
Amox/clavulanate	+	+	–	+	+	+	+	–	+	+	
Dicloxacillin	+	+	–	–	–	–	–	–	+	–	Drug of choice for MSSA
Nafcillin Oxacillin	+	+	–	–	–	–	–	–	+	–	Drug of choice for MSSA
Piperacillin/ tazobactam	+	+	–	+	+	+	+	+	+	+	

Cephalosporins

								Notes
Cefazolin	+	+	−	−	+	+	+	−	First generation
Cephalexin	+	+	−	−	+	+	+	−	First generation
Cefuroxime	+	+	−	+	+	+	+	−	Second generation
Cefoxitin	+	+	−	+	+	+	+	+	Second generation
Ceftriaxone Cefotaxime	+	+	−	+	+	+	+	−	Third generation
Ceftazidime	+/−	+/−	−	+	+	+	+/−	−	Third generation
Cefepime	+	+	−	+	+	+	+	−	Fourth generation

Aminoglycosides

								Notes
Gentamicin Tobramycin Amikacin	Syn	Syn	Not tested in vivo	Syn	+	+	−	−	Gentamicin is drug of choice for Gram-positive synergy Tobramycin and amikacin more potent against *Pseudomonas* *(continued)*

Table 15.4 SPECTRUM OF ANTIMICROBIAL ACTIVITY TO COMMON PATHOGENS *(continued)*

Fluoroquinolones	Gram Positive		Gram Negative		Anaerobes	Comments
Ciprofloxacin	–	+/–	+	+	–	–	Atypicals, poor Gram (+)
Levofloxacin	+	+	+	+	+/–	Atypicals
Moxifloxacin	+	+	+	–	+	Atypicals, most potent Gram (+)
Others						
Trimethoprim/ sulfamethoxazole	+	+/–	+	–	+	
Clindamycin	+	+	–	–	+	
Metronidazole	–	–	–	–	+	
Aztreonam	–	–	+	+	–	OK for beta-lactam allergy

Ertapenem	+	+	−	−	+	+	+	−	+	+	
Imipenem Meropenem	+	+	−	+/−	+	+	+	+	+	+	
Azithromycin Clarithromycin	+	+/−	−	−	−	+	+	−	+	−	Atypicals
Daptomycin	+	+	+	+	−	−	−	−	−	−	Activity against VRE
Linezolid	+	+	+	+	−	−	+/−	−	−	−	Activity against VRE
Tigecycline	+	+	+	+	+	+	+	−	+	+	Activity against VRE
Vancomycin	+	+	+	+	−	−	−	−	+	−	Activity against VRE

MSSA, methicillin-susceptible *Staphylococcus aureus*; MRSA, methicillin-resistant *Staphylococcus aureus*; Syn, synergy only, not likely to yield clinical cure as monotherapy; VRE, vancomycin-resistant *Enterococcus*; +, typically susceptible; −, typically resistant or no clinical activity

Note: Susceptibilities in this table are from national trends and should serve as a guide for selection of empiric antibiotics. Choice of initial antimicrobials should depend on local susceptibilities, presence of drug-resistance risk factors, previous susceptibilities and antimicrobial use, and severity of illness.

From Draghi DC, Sheehan DJ, Hogan P, et al. In vitro activity of linezolid against key Gram-positive organisms isolated in the United States: Results of the LEADER 2004 Surveillance Program. *Antimicrob Agents Chemother.* 2005;49(12):5024–5032; and Gales AC, Jones RN, Sader HS. Global assessment of the antimicrobial activity of polymyxin B against 54,731 clinical isolates of Gram-negative bacilli: report from the SENTRY Antimicrobial Surveillance Programme (2001–2004). *Clin Microbiol Infect.* 2006;12:315–321, with permission.

Table 15.5 ANTIFUNGAL SPECTRUM OF ACTIVITY AND CONCENTRATIONS IN THE URINE[15-17]

Drug	Activity Against *Candida* Species				Aspergillus Activity	Urine Concentrations	Comments
	C. albicans	*C. glabrata*	*C. parapsillosis*	*C. krusei*			
Azoles							
Fluconazole	+++	+	+++	−	−	Excellent	*C. glabrata* may need high doses
Itraconazole	+++	+	+++	+/−	+	Poor	Needs acidic environment for PO absorption, unless suspension is used
Posaconazole	+++	++	+++	++	+++	Poor	Activity against some zygomycetes
Voriconazole	+++	++	+++	+	+++	Poor	IV and PO

	C. albicans	C. glabrata	C. parapsillosis	C. krusei		
Echinocandins						
Anidulafungin	+++	+++	++	+++	Poor	Not metabolized
Caspofungin	+++	+++	++	+++	Poor	
Micafungin	+++	+++	++	+++	Poor	
Polyenes						
Amphotericin	+++	++	+++	++	Poor	Nephrotoxicity, electrolyte disturbances

From Kreiter P. Disposition of posaconazole following single-dose oral administration in healthy subjects. *Antimicrob Agents Chemother.* 2004;48(9):3543–3551; Pappas PG, et al. Guidelines for treatment of candidiasis. *Clin Infect Dis.* 2004;38:161–189; and Pfaller MA, Messer SA, Hollis RJ, et al. In vitro susceptibilities of *Candida* bloodstream isolates to the new triazole antifungal agents BMS-207147, Sch 56592, and voriconazole. *Antimicrob Agents Chemother.* 1998;43(12):3242–3244, with permission.

antimicrobial agent being used and take into account pharmacokinetics for the individual patient. Pharmacodynamics is the correlation of drug concentration and response, whereas pharmacokinetics describes absorption, distribution, metabolism, and elimination of the drug from the body. PK/PD parameters may be used to optimize clinical outcomes and avoid the development of antimicrobial resistance.[18,19] Overly simplified, an antimicrobial's effectiveness can be categorized as a concentration-dependent or time-dependent activity.

- Time-dependent killers: Frequent administration, prolonged infusion times, or continuous infusion are optimal. In cases of renal insufficiency, a dose reduction while maintaining a normal dosing interval is typically preferred.
- Concentration-dependent killers: Killing activity is related to peak:MIC or area under the curve (AUC):MIC ratios.[18,19] These antimicrobials may be dosed less frequently but in high doses. Once-daily aminoglycoside administration is an example of maximizing killing and postantibiotic effects. In patients with renal insufficiency, doses of concentration-dependent antimicrobials should generally be maintained while extending the dosing interval.

See Table 15.6 for PK/PD properties of antimicrobial drug classes.

Synergy and Double Coverage

Synergy occurs when the effects of two drugs combined are greater than the addition of the individual drug's effects acting separately. Although the term is used frequently in the infectious disease realm, it is clinically relevant in only a few circumstances. Some of the most popular drug combinations for synergy are beta-lactams and aminoglycosides or rifampin combinations.

- Aminoglycosides: Addition of gentamicin or streptomycin is essential when treating enterococcal endocarditis. Bactericidal effects of the penicillin or ampicillin are not seen in the absence of the aminoglycoside. Note: The dose of gentamicin is only 1 mg/kg every 8 hours in a patient with normal renal function, as gentamicin peaks of 3 to 5 mg/L have been studied for Gram-positive synergy. This is in contrast to once-daily administration mentioned previously in this chapter.
- Rifampin: Rifampin is frequently used in combination with other antibiotics for infections involving bone and prosthetic material. The dose

Table 15.6 PHARMACODYNAMIC PROPERTIES OF INDIVIDUAL ANTIMICROBIALS

Drug	PD Property	Notes
Aminoglycoside	Concentration-dependent	Peak:MIC, ideal Peak 4x MIC for GNB, 8x MIC for *Pseudomonas*
Fluoroquinolones	Concentration-dependent	AUC:MIC >100–125 for GNB, AUC:MIC >30 for *S. pneumoniae*
Metronidazole	Concentration-dependent	AUC:MIC, Cmax:MIC
Daptomycin	Concentration-dependent	AUC:MIC, Cmax:MIC
Cephalosporins	Time-dependent	50%–60% of T >MIC
Penicillins	Time-dependent	40%–50% of T >MIC
Carbapenems	Time-dependent	40%–50% of T >MIC
Macrolides	Time-dependent	T >MIC
Clindamycin	Time-dependent	T >MIC
Linezolid	Time-dependent	T >MIC
Vancomycin	Time-dependent	AUC:MIC
Tetracyclines	Time-dependent	AUC:MIC

PD, pharmacodynamic; MIC, minimum inhibitory concentration; GNB, Gram-negative bacilli; AUC, area under the curve; Cmax, maximum xoncentration.
From Ambrose PG, Bhavnani SM, Rubino CM, et al. Pharmacokinetics-pharmacodynamics of antimicrobial therapy: it's not just for mice anymore. *Clin Infect Dis.* 2007; 44:79–86; and Craig WA. Does the dose matter? *Clin Infect Dis.* 2001;33(Suppl 3):S233–237, with permission.

and timing of rifampin in therapy is somewhat questionable since large, randomized, placebo-controlled trials are lacking.

In the era of multidrug-resistant Gram-negative pathogens, it may be acceptable to use combination therapy empirically to provide appropriate antibiotic therapy to moderately to severely ill patients. In this circumstance, the clinician may choose drugs that may be additive or synergistic initially and adjust therapy when cultures and susceptibilities are available.

◼ IV or PO Therapy?

After choosing the correct antimicrobial spectrum and coverage, the next question is usually related to the appropriate route of administration.

Table 15.7 ORAL ANTIMICROBIALS WITH HIGH BIOAVAILABILITY

Antifungals	**Notes**
Fluconazole	—
Voriconazole	Take 1 h before or after a meal
Antibiotics	—
Clindamycin	Large oral doses may cause gastrointestinal (GI) distress
Doxycycline and minocycline	Absorption may be hindered by divalent and trivalent cations (calcium, iron, magnesium) in food or medication
Linezolid	—
Metronidazole	—
Quinolones	Absorption may be hindered by divalent and trivalent cations (e.g., aluminum, calcium, iron, magnesium) in food or medication
Trimethoprim/sulfamethoxazole	—

While it is appealing to maximize the oral route to minimize cost and risks of complications associated with intravenous access, in many clinical instances the intravenous route is preferred.

Oral medications are preferred for mild to moderate infections when adequate drug levels reach the site of infection. Oral formulations are acceptable in more severe infections if they have a high bioavailability (Table 15.7), the patient has a functioning gastrointestinal (GI) tract in which drug absorption can occur, and there is an absence of drug or food interactions that would interfere with drug absorption. Most oral antimicrobials, even with high bioavailability, have not been well studied and should not be used for endocarditis, meningitis, sepsis, or other life-threatening infections. Oral antimicrobials may serve a role in step-down therapy or initial therapy when no intravenous (IV) formulations are available.

HIV/AIDS

Treatment of the human immunodeficiency virus (HIV) has come a long way since the first antiretroviral (Retrovir or zidovudine or AZT) was approved by the U.S. Food and Drug Administration in 1987. Early antiretroviral (ARV) regimens presented many administration issues due to high pill burden and dosing frequencies greater than twice daily. Current ARV regimens require fewer tablets/capsules per day and once or twice daily dosing frequencies. However, the regimens remain complex due to the potential for severe medication toxicities, drug–drug interactions, and development of resistance.

As treatment has improved, survival has improved and the number of people living with HIV in the United States has increased dramatically. Terminology used in the area of HIV can be confusing and is not always intuitive. The following section includes explanations of terminology as well as basic medication and treatment information of which you should be aware.

Basic Terminology and Information

HIV Testing[20]

- The HIV test is an antibody test that must be followed by a confirmatory test (in the United States this is a Western blot).
- Antibodies to HIV are not present during early, acute infection but do appear in 97% of people within 3 months of infection.
- A person may test negative for HIV if testing is too soon following a potential exposure.

Viral Load (VL)

- The VL is a measure of the number of HIV viral RNA copies per mL of plasma and is used as a surrogate marker for measuring response to ARV treatment.
- One goal of ARV treatment is to achieve an undetectable viral load. This means that the number of HIV RNA copies per mL of plasma is less than the lower limit of detection of the process being used. "Undetectable" is reported as either <50 copies/mL or <75 copies/mL depending on the assay used.

CD4 Cell Count (CD4)[20]

- The CD4 cell count is an absolute measurement of CD4 cells (also known as T cells or helper T cells).
- The CD4 cell count is used as a measure of the immune system's competency.
- CD4 cell count cutoffs are used to determine when to begin ARV treatment as well as when patients should receive prophylaxis for specific opportunistic infections.

Highly Active Antiretroviral Therapy (HAART)

- HAART refers to combination antiretroviral therapy (i.e., using more than one class of ARV medication in the regimen). It is now the standard of treatment.
- When people refer to plain old "antiretroviral therapy" or ART, combination treatment is implied.

Boosting

- A boosted ARV regimen refers to a protease inhibitor (PI)-based regimen including ritonavir (Norvir).
- In this situation the ritonavir is being used for its strong CYP P450 3A4 inhibitory properties to increase trough levels of the active ARV. Ritonavir is *not* being used for its ARV effects.
- Boosted PI regimens are often preferred to unboosted (i.e., a PI-based regimen that does not include ritonavir) regimens.[21]
- Nelfinavir is the only PI that is never given with ritonavir.

Opportunistic Infections (OI)

- An OI is an infection that affects only people who have a dysfunctional immune system.
- OIs may be due to a new exposure to the pathogen (such as with *Mycobacterium avium* complex) or may be due to reactivation of latent infection (such as with cytomegalovirus).[22]
- Common OIs affecting patients with HIV/AIDS include the following: *Pneumocystis jirovecii* pneumonia (PCP; formerly *Pneumocystis carinii* pneumonia), *Mycobacterium avium* complex (MAC), oral candidiasis, toxoplasmosis.

HIV versus AIDS Diagnosis

- HIV is the virus that causes the acquired immunodeficiency syndrome (AIDS).
- HIV diagnosis is based on HIV antibody and confirmatory follow-up testing.
- AIDS is a syndrome of immunodysfunction. AIDS diagnosis is based on the following:
  1. Having tested positive for HIV, and
  2. Signs of severe immunodeficiency are present.[23]
- Signs of AIDS immunodeficiency may be based on laboratory data (such as a CD4 cell count <200 cells/mm^3) and/or clinical consequences due

to immunodeficiency (such as infection with an OI or development of Kaposi's sarcoma or other types of malignancies).[23]

Genotype and Phenotype Testing

- The genotype reports the genetic sequence of the HIV viral genome to detect any genetic mutations that may result in decreased or increased ARV susceptibilities.
- See the International AIDS Society-USA (IAS-USA) and the Stanford Resistance Database references listed in the recommended Web sites list at the end of this chapter to help interpret the significance of specific HIV mutations.
- Phenotypic testing is similar to a bacterial culture susceptibility test. Results are reported based on how well the patient's virus survives and replicates in the presence of each ARV medication. The phenotype may be the preferred method of evaluating treatment options in highly treatment-experienced patients.
- Note: Both tests require that the HIV plasma viral load be $\geq$500 to 1,000 copies/mL at the time the sample is collected for testing.

Antiretroviral Information

- See Table 15.8 for a list of currently available ARV medication brand names, generic names, three-letter abbreviations, and the ARV class designated for each ARV.
- Didanosine EC and zidovudine are currently the only ARVs available in the United States as generic products.

Common Drug–Drug Interactions to Watch for (Note: See the Department of Human Health Services, DHHS, guidelines in the recommended Web sites list at the end of this chapter for more detailed information regarding these and other ARV drug–drug interactions):

In general:

- PIs (except tipranavir): *inhibition* of CYP 3A4 and
- Nonnucleoside reverse transcriptase inhibitors (NNRTIs) (plus tipranavir): *induction* of CYP 3A4.

Atazanavir (Reyataz)[24]

- Dose times must be spaced with dose times of H2 blockers and antacids that a patient may be taking.

Table 15.8 ANTIRETROVIRAL (ARV) NAMES, CLASSES, AND DOSING FREQUENCIES

Brand Name	Generic Name	3-Letter Abbreviation	ARV Class	Dosing
Aptivus	Tipranavir	TPV	PI	bid
Atripla	Emtricitabine/ Tenofovir / Efavirenz	FTC/TDF/EFV	NRTI + NNRTI	qday
Combivir	Lamivudine/ Zidovudine	3TC/AZT	NRTI	bid
Crixivan	Indinavir	IDV	PI	bid–tid
Emtriva	Emtricitabine	FTC	NRTI	qday
Epivir	Lamivudine	3TC	NRTI	qday–bid
Epzicom	Lamivudine/ Abacavir	3TC/ABC	NRTI	qday
Fuzeon	Enfuvirtide	T20	EI	bid
Intelence	Etravirine	ETV (or TMC-125)	NNRTI	bid
Invirase	Saquinavir	SQV	PI	bid
Isentress	Raltegravir	RAL	InSTI	bid
Kaletra	Lopinavir/ Ritonavir	LPV/r	PI	qday–bid
Lexiva	Fosamprenavir	FPV (or LXV)	PI	qday–bid
Norvir	Ritonavir	RTV	PI	See note[a]
Prezista	Darunavir	DRV (or TMC 114)	PI	bid[b]
Rescriptor	Delavirdine	DLV	NNRTI	tid
Retrovir	Zidovudine	AZT (or ZDV)	NRTI	bid
Reyataz	Atazanavir	ATV	PI	qday
Selzentry	Maraviroc	MVC	EI	bid
Sustiva	Efavirenz	EFV	NNRTI	qday
Trizivir	Lamivudine/ Zidovudine/ Abacavir	3TC/AZT/ABC	NRTI	bid

(continued)

Table 15.8 ANTIRETROVIRAL (ARV) NAMES, CLASSES, AND DOSING FREQUENCIES *(continued)*

Brand Name	Generic Name	3-Letter Abbreviation	ARV Class	Dosing
Truvada	Emtricitabine/ Tenofovir	FTC/TDF	NRTI	qday
Videx EC	Didanosine EC	ddI (or ddI-EC)	NRTI	qday
Viracept	Nelfinavir	NFV	PI	bid
Viramune	Nevirapine	NVP	NNRTI	bid
Viread	Tenofovir	TDF	NtRTI	qday–bid
Zerit	Stavudine	d4T	NRTI	bid
Ziagen	Abacavir	ABC	NRTI	qday–bid

PI, protease inhibitor; NRTI, nucleoside reverse transcriptase inhibitor; NNRTI, nonnucleoside reverse transcriptase inhibitor; EI, entry inhibitor; InSTI, integrase inhibitor; NtRTI, nucleotide reverse transcriptase inhibitor.

[a]Bid dosing if used for treatment (very rare); qday to bid dosing as booster with another PI.

[b]Currently being studied for qday dosing.

Adapted from Panel on Antiretroviral Guidelines for Adult and Adolescents. Guidelines for the use of antiretroviral agents in HIV-infected adults and adolescents. Department of Health and Human Services. December 1, 2007:1–136, with permission.

- Proton pump inhibitors (PPIs) should be avoided altogether in highly treatment-experienced patients taking atazanavir but may be used (up to a maximum dose equivalent of omeprazole, 20 mg) in treatment-naïve patients taking boosted atazanavir.
- Patients taking antacids, H2 blockers, or a PPI with atazanavir should be taking the atazanavir with ritonavir (Norvir) (i.e., the atazanavir should be boosted).
- Be aware of patients admitted to the hospital and administered an H2 blocker or PPI for stress ulcer prophylaxis.
- Be aware of patients taking over-the-counter acid-reducing products.

HMG-Coenzyme Inhibitor (Statin) Interactions with PIs (Especially with Regimens Containing Ritonavir)

- Simvastatin and lovastatin are contraindicated for use with regimens containing ritonavir.[21]

- Be aware of patients with HIV who may have been admitted to the hospital with a myocardial infarction (MI)—they may be placed on high-dose simvastatin post MI.
- Atorvastatin may be used but initiated at lower doses.[21]
- Pravastatin is another option (use caution with darunavir).[21]
- Data are limited regarding rosuvastatin use with the PIs.

Oral Contraceptives
- Many NNRTIs and PIs reduce the levels of ethinyl estradiol in oral contraceptives.[21]
- Medroxyprogesterone injection may be an option.
- Women of childbearing age should be counseled regarding the risk of pregnancy and additional contraception techniques when taking oral contraceptives for birth control.

Tuberculosis
Tuberculosis (TB) and other mycobacterial treatment regimens should be carefully selected in patients also taking ARV medications.

- Rifampin is contraindicated for use with many ARVs, and rifabutin is often used in its place.
- The dosing of rifabutin and ARVs (NNRTIs, PIs, and maraviroc) are often different from standard doses when used concomitantly. Double-check doses of both the TB regimen and the ARV regimen to ensure that the patient receives optimal treatment for both TB and HIV.

Methadone
- Some ARVs (especially efavirenz, nevirapine, and some PIs) may decrease levels of methadone and cause signs/symptoms of opiate withdrawal.[21]

Laboratory Interference
- Efavirenz (Sustiva) may cause a false-positive result on some cannabinoid urine drug assays.[25] Be aware of this counseling point for patients who may be involved in addiction recovery programs that require periodic urine drug tests.

Renal Dosing[21]
- Renal dosing is required for all of the nucleoside reverse transcriptase inhibitors (NRTIs) (zidovudine, stavudine, didanosine, tenofovir, lamivudine, and emtricitabine), *except* abacavir.
- Combination tablets should be avoided when renal dosing is required.

Weight-Based Dosing

- Weight-based dosing is required for stavudine and didanosine.[21]
- Zidovudine is dosed by weight when being used intravenously during labor and delivery for prevention of mother-to-child-transmission (MTCT).[26]

Antiretroviral Regimens[21]

- In general, an antiretroviral (ARV) treatment regimen should include *either* one NNRTI *or* one PI in addition to two NRTIs for a total of three different medications from at least two different classes of ARVs.
  - ‣ Two NRTIs + one NNRTI *or*
  - ‣ Two NRTIs + one PI. Note: "One PI" includes boosted PI regimens (see "boosting" explanation above).
- More highly treatment-experienced patients may take ARV regimens that do not look like the above formulas.

Dosing Matters!

- Pay attention to ARV dosing, especially during medication reconciliation and when ARVs are ordered in the hospital setting.
- Pay close attention to timing of doses and food requirements, as they may differ from the hospital's standard meal and dose times and are important to achieve and maintain adequate ARV blood levels.
- ARV doses may be different when used with other specific ARVs. For example, the recommended dose for lopinavir/ritonavir (Kaletra) when given with efavirenz (Sustiva) is three tablets twice a day instead of just two tablets twice a day when efavirenz is not a component of the regimen. See the DHHS guidelines in the recommended Web sites list at the end of this chapter for more information.

Patients Coinfected with Hepatitis B

- Many of the medications used to treat hepatitis B are also active against HIV (lamivudine and tenofovir).
- If the patient is treated only for the hepatitis B with one of these medications, there is a risk of HIV resistance developing during hepatitis B treatment. Adefovir continues to have a theoretical risk for promoting HIV resistance (especially to tenofovir) due to its anti-HIV activity at high doses. However, adefovir is active against HIV only at doses much higher than those indicated for treatment of hepatitis B.
- Case reports of HIV resistance developing with entecavir (previously thought to have no activity against HIV) have been reported.

- It is recommended that if a patient requires treatment for hepatitis B, he or she should be treated with a fully suppressive HIV regimen that (preferably) includes either lamivudine or emtricitabine and tenofovir.[21]
- Keep in mind that patients with hepatitis B who are taking an HIV regimen that includes lamivudine, emtricitabine (a close relative of lamivudine), or tenofovir may experience an acute flare, or worsening, of hepatitis B if the HIV regimen is discontinued.

Discontinuation of ARVs

- If one drug of the ARV regimen needs to be stopped, it must be replaced with another ARV medication or *all* of the ARV medications need to be stopped together.
- Note that the half-life of efavirenz (Sustiva) is 40 to 55 hours, making it take longer to clear efavirenz from the blood after stopping the medication. Therefore, the other ARVs in the regimen may be continued for 7 to 10 days after stopping efavirenz to avoid exposing the patient to monotherapy that may promote resistance. This is referred to as providing an ARV "tail."
- Nevirapine (Viramune) may also require an ARV tail of 3 to 7 days when the ARV regimen is discontinued.

Use of Enfuvirtide (Fuzeon) in the Hospital Setting

- Enfuvirtide presents many preparation, stability, and administration issues.
- Consultation with pharmacy and hospital administrators to determine the best way to maintain a patient on enfuvirtide treatment during his or her hospital stay is advised.
- The best solution may include allowing the patient to prepare and administer his or her own supply of medication if possible.

ARV Treatment During Pregnancy[26]

- *All* pregnant women with HIV should be treated for HIV regardless of CD4 cell count and viral load.
- A three-medication regimen should be used, as discussed above. It is preferable to include zidovudine as one of the medications in the ARV regimen.
- If the mother is on an ARV regimen at the time she becomes pregnant, assess the regimen for safety in pregnancy and continue the regimen.
- If the mother is not on ARV treatment at the time of pregnancy, it is recommended to wait until 14 to 16 weeks gestation to begin an ARV regimen compatible with pregnancy.

- PIs in pregnancy: Levels of lopinavir/ritonavir (Kaletra) may be decreased during the third trimester and require increased dosing.
- NNRTIs in pregnancy: nevirapine (Viramune) may be used, although, there is an increased risk of hepatotoxicity in pregnant women. Efavirenz (Sustiva) is U.S. FDA pregnancy category D and should not be used in pregnant women or women planning to become pregnant.
- NRTIs in pregnancy: Tenofovir (Viread) use should be avoided due to theoretical risks of skeletal defects. Pregnancy registry data have not shown the risks of birth defects with tenofovir use during the first trimester to be greater than in the general population.
- Zidovudine should be administered intravenously during labor and delivery. The infant should receive zidovudine treatment for 6 weeks postpartum. In some instances, single-dose nevirapine may be used during the intrapartum period; however, the risk of nevirapine resistance is high. The mother should receive a tail of ARVs for 3 to 7 days postpartum if she received single-dose nevirapine.

Table 15.9 CD4 CELL COUNT AND PREFERRED PRIMARY PROPHYLACTIC REGIMENS FOR PREVENTION OF OPPORTUNISTIC INFECTIONS

CD4 Cell Count	OI Risk	Preferred Prophylaxis
<200 cells/mm^3	*Pneumocystis jirovecii* pneumonia (PCP)	TMP/SMX DS 1 daily or SS 1 daily
<100 cells/mm^3	Toxoplasmosis	TMP/SMX DS 1 daily
<50 cells/mm^3	Mycobacterium avium complex	Azithromycin, 1,200 mg weekly (may be once weekly or 600 mg twice weekly) or clarithromycin, 500 mg twice daily (not often used because of drug–drug interactions and less advantageous dosing schedule)

OI; opportunistic infection; TMP/SMX, trimethoprim/sulfamethoxazole.
Note: This table is *not* all-inclusive. OIs listed above are those that require primary prophylaxis only. Patients are at risk for other acquired or reactivated OIs at the CD4 cell counts listed above; however, primary prophylaxis is not routinely recommended for these other OIs. See the references listed at the end of this chapter for further information regarding OIs and risk.
Adapted from Guidelines for Prophylaxis and Treatment of Opportunistic Infections in HIV-infected Adults and Adolescents. 2008 June 18. Available at www.aidsinfo.nih.gov.

Table 15.10 HELPFUL INFECTIOUS DISEASES WEB SITES

Web Site	Contents
Centers for Disease Control and Prevention—Sexually Transmitted Diseases (www.cdc.gov/std/)	Sexually transmitted diseases guidelines and updates
Centers for Disease Control and Prevention—Travel (www.cdc.gov/travel)	Travel-related immunizations and travel medicine
Centers for Disease Control and Prevention—Vaccine Schedules (www.cdc.gov/vaccines/recs)	Adult and pediatric vaccination schedules and resources
Doctor Fungus (www.doctorfungus.org)	Source for fungal infections and treatment strategies
Infectious Diseases Society of America (www.idsociety.org)	Primary site for clinical guidelines for numerous infections and pathogens
Society of Infectious Diseases Pharmacists (www.sidp.org)	Pharmacist training, research, antibiotic stewardship
Department of Health and Human Services: AIDS info web site (www.aidsinfo.nih.gov)	Adult, adolescent, pediatric, and perinatal HIV/AIDS treatment guidelines as well as opportunistic infections prophylaxis and treatment guidelines
International AIDS Society—USA (www.iasusa.org)	HIV/AIDS treatment guidelines and great HIV mutation database with ARV resistance information
University of California, San Francisco–National HIV/AIDS Clinician's Consultation Center (www.ucsf.edu/hivcntr) UCSF HIV InSite web site (www.hivinsite.ucsf.edu/insite)	General HIV/AIDS information, hotline information, great resource for ARV tablet crushing/capsule opening information General HIV/AIDS information and extensive links to other resources
Stanford University HIV Resistance Database (hivdb.stanford.edu)	Great resource to help in evaluating genotype results
Johns Hopkins (www.hopkins-aids.edu)	Patient case discussions, medication reviews, general information about HIV and OIs

HIV/AIDS, human immunodeficiency virus/acquired immunodeficiency syndrome; ARV, antiretroviral; OIs, opportunistic infections.

Opportunistic Infections Prophylaxis

- Preventive medications for opportunistic infections are indicated based on CD4 cell count. See Table 15.9 for CD4 cell count cutoffs for specific OI prophylaxis and the preferred regimens for prophylaxis.

▨ Helpful Infectious Diseases Web Sites

Table 15.10 includes several electronic links to important infectious diseases–related Web sites commonly visited by practicing infectious diseases pharmacists.

References

1. Mackowiak PA, Bartlett JG, Borden EC, et al. Concepts of fever: recent advances and lingering dogma. *Clin Infect Dis.* 1997;25:119–138.
2. Koneman EW, Allen SD, Janda WM, et al. Color Atlas and Textbook of Diagnostic Microbiology. 5th Ed. Philadelphia, PA: Lippincott-Raven; 1997:2.
3. American Academy of Family Physicians and American Academy of Pediatrics. Diagnosis and Management of Acute Otitis Media 2004. Available at www.aafp.org/x26481.xml.
4. Bisno AL, et al. Practice guidelines for the diagnosis and management of group A streptococcal pharyngitis. Clin Infect Dis. 2002;35:113–125.
5. Guidelines for the management of adults with hospital-acquired, ventilator-associated, and healthcare-associated pneumonia. *Am J Respir Crit Care Med.* 2005;171:388–416.
6. Lipsky BA, Berendt AR, Deery HG, et al. Diagnosis and treatment of diabetic foot infections. *Clini Infect Dis.* 2004;39:885–910.
7. Mandell LA, Wunderink RG, Anzueto A, et al. Infectious Diseases Society of America/American Thoracic Society consensus guidelines on the management of community-acquired pneumonia in adults. *Clin Infect Dis.* 2007;44: S27–72.
8. Rosenfeld RM. Clinical practice guideline on adult sinusitis. Otolaryngol Head Neck Surg. 2007;137:365–377.
9. Solomkin JS, Mazuski JE, Baron EJ, et al. Guidelines for the selection of anti-infective agents for complicated intra-abdominal infections. *Clin Infect Dis.* 2003;37: 997–1005.
10. Stevens DL, Bisno AL, Chambers HF, et al. Practice guidelines for the diagnosis and management of skin and soft-tissue infections. *Clin Infect Dis.* 2005;41:1373–1406.
11. Tunkel AR, Hartman BJ, Kaplan SL, et al. Practice guidelines for the management of bacterial meningitis. *Clin Infect Di.* 2004;39:1267–8124.
12. Warren JW, Abrutyn E, Hebel JR, et al. Guidelines for antimicrobial treatment of uncomplicated acute bacterial cystitis and acute pyelonephritis in women. *Clin Infect* Dis. 1999;29:745–758.
13. Draghi DC, Sheehan DJ, Hogan P, et al. In vitro activity of linezolid against key Gram-positive organisms isolated in the United States: Results of the

LEADER 2004 Surveillance Program. Antimicrob Agents Chemother. 2005;49(12): 5024–5032.

14. Gales AC, Jones RN, Sader HS. Global assessment of the antimicrobial activity of polymyxin B against 54,731 clinical isolates of Gram-negative bacilli: report from the SENTRY Antimicrobial Surveillance Programme (2001–2004). Clin Microbiol Infect. 2006;12:315–321.

15. Kreiter P. Disposition of posaconazole following single-dose oral administration in healthy subjects. *Antimicrob Agents Chemother*. 2004;48(9):3543–3551.

16. Pappas PG, et al. Guidelines for treatment of candidiasis. Clin Infect Dis. 2004;38:161–189.

17. Pfaller MA, Messer SA, Hollis RJ, et al. In vitro susceptibilities of Candida bloodstream isolates to the new triazole antifungal agents BMS-207147, Sch 56592, and voriconazole. Antimicrob Agents Chemother. 1998;43(12):3242–3244.

18. Ambrose PG, Bhavnani SM, Rubino CM, et al. Pharmacokinetics-pharmacodynamics of antimicrobial therapy: it's not just for mice anymore. *Clin Infect Dis.* 2007; 44:79–86.

19. Craig WA. Does the dose matter? *Clin Infect Dis.* 2001;33(Suppl 3):S233–237.

20. *AAHIVM Fundamentals of HIV Medicine*, 2007 ed. Washington, D.C: American Academy of HIV Medicine; 2007.

21. Panel on Antiretroviral Guidelines for Adult and Adolescents. Guidelines for the use of antiretroviral agents in HIV-infected adults and adolescents. Department of Health and Human Services. December 1, 2007:1–136.

22. Mandell LA, Bennett JE, Dolin R, eds. *Principles and Practice of Infectious Diseases.* 6th ed. Vol. 2, Part III: Infectious Diseases and Their Etiologic Agents. Philadelphia, PA: Churchill Livingstone, 2005.

23. 1993 Revised classification system for HIV infection and expanded surveillance case definition for AIDS among adolescents and adults. Centers for Disease Control and Prevention, National Center for Infectious Diseases Division of HIV/AIDS. *MMWR Recomm Rep*. 1992 Dec 18;41(RR-17):1–19.

24. Atazanavir [package insert]. Princeton, NJ: Bristol-Myers Squibb Company; December 2007.

25. Sustiva [package insert]. Princeton, NJ: Bristol-Myers Squibb Company; January 2007.

26. Perinatal HIV Guidelines Working Group. Public Health Service Task Force. Recommendations for Use of Antiretroviral Drugs in Pregnant HIV-Infected Women for Maternal Health and Interventions to Reduce Perinatal HIV Transmission in the United States. November 2, 2007:1–96.

27. Guidelines for the prevention of opportunistic infections among HIV-infected persons—2002. Recommendations of the U.S. Public Health Service and the Infectious Diseases Society of America. *MMWR Recomm Rep*. 2002 Jun 14;51(RR-8):1–52.

16

Pain Management

Kenneth C. Jackson II

Pain Defined

Pain is often the primary complaint noted by patients and clinicians during the initial health care interview. Pain is the primary motivator for many patients to seek health care, and is often the impetus for patients seeking health care advice from pharmacists. Pain is defined by the International Association for the Study of Pain (IASP) as an unpleasant sensory and emotional experience associated with actual or potential tissue damage, or described in terms of such damage.[1]

Pain Differentiation

Pain, like most conditions, is often categorized into acute and chronic presentations. A consensus panel commissioned by The National Institute of Health used this as the basis for categorizing pain, providing for three discreet types of pain:[2]

- Acute—primarily the consequence of physical injury, often related to traumatic situations such as accidents or surgical procedures. Acute pain is time limited and often lasts only hours to days. In some situations the pain may last several weeks as a consequence of the clinical paradigm that has initiated the pain experience.
- Chronic cancer or malignant pain—persistent pain (e.g., >3 months) that is the consequence of an underlying neoplasm or the result of cancer treatment.
- Chronic nonmalignant pain—a diverse group of pain conditions that are unrelated but share the common thread that the pain is ongoing

(e.g., >3 months) and typically does not have any useful biologic value to patients or clinicians.

All chronic pain is pain that lasts longer than would be normally anticipated or is associated with a chronic condition that produces persistent ongoing pain. The length of time for chronic pain is difficult to ascertain, but many would consider persistent pain that lasts >3 months to be chronic in nature. In the setting of chronic pain, it should be noted that the intensity of pain can have a waxing and waning over time. This is an especially useful construct to understand as many patients can have various pain experiences that can be affected by several factors that may include daily activity, pain treatments (e.g., pharmacologic, physical, and psychological), and/or diurnal variation. Moreover, patients may have additional pain experiences in addition to their underlying persistent pain. This additional pain experience is often defined as breakthrough pain. This additional pain experience is often severe and can become debilitating.[3,4]

▣ Pathologic Differentiation

Pain is often described clinically in relation to the underlying pathologic properties, where in essence the pain signaling process is initiated. It should be noted that regardless of the initiating mechanism, pain as a construct does not occur until a patient's somatosensory cortex receives and recognizes the pain signal. Although nociceptive and neuropathic pain are described below as separate entities, it should be remembered that patients can manifest both pain types concurrently.

Nociceptive Pain

Nociceptive pain is pain signaling emanating from activation of peripheral receptors that propagate pain along undamaged neuronal tissue.

- Somatic pain (also known as [AKA] musculoskeletal pain) involves tissues such as skin, soft tissues, muscle, and bone structures. Pain results from stimulation of "normal" peripheral nociceptors within the somatic nervous system. Pain may be described as sharp, aching, and/or throbbing. Often this type of pain is easily localized by patient report.
- Visceral pain (AKA organ pain) involves organ systems such as the heart, lungs, and gastrointestinal and genitourinary tracts). This type of pain emanates from stimulation of the autonomic nervous system. Pain may be described as sharp, aching, and/or throbbing but is often difficult to describe in relation to a specific location.

Neuropathic Pain

Neuropathic pain is pain that results from damage to nerve tissue in the peripheral nervous system, the central nervous system, or sometimes both concurrently. Pain descriptors for neuropathic pain include burning, tingling, numbness, shooting, stabbing, and electrical.

- Peripheral neuropathic pain includes malignant plexopathies, painful polyneuropathy, postherpetic neuropathy, and diabetic peripheral neuropathy.
- Central neuropathic pain includes phantom pain and poststroke/thalamic pain.
- Mixed neuropathic pain includes CRPS (complex regional pain syndromes AKA causalgia or reflex sympathetic dystrophies).

Consequences of Pain

Poorly treated or untreated pain has many negative consequences as described in Table 16.1.[5,6] These consequences range from the more obvious physiologic issues to more overt issues that affect not only the patient but our larger society. Pharmacists should be vigilant in assessing these issues, both in the setting of prevention and aggressive treatment to reverse these sequelae.

Barriers to Pain Management

Table 16.2 provides an overview of the common issues that serve to preclude effective and necessary pain management. These issues span the entire health care spectrum. Patients, clinicians, health care systems, health care educational units, and the various regulatory bodies all play a part in the poor delivery of pain management.[7] It is incumbent on the practicing pharmacist to understand good analgesic pharmacotherapy and the potential impact of each of these areas of potential conflict in providing analgesia to patients.

Pain Assessment

Patient self-report should be the primary source of pain assessment whenever feasible or possible.[8,9] Clinician observations and physiologic

Table 16.1	POTENTIAL CLINICAL CONSEQUENCES RELATED TO PAIN		
Physical	**Psychological**	**Immunologic**	**Sociologic**
Increased catabolic demands: • Poor wound healing • Asthenia, fatigue	Mood disorders • Anxiety • Depression	Decreased host defenses: • Decreased natural killer cell function • Increased risk of infection • Poor response to chemotherapy	Increased health care use: • Increased ED visits • Increased use of pharma-cotherapy
Respiratory effects: • Shallow breathing • Tachypnea (acutely) • Atelectasis • Pneumonia	Sleep disorders		Decreased productivity: • Decreased performance • Lost work days
Gastrointestinal • Decreased GI motility • Constipation • Nausea • Vomiting	Existential suffering		Societal interaction: • Lack of family involvement • Decreased ability to interact in society
Cardiorenal: • Tachycardia • Hypertension • Increased sodium and water retention			

ED, emergency department; GI, gastrointestinal.

parameters or measurements may provide additional information but should be avoided as the primary pain assessment. Two exceptions may include preverbal children and nonverbal, cognitively impaired individuals. In these cases behavioral observations may be required to function as the primary source of pain assessment.

The most common and easiest method for assessing pain intensity in adults is the numeric rating scale (NRS). On the NRS the patient is asked to select a number (e.g., from 0 = no pain to 10 = pain as bad as it can be) that

Table 16.2 BARRIERS TO PAIN MANAGEMENT

Patient-related Barriers	• Reluctance to report pain
	• Reluctance to take certain medications
	    Fear of adverse effects
	    Fear of social stigma
	• Poor adherence

Clinician-related Barriers	• Lack of training • Lack of pain-assessment skills • Insufficient attention to patients • Difficulty in assessing pain • Rigidity or timidity in prescribing practices • Regulatory oversight
System-related Barriers	• Low institutional priority • Medication availability • Issues related to cost • Poor access to pain specialists • Regulatory inconsistency

best describes the intensity of the pain. To obtain an accurate assessment of variations in pain, it is often useful to have patients rate the intensity of current pain, as well as the worst pain, least pain, and average pain the person has experienced in a given time frame. This time frame may be the over the past 24 hours in the setting of acute pain, to several weeks for patients with chronic pain. Pain intensity measures such as the NRS are easy to use and can be used repeatedly over the course of treatment to monitor progress.

The NRS is based on an older scale known as the visual analog scale (VAS). The NRS and VAS correlate well with one another and can be used at the discretion of a clinician for an individual patient. The VAS requires the patient to make a mark representing his or her pain intensity on a 10-cm line with the same anchors used on the NRS. The VAS may be useful for patients who are more visually oriented. The VAS can prove challenging, if not inappropriate, for patients with poor vision or manual dexterity.

The Wong-Baker Faces scale (Fig. 16.1) is another commonly used assessment tool that has been validated for use with children and cognitively impaired adults.[10] The basic premise is similar to that discussed above with the NRS and VAS.

Good analgesic pharmacotherapy requires thorough patient assessment. The best approach to accomplishing this goal is the use of the

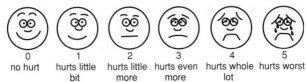

0	1	2	3	4	5
no hurt	hurts little bit	hurts little more	hurts even more	hurts whole lot	hurts worst

FIGURE 16.1 The Wong-Baker FACES Pain Rating Scale. (Reprinted with permission from Hockenberry MJ, Wilson D, Winklestein ML: *Wong's Essentials of Pediatric Nursing*, 7th ed. St. Louis, MO: 2005;1259. Copyright, Mosby.)

interdisciplinary team, where physicians, nurses, social workers, psychologists, therapists, and pharmacists each contribute their expertise to understanding the multidimensional nature of a patient's pain experience. The interdisciplinary approach affords each member of the team to have access to a comprehensive assessment that includes the medical history, physical and psychological pain assessments and access to appropriate laboratory and imaging studies.[11] The pain-specific components of the history include those components in Table 16.3.

Medication History

An accurate and organized medication history is an area where the pharmacist can provide great utility to the health care team.[11] This is especially

Table 16.3 COMPONENTS OF PAIN ASSESSMENT

- ❏ Pain type (nociceptive vs. neuropathic)
- ❏ Pain intensity (numeric rating scale)
- ❏ Pain source (if known—e.g., tumor, arthritis, etc.)
- ❏ Pain location (can use body map)
- ❏ Pain duration (hours, days, weeks, months, years)
- ❏ Time course (persistent, intermittent, fluctuating)
- ❏ Alleviating factors (specific medications, positioning, heat, cold, etc.)
- ❏ Aggravating factors (walking, sitting, lying on back, etc.)
- ❏ Pain affect (depression, anxiety, etc.)
- ❏ Effects on activities of daily life (e.g., unable to bathe)
- ❏ Effects on quality of life
- ❏ Effects on functional capacity (e.g., unable to perform certain tasks)
- ❏ Presence of common barriers
- ❏ Patient's goal

Table 16.4 COMPONENTS OF A PAIN
MEDICATION HISTORY

- *All* current medication use
- *All* medications used in the past 6 months
- *All* current analgesic use
- *All* pertinent past analgesic use
- *All* drug-related problems related to current regimen
- Social substance use (current and historical)
  ○ Caffeine, alcohol, tobacco, recreational drugs
- Nutritional dietary supplements

salient for patients with multiple chronic conditions and pharmacotherapies, which is often the case for patients with chronic pain. Drug–disease
and drug–drug interactions are common in this patient population. Another confounder is that many patients may seek health care from multiple
sources, including multiple prescribers and pharmacies. In recent years
this issue has been further compounded by the increased use of over-the-
counter medications and complementary medicinal agents. A thorough
medication history will allow the pharmacist to identify both actual and
potential drug-related problems. When interviewing the patient, a number of facets related to the patient's pharmacotherapy must be evaluated.
For each drug assessed, the length of therapy, dose, duration, indication,
and reason for discontinuation should be documented. Any pertinent information related to the effects of pain pharmacotherapy, both analgesic
and adverse, should be noted as well. The components of pain medication
history are presented in Table 16.4.

Pharmacist Role

Pharmacists play a significant role in the management of pain across the
entire health care continuum. This is in large part because pharmacotherapy is such a central component to most analgesic regimens. In addition, within the community practice setting pharmacists are recognized as
easily accessible and trusted advisors for pain issues. In the institutional
setting pharmacists are often members of clinical services that deal with
various pain management issues and may be responsible for implementing analgesic pharmacotherapy in accordance with institutional guidelines. In a number of hospitals, pharmacists are primarily responsible for
managing patient-controlled analgesia (PCA) programs. Pharmacists play

various other roles including development of guidelines, formulary management, and educating patients as well as other health care providers.[12]

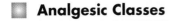 Analgesic Classes

Acetaminophen

Acetaminophen is an effective step 1 analgesic that is often useful as a coanalgesic but does not have any significant anti-inflammatory effect. Caution is needed to not exceed 4 g/24 hours as this may lead to hepatotoxicity. This appears to be more problematic for patients with prior hepatic disease, poor nutritional status, or with heavy alcohol use. Acetaminophen does maintain an analgesic ceiling, such that doses >4 g/24 hours do not provide additional analgesia.

Nonsteroidal Anti-inflammatory Drugs

Nonsteroidal anti-inflammatory drugs (NSAIDs, including aspirin) are effective step 1 analgesics and like acetaminophen are often useful as coanalgesics. They differ from acetaminophen in that they do maintain anti-inflammatory properties. Several classes of NSAIDs exist (Table 16.5), and some patients may respond better to one class than another. There is no a priori test to determine which NSAID a patient may benefit from, and as such, serial trials may be necessary to determine efficacy with this drug class. NSAIDs can have significant adverse effects, especially from a gastrointestinal standpoint. All NSAIDs maintain an analgesic ceiling, so exceeding the maximum listed doses only promotes adverse effects.

Opioids

Opioids are effective analgesics for steps 2 and 3 type pain (Table 16.6). Indeed, opioids are useful for most nociceptive pain and can be useful for some patients with neuropathic pain.[13] Opioid analgesics have traditionally been classified into three pharmacologic classes: the full agonists, partial agonists, and mixed agonist-antagonists. A more detailed description of opioid pharmacotherapy follows later in this chapter.

Adjuvant Analgesics

Adjuvant analgesics constitute a diverse group of medications that are effective for pain at all three steps that is neuropathic in origin. These substances are considered to provide analgesia in addition to or that improves pain treated with acetaminophen, NSAIDs, or opioids. Common adjuvant

Table 16.5 ORAL NONSTEROID ANTI-INFLAMMATORY DRUGS (NSAIDs)

Drug	Average Analgesic Dose (mg)	Dose Interval (h)	Maximal Daily Dose (mg)	Comments
Aspirin	500–1,000	4–6	4,000	Due to risk of Reye syndrome should not be used in children <12 y of age with possible viral illness
Diflunisal	1,000 initial, 500 subsequent	8–12	1,500	Dose in elderly 500–1,000 mg/day does not yield salicylate
Choline magnesium trisalicylate	1,000–1,500	12	2,000–3,000	Unlike aspirin and NSAIDs, does not increase bleeding time
Ibuprofen	200–800	4–8	2,400	Available OTC
Naproxen	250–500	6–8	1,500	—
Naproxen sodium	275–550	6–8	1,650	Available OTC
Fenoprofen	200	4–6	3,200	—
Ketoprofen	25–50	6–8	300	Available OTC
Oxaprozin	600	12–24	1,200	—
Indomethacin	25	8–12	200	Rectal, IV, and sustained-release forms available for adults.

(continued)

531

Table 16.5 ORAL NONSTEROID ANTI-INFLAMMATORY DRUGS (NSAIDs) *(continued)*

Drug	Average Analgesic Dose (mg)	Dose Interval (h)	Maximal Daily Dose (mg)	Comments
Sulindac	150	12	400	—
Etodolac	300–400	8–12	1,000	—
Ketorolac	10	6	40	Also available in parenteral dosage form. Limit treatment to 5 days. Caution: may precipitate renal failure in dehydrated patients.
Tolmetin	200–600	8	1,800	—
Mefenamic acid	500 initial, 250 subsequent	6	1,500	—
Diclofenac potassium	25–75	8–12	150	—
Meloxicam	7.5–15	24	15	—
Piroxicam	20–40	24	40	—
Nabumetone	500–750	8–12	2,000	—
Celecoxib	100–200	12–24	400	—

OTC, over the counter; IV, intravenous.

Table 16.6 COMMON OPIOID ANALGESICS

Generic Name	Common Available Dosage Forms and Strengths	Comments
	Full Agonists	
Codeine	*Injectable:* 50 μg/mL *Tablets:* 15, 30, and 60 mg	Available as combination product with either APAP (Tylenol with Codeine #1–4 or ASA
Fentanyl	*Injectable:* 50 μg/mL *Transdermal patch (Duragesic):* 25, 50, 75, 100 μg/h *Buccal effervescent (Fentora):* 100, 200, 400 μg *Transmucosal (Fentanyl Oralet):* 100, 200, 300, 400 μg *Transmucosal (Actiq):* 200, 400, 600, 800, 1,200, 1,600 μg	
Hydrocodone	*Tablets with APAP:* 2.5 mg + 500 mg APAP (Lortab) 5 mg + 325 mg APAP (Norco) 5 mg + 500 mg APAP (Lortab, Vicodin, Lorcet HD) 7.5 mg + 325 mg APAP (Norco) 7.5 mg +500 mg APAP (Lortab) 7.5 mg + 650 mg APAP (Lorcet Plus) 7.5 mg + 750 mg APAP (Vicodin ES) 10 mg + 325 mg APAP (Norco) 10 mg + 500 mg (Lortab) 10 mg + 650 mg APAP (Lorcet) 10 mg + 660 mg APAP (Vicodin HP) *Oral elixir with APAP:* 7.5 mg + 500 mg APAP per 15 mL (Lortab) *Tablets with ibuprofen:* 7.5 mg + 200 mg (Vicoprofen)	Available only as combination product in United States
Hydromorphone	*Injectable:* 1, 2, 3, 4, 10 mg/mL *Tablets:* 1, 2, 3, 4, 8 mg *Oral liquid:* 5 mg/5 mL *Suppositories:* 3 mg	
Levorphanol	*Injectable:* 2 mg/mL *Tablets:* 2 mg	—

(continued)

Table 16.6 COMMON OPIOID ANALGESICS (continued)

Generic Name	Common Available Dosage Forms and Strengths	Comments
Methadone	*Injectable:* 10 mg/mL *Tablets:* 5, 10 mg *Dispersable tablets:* 40 mg *Oral liquid:* 5 mg/5 mL, 10 mg/5 mL, 10 mg/10 mL *Oral concentrate:* 10 mg/mL	—
Morphine	*Injectable:* 0.5, 1, 2, 3, 4, 5, 8, 10, 15, 25, 50 mg/mL *Immediate release tablets:* 15, 30 mg *Soluble tablets:* 10, 15, 30 mg *Controlled release tablets (MS Contin):* 15, 30, 60, 100, 200 mg *Controlled release tablets (Kadian):* 15, 30, 60, 100, 200 mg *Controlled release tablets (Avinza):* 15, 30, 60, 100, 200 mg *Oral liquid:* 10 mg/5mL, 10 mg/2.5mL, 20 mg/5mL, 20 mg/mL, 100 mg/5mL *Suppositories:* 5, 10, 20, and 30 mg	Avinza dosing interval every 24 h; Kadian dosing intervals every 12–24 h; MS Contin dosing intervals every 8–12 h
Oxycodone	*Immediate release tablets:* 5 mg *Controlled release tablets (OxyContin):* 10, 20, 40 mg *Oral liquid:* 5 mg/5 mL *Oral concentrate :* 20 mg/mL	Available as combination product with either APAP or ASA.
Oxymorphone	*Injectable:* 1, 1.5 mg/mL *Suppository:* 5 mg *Immediate release tablets (Opana):* 5 mg, 10 mg *Controlled-release tablets (Opana ER):* 5, 10, 20, 40 mg	—

Table 16.6 COMMON OPIOID ANALGESICS
(continued)

Generic Name	Common Available Dosage Forms and Strengths	Comments
Partial Agonists		
Buprenorphine	_Injectable:_ 0.3 mg/mL	Has been used sublingually; tablets available for opioid detoxification
Mixed Agonist-Antagonists		
Butorphanol	_Injectable:_ 1, 2 mg/mL _Nasal Spray:_ 10 mg/mL	—
Nalbuphine	_Injectable:_ 10, 20 mg/mL	—
Pentazocine	_Injectable:_ 30 mg/mL _Tablet:_ 50 mg (with 0.5 mg naloxone)	Also in combination with ASA or APAP

APAP, acetaminophen; ASA, acetylsalicylic acid (aspirin).

medications include tricyclic antidepressants (e.g., amitriptyline, desipramine) and anticonvulsants (e.g., gabapentin). Other medications may include bisphosphonates (e.g., alendronate, pamidronate), calcitonin, radiopharmaceuticals, steroids, psychostimulants (e.g., methylphenidate).

Pain Pharmacotherapy

Selection of the appropriate pharmacotherapy is predicated on two primary issues, pain intensity and presentation. Using the numeric rating scale, a clinician can choose the appropriate set of medication classes to evaluate. Then depending on the pain presentation (e.g., nociceptive, neuropathic, or both) the regimen can be tailored to the patients' needs. It is important to remember that this approach is fluid, and as such, it is often necessary to make adjustments throughout the course of an individual patient's care. Additionally, patient care is not a static process. As such it may be appropriate to titrate patients as indicated. As previously discussed,

Table 16.7	THE WORLD HEALTH ORGANIZATION (WHO) ANALGESIC LADDER

Step 1. Mild pain: pain intensity 1–3 on the numeric rating scale.
   Acetaminophen, nonsteroidal anti-inflammatory drugs (NSAIDs)
   +/− adjuvant analgesics

Step 2. Moderate pain: pain intensity of 4–6 on the numeric rating scale
   Simple analgesics (acetaminophen, NSAIDs)
   plus weaker opioids (codeine, hydrocodone, oxycodone)
   +/− adjuvant analgesics

Step 3. Severe pain: pain intensity of 7–10 on the numeric rating scale
   Simple analgesics (acetaminophen, NSAIDs)
   plus stronger opioids (morphine, oxycodone, hydromorphone,
      fentanyl, methadone, levorphanol)
   +/− adjuvants

patient assessment and reassessment is a priority in providing good analgesic care.

In 1986, the World Health Organization (WHO) developed a simple three-step approach to the management of cancer pain (Table 16.7).[14] This approach is often referred to as the WHO analgesic ladder. This simple and well-tested approach to the rational selection, administration, and titration of analgesics is commonly used in pain management. Although designed initially for cancer pain, the general tenets of this approach can be useful when considering drug therapy for patients with other pain presentations.

Opioid Pharmacotherapy

As noted above, opioid analgesics are classified into three classes that arise from our understanding of how these substances occupy and activate primarily the mu and kappa regions of the opioid receptor complex.[15] Full agonists fully occupy and activate the mu and kappa regions of the opioid receptor complex and as such have the potential for an unlimited dose/analgesic response. Partial agonists function by occupying only part of the mu region of an opioid receptor and produce a lesser degree of analgesia than a full agonist. Mixed agonist-antagonist opioids activate kappa receptors and either block or antagonize the mu receptor region, yielding a lesser degree of analgesia than full agonists. In the case of partial agonists and mixed agonist-antagonists, a dose ceiling effect occurs. These two classes are known clinically to have a maximal analgesic effect at their FDA-labeled maximum doses. Unfortunately the adverse effect profile for these two classes continues to worsen when patients use doses in excess of the listed maximum dose. Clinicians should avoid using mixed agonist-antagonists or partial agonists in combination with full agonist opioids, as this combination can lead to an opioid withdrawal and worsening of the patient's pain situation.

Opioid pharmacotherapy is often complicated by various issues related to misunderstanding the actual pharmacologic basis for their use. Understanding the following terms will enable clinicians to better provide analgesic care to their patients:

- Opiophobia—the irrational fear by clinicians and/or patients related to appropriate opioid use for analgesic purposes. This phenomenon appears to be due in part to misunderstanding such terms as addiction, dependence, and tolerance.[16]
- Narcotic—a term many clinicians still inappropriately use when they refer to opioid analgesics. This archaic term was used to describe opium and its derivatives in prior generations. Today the word *narcotic* is a legal term that includes a wide range of sedating and potentially abused substances and is no longer limited to opioid analgesics.[17]
- Addiction—the use of a substance that causes the user harm, yet the user continues to use the substance. Iatrogenic addiction as a consequence of opioid exposure for analgesic purposes is extremely rare.[18,19]
- Dependence—a pharmacologic situation where removal of a substance from a patient will induce a withdrawal reaction. This phenomenon is common with many medications and is to be expected for all patients with repeated exposure to opioid analgesics.[19]
- Tolerance—a state of adaptation in which exposure to a drug induces changes in the central nervous system (CNS) that result in diminution of one or more of the drug's effects over time. Tolerance is a variable experience for patients using opioids and is more pronounced during acute and subacute administration.[19]
- Pseudoaddiction—a behavior defined in terms of patients who have appropriate drug-seeking behavior for the purpose of pain relief, not for abuse or substance misuse.[20] This type of presentation occurs when a patient requests more opioid for analgesic purposes but has behaviors (e.g., anger, hostility) that are attributed incorrectly to addiction. Appropriate attention to analgesia will unmask this situation.
- Pseudotolerance—a situation where opioid dose escalation occurs and appears consistent with pharmacologic tolerance.[21] However,

following careful assessment, this is better attributed to other variables such as progressive disease, the presence of new pathology, or increased or excessive physical activity. Other issues that can manifest as pseudo-tolerance are nonadherence, drug interactions, or when patients divert medications.

Oral Opioid Pharmacotherapy

Persistent ongoing pain is often best approached by using oral long-acting opioids to provide for a patient's pain requirements throughout the day.[22] This approach is consistent with the WHO guidelines, facilitates compliance, and minimizes the potential for toxicity. Long-acting opioids can be separated into those that are pharmaceutically enhanced to deliver shorter half-life agents over a longer time period (e.g., MS Contin, OxyContin), or the agents with inherently long-acting pharmacokinetic profiles (e.g., methadone). In general, the pharmaceutically modified agents are much easier to dose and titrate. These agents typically can be managed in most primary care settings with little special training. Methadone pharmacokinetics are more complicated, especially in patients with renal clearance concerns. As a consequence, dosing becomes more problematic for those not accustomed to monitoring this therapy. The reader is referred to other sources for a more detailed discussion.[23,24]

Opioid PCA Pharmacotherapy

Opioids are also commonly used in the setting of various pain presentations using an approach called patient-controlled analgesia (PCA).[25] In general terms, this approach uses intravenous or epidural (PCEA) opioids in a manner that allows the patient to help titrate the dose they need to manage their pain. PCAs have become commonplace in most hospitals, and pharmacy services are often responsible for many of the components of delivering this type of analgesia. Depending on the patient's presentation, the variables associated with PCA delivery can include a patient-directed dose at clinician preselected time points. Typically this involves prescribing a set mg dose, a dosing interval, and maximum or lockout amount per larger time frame. At times this as-needed component can be augmented by a basal or continuous infusion where warranted. For many patients during the initial phase of acute pain management, it is probably wise to avoid initiating a basal infusion. Table 16.8 lists examples of data found on a typical PCA order sheet.

Table 16.8 OPIOID PCA SETTING INFORMATION

Drug	Typical Drug Concentration for PCA	Typical Starting Demand Dose (Range)	Typical Lockout Demand Dose Interval (Range)
Fentanyl	50 μg/mL	10 μg (10–50 μg)	6 minutes (5–8 minutes)
Hydromor-phone	0.2 mg/mL	0.2 mg (0.05–0.4 mg)	8 minutes (5–10 minutes)
Morphine	1 mg/mL	1 mg (0.5–2.5 mg)	8 minutes (5–10 minutes)

PCA, patient-controlled analgesia.
Adapted with permission from Ashburn MA, Lipman AG, Carr D, et al. *Principles of Analgesic Use in the Treatment of Acute Pain and Cancer Pain.* Glenview, IL: American Pain Society; 2003.

Opioid Pharmacotherapy Pearls

- Patients already receiving opioid pharmacotherapy for persistent pain: If the patient uses short-acting opioids on a regular basis and it is appropriate to continue with opioid pharmacotherapy, calculate the average 24-hour opioid dose and then consider using a long-acting opioid alternative to provide around-the-clock analgesia where appropriate. When using long-acting opioid, continue using breakthrough short-acting doses when indicated.

- Opioid-naïve patients with episodic or fluctuating pain: Consider using an opioid analgesic based on the WHO analgesic ladder and level of pain. Reassess routinely to determine if pain is appropriately treated, and when indicated, determine if chronic/persistent pain will be better managed with long-acting formulations. If pain remains uncontrolled after 24 hours, increase the routine dose by 25% to 50% for reports of mild to moderate pain, by 50% to 100% for severe to uncontrolled pain, or by an amount at least equal to the total dose of as-needed (PRN) medication used during the previous 24 hours. If pain is severe and uncontrolled after 1 or 2 doses (e.g., crescendo pain), increase the dose by 50% to 100%.

- Breakthrough or PRN analgesia: In most situations, patients using long-acting opioids should also be offered rescue analgesia for breakthrough pain in the event of worsening pain, episodic pain, or pain that is inadequately controlled by the long-acting opioid regimen. A simple approach is to provide doses that are 5% to 15% of the total 24-hour long-acting opioid dose in use.[27] Normally these doses are offered to the patient on a PRN basis every 3 or 4 hours. *Always* recalculate the breakthrough opioid dose after changing the long-acting regimen so that it is always 5% to 15% of this total daily dose.

- Opioid dose escalation: Patients requiring more than two to four daily breakthrough doses on a routine basis may need to have their long-acting opioid regimen increased.[18,27] A simple approach is to determine the total amount of opioid used in an average 24-hour period (routine plus breakthrough) and administer this new total in divided doses as indicated by the product used.

- Equianalgesic conversion: At times it is necessary to stop one opioid and initiate an alternative. This can be due to suboptimal relief or the presence of adverse effects. Traditionally clinicians have used published equianalgesic dose charts (Table 16.9) to determine the effective

Table 16.9 ADULT EQUIANALGESIC DOSE COMPARISON

Name	Equianalgesic Dose (mg)	
	Oral	Parenteral
Full Agonists		
Morphine	30	10
Hydromorphone	7.5	1.5
Oxycodone	20	—
Oxymorphone	10	1
Meperidine	300	75
Mixed Agonist-antagonists		
Nalbuphine	—	10
Butorphanol	—	2
Pentazocine	50	30
Partial Agonist		
Buprenorphine	—	.4

Adapted with permission from Ashburn MA, Lipman AG, Carr D, et al. *Principles of Analgesic Use in the Treatment of Acute Pain and Cancer Pain.* Glenview, IL: American Pain Society; 2003.

equianalgesic dose conversion for many commonly prescribed opioids (26,28). Unfortunately, these tables are based on older data that are primarily associated with single-dose studies and do not compensate for incomplete cross-tolerance and individual variation. In recent years it has been suggested that for patients with well-controlled pain, it is advisable to use 50% to 75% of the published equianalgesic dose of the new opioid to compensate for incomplete cross-tolerance and individual variation. If the patient has moderate to severe pain, 25% or less dose reduction is advised. An important exception to this paradigm is methadone, which appears to have higher-than-expected potency during chronic dosing compared with published equianalgesic doses for acute dosing. The reader is referred to other resources for methadone dosing.

- Opioids to avoid: Meperidine is an opioid analgesic that has proven extremely problematic over the years. The principal metabolite is normeperidine, which produces significant adverse effects such as tremulousness, dysphoria, myoclonus, and seizures. Many hospitals and health systems either severely restrict its use or have banned it from their formulary. Propoxyphene is another agent with a checkered past but does not maintain the same stigma as meperidine. Propoxyphene provides minimal analgesia, and chronic use can lead to accumulation of a toxic metabolite. The analgesic efficacy of propoxyphene has been called into question in recent years. There appears to be no significant value in promoting the use of this suboptimal agent.

Common Opioid Adverse Reactions

- Constipation due to opioids is almost universal, and tolerance very rarely, if ever, develops. Management should be proactive, using stimulant laxatives (e.g., senna, bisacodyl, glycerin, casanthranol, etc.) that are titrated to effect. Stool softeners (e.g., docusate sodium) are not usually effective by themselves but can prove useful in addition to the stimulant laxative for patients with dry hard stools. Bulk-forming agents (e.g., psyllium) should be avoided in the vast majority of patients since they require substantial fluid intake and are poorly tolerated in patients with advanced disease and poor gastrointestinal mobility. For patients unable or unwilling to use a stimulant laxative, the addition of an osmotic agent (e.g., milk of magnesia, lactulose, or sorbitol) may be useful.

- Nausea and vomiting due to opioids usually disappears as tolerance develops during the first few days of therapy. Effective pharmacotherapies used to treat this problem include prochlorperazine, haloperidol, and metoclopramide. Patients not responding to these agents may require changes in the opioid used, the route the opioid is administered, or both.

- Sedation and/or mental clouding is often an issue during opioid initiation or during dose escalation. Sedation may be the result of prior inadequate sleep due to poor pain control. If the sedation is due to the opioid and continues to be problematic, a different opioid and/or alternate route may improve the problem. However this may not be in the best interest of the patient if he or she has achieved good analgesia. In this setting, the use of a psychostimulant (e.g., methylphenidate) may be a consideration.

- Agitation, confusion, excessive sedation, hallucinations, myoclonus, nightmares, or seizures may imply that too much opioid is on board or that the patient is unable to effectively eliminate toxic metabolites. Opioid use is often complicated by buildup of metabolites in patients who are dehydrated or have poor renal function. If metabolite buildup is suspected, it is advisable to consider switching the patient to another opioid. If buildup of an opioid metabolite is not suspected (e.g., excessive dosing) re-evaluation and titration of the opioid should take precedence.

References

1. Merskey H, Bogduk N. *Classification of Chronic Pain*. 2nd ed. Seattle, WA: IASP Press; 1994.
2. National Institutes of Health Consensus Development Conference. The integrated approach to the management of pain. *J Pain Symptom Manage*. 1987;2:35–44.
3. Portenoy R, Hagen N. Breakthrough pain: definition, prevalence and characteristics. *Pain*. 1990;41:273–281.
4. Cleary J. Pharmacokinetic and pharmacodynamic issues in the treatment of breakthrough pain. *Semin Oncol*. 1997;214:13–19.
5. Siddall PJ, Cousins MJ. Persistent pain as a disease entity: implications for clinical management. *Anesth Analg*. 2004;99(2):510–520.
6. Gloth FM 3rd. Principles of perioperative pain management in older adults. *Clin Geriatr Med*. 2001;17(3):553–573.
7. Gilson AM, Joranson DE. U.S. policies relevant to the prescribing of opioid analgesics for the treatment of pain in patients with addictive disease. *Clin J Pain*. 2002; 18(4 Suppl):S91–98.
8. Acute Pain Management Guideline Panel. Acute Pain Management: *Operative or Medical Procedures and Trauma. Clinical Practice Guideline*. AHCPR Pub. No. 92-0032. Rockville, MD: Agency for Health Care Policy and Research, Public Health Service, U.S. Department of Health and Human Services. 1992 (Feb).

9. Jacox A, Carr DB, Payne R, et al. *Management of Cancer Pain. Clinical Practice Guideline Number 9.* AHCPR Publication No. 94-0592. Rockville, MD: Agency for Health Care Policy and Research, US Department of Health and Human Services, Public Health Service. 1994 (Mar).

10. Wong DL, Baker CM. Smiling faces as anchor for pain intensity scales. *Pain.* 2001;89(2–3):295–300.

11. Hadjistavropoulos T, Herr K, Turk DC, et al. An interdisciplinary expert consensus statement on assessment of pain in older persons. *Clin J Pain.* 2007;23(1 Suppl): S1–43.

12. Strassels SA, McNicol E, Suleman R. Postoperative pain management: a practical review, Part 1. *Am J Health Syst Pharm.* 2005; 62(18):1904–1916.

13. Eisenberg E, McNicol E, Carr DB. Opioids for neuropathic pain. *Cochrane Database Syst Rev.* 2006;19;3:CD006146.

14. World Health Organization (WHO). Cancer pain relief and palliative care: report of a WHO expert committee. Geneva, Switzerland: WHO; 1990.

15. Hare B. The opioid analgesics: rational selection of agents for acute and chronic pain. *Hosp Formul.* 1987;22:64–86.

16. Rhodin A. The rise of opiophobia: is history a barrier to prescribing? *J Pain Palliat Care Pharmacother.* 2006;20(3):31–32.

17. Jackson KC, Lipman AG. Opioid analgesics. In: Tollison CD, Satterwhite JR, Tollison JW, eds. *Practical Pain Management*, 3rd ed. Philadelphia, PA: Lippincott Williams & Wilkins; 2002.

18. The American Society of Addiction Medicine. Public Policy Statement on Definitions Related to the Use of Opioids in Pain Treatment. www.asam.org, 1997 (April).

19. Rinaldi R, Steindler E, Wilford B, et al. Clarification and standardization of substance abuse terminology. *JAMA.* 1988;259:555–557.

20. Weissman DE, Haddox JD. Opioid pseudoaddiction—an iatrogenic syndrome. *Pain.* 1989;36:363–366.

21. Pappagallo M. The concept of pseudotolerance to opioids. *J Pharm Care Pain Symptom Control.* 1998;6:95–98.

22. Pillai Riddell RR, Craig KD. Time-contingent schedules for postoperative analgesia: a review of the literature. *J Pain.* 2003;4(4):169–175.

23. www.cancer.gov/cancertopics/pdq/supportivecare/pain/HealthProfessional/page4.

24. Lugo RA, Satterfield KL, Kern SE. Pharmacokinetics of methadone. *J Pain Palliat Care Pharmacother.* 2005;19(4):13–24.

25. Beeton A, Upton P, Shipton E. The case for patient-controlled analgesia. Inter-patient variation in postoperative analgesic requirements. *S Afr J Surg.* 1992;30:1–6.

26. Ashburn MA, Lipman AG, Carr D, et al. *Principles of Analgesic Use in the Treatment of Acute Pain and Cancer Pain.* Glenview, IL: American Pain Society; 2003.

27. Indelicato RA, Portenoy RK. Opioid rotation in the management of refractory cancer pain. *J Clin Oncol.* 2003;21(9 Suppl):87s–91s.

28. Prommer E. Oxymorphone: a review. *Support Care Cancer.* 2006;14:109–115.

17 Over-the-Counter Drug Therapy and Dietary Supplements/ Complementary Care

Patricia M. Mossbrucker and Ty Vo

◼ Over-the-Counter Drug Therapy

The prevalence of over-the-counter (OTC) drug use has increased significantly over the past 25 years. In 2000, its sales including dietary supplements exceeded > $30 billion.[1] As a growing number of drugs are switched from prescription to OTC status, the OTC drug market has become complex. It has been estimated that 57% of all health problems can be treated with OTC products.[1] The growing demand for OTC drug therapy may be attributed to patients becoming empowered to take ownership of their own health care and feeling more confident in self-treating their illnesses. This demonstrates a need and an opportunity for pharmacist intervention.[1,2] The pharmacist is viewed by patients as the most accessible health care provider and a good source of drug information. This provides the pharmacist with an excellent opportunity to provide patient education and assist with product selection to ensure safe, appropriate, and effective use.

Role of the Pharmacist

- Be familiar with currently available products and product labels.
- Gather patient-specific information to make an assessment.
- Determine if self-treatment is appropriate.
  - ‣ Refer to primary care clinician as appropriate.
- Develop an individualize action plan.
  - ‣ Select the OTC product(s).
  - ‣ Set therapeutic goals.
  - ‣ Set therapeutic end points.

- Provide patient education.
- Provide patient follow-up.
- Document encounter.

In the process of gathering information, the pharmacist can pose the following open-ended questions or queries:[3]

- Describe your problem.
- Describe to me how your problem has changed over time.
- How does the problem limit your daily activities?
- How has this problem affected you in the past?
- Tell me about any food, drugs, and/or physical activities that make the problem worse.
- What have you done to relieve this problem in the past?
- What have you been doing so far to treat the problem?

The pharmacist should selectively elicit the following information:[3]

- Who is the patient? Is the patient the person in the pharmacy or someone else?
- How old is the patient?
- Is the patient male or female? If the patient is female, is she pregnant or breast-feeding?
- Does the patient have any other medical problems that may alter the expected effects of a nonprescription drug or be aggravated by the drug's effects? Is the complaint related to a chronic illness?
- Does the patient have any allergies?
- Is the patient on a special diet? Does the patient have special nutritional requirements?
- Is the patient using any prescription, nonprescription, or social drugs? How long has the patient been taking the drugs?
- Has the patient experienced adverse drug reactions in the past?
- Who is responsible for administering medication?

Refer patient to the primary care clinician when:[3]

- Symptoms are too severe to be endured by the patient without definitive diagnosis and treatment.
- Symptoms are minor but persistent and do not appear to be the result of some easily identifiable cause.
- Symptoms have repeatedly returned with no readily recognizable cause.
- The pharmacist is in doubt about the patient's medical condition.

Special Populations

Pediatric[4]

- It is important to note the recommendation by Food and Drug Administration against self-medication in infants and children under the age of 2 years.
- OTC cough and cold products have not been shown to be more effective than placebo by systematic reviews of controlled trials in this age group.
- Parents should be educated regarding the lack of antitussive effects, risk for adverse events, and potential for overdose in children from OTC cough and cold medications.
- Consult the *Harriet Lane Handbook* for guidance on specific dosing.

Pregnancy and Lactation

- Be familiar with the risk factors assigned to all drugs based on the level of risk to the fetus.[5]
  - A: Adequate and well-controlled studies in pregnant women have not shown an increased risk to the fetus in any trimester of the pregnancy.
  - B: Animal studies have shown no evidence of harm to the fetus, but there are no adequate and well-controlled studies in pregnant women; or animal studies have shown an adverse effect, but adequate and well-controlled studies in pregnant women have failed to demonstrate a risk to the fetus in any trimester.
  - C: Animal studies have shown an adverse effect, and there are no adequate and well-controlled studies in pregnant women; or no animal studies have been conducted and there are no adequate and well-controlled studies in pregnant women.
  - D: Evidence of harm to the fetus has been shown in studies, but the benefits of therapy may outweigh the risk. For example, if the drug is needed in a life-threatening situation or for a serious disease for which safer drugs cannot be used or are ineffective.
  - X: Evidence of harm to the fetus has been shown in studies. The use of the drug outweighs any possible benefit. The drug is contraindicated in women who are or may become pregnant.
- Consult *Drugs in Pregnancy and Lactation* by Briggs for guidance.

Geriatric[6]

- Age 65 years or older.
- May predispose patients to potential problems with nonprescription drugs due to.
  - Altered pharmacokinetic and pharmacodynamic profile.

- Pre-existing medical conditions.
- Duplicate therapy or polypharmacy.
- Increased sensitivity to anticholinergic drugs.

Common Conditions Treated with OTC Drugs[7]

- Cough and cold.
- Headache.
- Muscle aches/pain.
- Heartburn.
- Constipation.
- Fever.
- Allergic rhinitis.
- Insomnia.
- Premenstrual and menstrual symptoms.
- Smoking cessation.
- Minor wounds.
- Dermatologic conditions.

Recommended Pediatric Dosages of Nonprescription Drugs[8,9]

Pediatric Age Groups[10]

- Neonates: 1 day to 1 month.
- Infants: 1 month to 1 year.
- Children: 1 year to 11 years.
- Adolescents: 12 years to 16 years.

Analgesics

- Acetaminophen.
  - Infants and children.
- Use caution with different dosage forms: infant drops versus children's suspension.
  - Orally: 10–15 mg/kg every 4 to 6 hours as needed (PRN). Maximum 75 mg/kg per 24 hours.
  - Rectally: 10–20 mg/kg every 4 to 6 hours PRN. Maximum 75 mg/kg per 24 hours.
- Ibuprofen.
  - Infants and children.
- Use caution with different dosage forms: infant drops versus children's suspension.
  - 5–10 mg/kg every 6 to 8 hours PRN. Maximum 1,200 mg per 24 hours.

Antihistamines

- Brompheniramine.
  - Not recommended in infants and children younger than 2 years of age.
  - Ages 2 to 6 years: 1 mg every 6 to 8 hours PRN. Maximum 6 mg per 24 hours.
  - Ages 6 to 12 years: 2–4 mg every 6 to 8 hours PRN. Maximum 12 mg per 24 hours.
- Chlorpheniramine.
  - Not recommended in infants and children younger than 2 years of age.
  - Ages 2 to 6 years: 1 mg every 4 to 6 hours PRN. Maximum 6 mg per 24 hours.
  - Ages 6 to 12 years: 2 mg every 4 to 6 hours PRN. Maximum 12 mg per 24 hours.
- Diphenhydramine.
  - Not recommended in infants and children younger than 2 years of age.
  - Ages 2 to 6 years: 6.25 mg every 4 to 6 hours PRN. Maximum 37.5 mg per 24 hours.
  - Ages 6 to 12 years: 12.5–25mg every 4 to 6 hours PRN. Maximum 150 mg per 24 hours.
- Cetirizine.
  - Ages 2 to 5 years: 2.5 mg once or twice a day. Maximum 5 mg per 24 hours.
  - Ages 6 years or older: 5–10 mg once a day or divided into two doses.
- Loratadine.
  - Ages 2 to 5 years: 5 mg once a day. Maximum 5 mg per 24 hours.
  - Ages 6 years or older: 5–10 mg once a day. Maximum 10 mg per 24 hours.

Decongestants

- Phenylephrine.
  - Not recommended in infants and children younger than 2 years of age.
  - Ages 2 to 5 years: 2.5 mg every 4 hours PRN. Maximum 15 mg per 24 hours.
  - Ages 6 to 12 years: 5 mg every 4 hours PRN. Maximum 30 mg per 24 hours.
- Pseudoephedrine.
  - Note legal requirements for the sale and purchase for individual state.
  - Not recommended in infants and children younger than 2 years of age.

- Ages 2 to 5 years: 15 mg every 4 to 6 hours PRN. Maximum 60 mg per 24 hours.
- Ages 6 to 12 years: 30 mg every 4 to 6 hours PRN. Maximum 120 mg per 24 hours.

Expectorants
- Guaifenesin.
  - Consult a physician.
  - Ages 2 to 5 years: 50–100 mg every 4 hours PRN. Maximum 600 mg per 24 hours.
  - Ages 6 to 11 years: 100–200 mg every 4 hours PRN. Maximum 1,200 mg per 24 hours.

Cough Suppressants
- Dextromethorphan.
  - Not recommended in infants or children younger than 2 years of age.
  - Ages 2 to 6 years: 2.5–7.5 mg every 4 to 8 hours PRN or 15 mg every 12 hours PRN (sustained release suspension).
  - Ages 6 to 12 years: 5–10 mg every 4 hours PRN or 30 mg every 12 hours PRN (sustained release suspension).
  - Note: The American Academy of Pediatrics recommends against its use in children due to lack of proven benefit.[11]

Recommend Adult Dosages of Nonprescription Drugs[12]
Analgesics
- Acetaminophen.
  - 325–1,000 mg every 4 to 6 hours PRN. Maximum 4,000 mg per day.
- Ibuprofen.
  - 200–400 mg every 4 to 6 hours PRN. Maximum 1,200 mg per day.
- Naproxen sodium.
  - 220 mg every 8 to 12 hours PRN. Maximum 660 mg per day.
- Ketoprofen.
  - 12.5–25 mg every 4 to 6 hours PRN. Maximum 75 mg per day.

Antihistamines
- Chlorpheniramine: 4 mg every 4 to 6 hours PRN. Maximum 24 mg per 24 hours or 12 mg every 12 hours PRN (sustained release tablet).
- Diphenhydramine: 25–50 mg every 4 to 6 hours PRN. Maximum 300 mg per 24 hours.

- Loratadine: 10 mg once a day. Maximum 10 mg per 24 hours.
- Cetirizine: 5–10 mg once a day. Maximum 10 mg per 24 hours.

Cough Suppressants
- Dextromethorphan: 10–20 mg every 4 hours PRN or 30–60 mg every 12 hours (sustained release suspension).

Decongestants
- Phenylephrine: 10–20 mg every 4 hours PRN.
- Pseudoephedrine: 30–60 mg every 4 to 6 hours PRN. Maximum 240 mg per 24 hours.

Expectorants
- Guaifenesin: 200–400 mg every 4 hours. Maximum 2,400 mg per 24 hours.

Useful Resources

1. Berardi RR, Kroon LA, McDermott JH, et al., eds. *Handbook of Nonprescription Drugs: An Interactive Approach to Self-Care*. 5th ed. Washington, DC: American Pharmacists Association; 2006.
2. Gunn VL, Nechyba C, eds. *The Harriet Lane Handbook*. 17th ed. Philadelphia, PA: Mosby; 2005.
3. Briggs GG, Freeman RK, Yaffe SJ. *Drugs in Pregnancy and Lactation*. 7th ed. Philadelphia, PA: Lippincott Williams & Wilkins;, 2005.
4. Consumer Education: Over-the-Counter Medicine. U.S. Food and Drug Administration page. Available at www.fda.gov/cder/consumerinfo/otc_text.htm.

▪ Dietary Supplements/ Complementary Care

It is estimated that 38 million adults in the United States use herbal and other dietary supplement products, but only one third share this information with their health care clinicians.[13] Pharmacists can play a unique role in helping patients make appropriate decisions about supplement use. Reasons for using dietary supplements can vary, including belief that conventional medicine is ineffective, too expensive, or will work better in combination with supplements.[14] Although the focus may be on herbs, dietary supplements also include a wide range of vitamins, minerals, amino acids, enzymes, organ tissues, metabolites, and hormones. This section focuses on the dietary supplements.

Because supplements are derived originally from natural sources, patients may feel that they are safe. It is important for them to understand that there is currently no government regulation of supplements. The manufacturer is responsible for ensuring that a product is safe before it is marketed under the Dietary Supplement Health and Education Act of 1994 (DSHEA). The Food and Drug Administration is responsible for taking actions against any unsafe product after it reaches the market.[15] In 2009, the FDA will phase in a program requiring manufacturers of supplements to certify good manufacturing processes and verify that listed label ingredients match package contents.[16]

Role of the Pharmacist

Patients often seek advice in product selection from pharmacists. Key considerations to inform patients in selection and use of dietary supplements include the following:[17]

- Use products with labels containing symbols of USP (United States Pharmacopoeia), NF (National Formulary), and/or GMP (Good Manufacturing Practice).
- Use products that identify the following:
  - Source (i.e., the botanical name and part of the plant used).
  - Strength of the preparation or dose.
  - Lot number and expiration date.
  - Name, address, and phone number of manufacturer.
- Use supplements containing only one ingredient.
- Use a low, usual dose.
- Limit how long you take the supplement.
- Tell your health care providers you are using this supplement.
- Report side effects related to the supplement to the FDA by calling 1-800-332-1088 or online at www.fda.gov/medwatch.

Medical Condition Considerations

Pharmacists should make note of the individual patient's history before making a recommendation to use dietary supplements. If possible, including the patient's supplement use in his or her medication profile can prevent future adverse outcomes. Before using a dietary supplement, patients should discuss use with their clinicians if they[17]

1. Plan to become pregnant, are pregnant, or are breast-feeding.
2. Plan to use the supplement for a child.

Table 17.1 TOP 10 SUPPLEMENTS USED BY ADULTS IN THE UNITED STATES IN 2002

1. Echinacea
2. Ginseng
3. Gingko
4. Garlic
5. Glucosamine
6. St. John's Wort
7. Peppermint
8. Fish oil/omega-3 fatty acids
9. Ginger
10. Soy

From Consumer Reports. "Dangerous supplements, 12 supplements to avoid." May, 2004, with permission.

3. Have a serious medical condition such as diabetes; heart, kidney, or liver disease; or cancer.
4. Take prescription or over-the-counter medications regularly.
5. Have a history of allergic reaction to a specific dietary supplement.
6. Have surgery or other procedure scheduled. Some dietary supplements may cause bleeding or interfere with anesthesia. Stop taking dietary supplements 2 weeks before any procedure.'

With an estimated 18% of the U.S. population using supplements on a regular basis,[18] it is important for pharmacists to be familiar with commonly used products. Table 17.1 lists the top 10 supplements used by adults in the United States in 2002.[19] Likewise, some supplements present risk to anyone using them and should be avoided.[17,20] Table 17.2 lists these supplements.

Caution is advised against use of multiple products or products containing multiple ingredients. Recommend patients use care or avoid using the following: products with multiple sedating effects (valerian, chamomile, hops, kava); energy or weight loss products with stimulating effects (ginseng, green tea, cola nut, guarana, mate); products that lower blood glucose levels (bitter melon, cinnamon, fenugreek, garlic); or products that may alter liver function (black cohosh, green tea, kava, red yeast).[17,20]

The following list of frequently used supplements includes some considerations for their use.[21–23] It is important to note that this is not a comprehensive listing of all indications, side effects, or interactions, but is

Table 17.2 SELECTED SUPPLEMENTS TO AVOID[18,21]

Aconite
Androstenedione
Aristolochic acid
Bitter orange
Chaparral
Comfrey
Ephedra (Ma Huang)
Germander
Kava
Lobelia
Organ/glandular extracts
Pau d'arco
Pennyroyal oil
Sassafras
Skullcap
Yohimbe

From Tindle HA, Davis RB, Phillips RS, et al. Trends in use of complementary and alternative medicine by US adults: 1997–2002. *Altern Ther Health Med.* 2005;11:42–49; and Natural Medicine Comprehensive Database. Available at *www.naturaldatabase.com*, with permission.

intended as a starting point for pharmacists in answering patients' questions and guiding appropriate use.

Black Cohosh

- Do not confuse with blue cohosh.
- Has estrogenic effects.

Used for:

- Menopausal symptoms (possibly effective).

Common side effects:

- Bradycardia, dizziness, headache, tremors, nausea and vomiting.

Possible drug interactions:

- Cisplatin: may decrease cytoxic effect.
- Hepatotoxic drugs: may increase risk of liver damage.

Possible lab changes:

- May cause changes in liver function tests.

Avoid or use precaution in patients with:

- Pregnancy and lactation, breast and other hormone-sensitive cancers, kidney transplant, liver disease.

Coenzyme Q-10 (Ubiquinone)

Used for:

- Improving immune function in HIV/AIDS (possibly effective).
- Migraine headache prevention (possibly effective).
- Hypertension (possibly effective).
- Statin-induced myopathy (insufficient reliable evidence).

Common side effects:

- Nausea, vomiting, appetite suppression, heartburn, rash.

Possible drug interactions:

- Antihypertensive drugs: may have additive blood pressure lowering.
- Chemotherapy: antioxidant effects may protect tumor cells from chemotherapeutic agents.
- Warfarin: may have vitamin K–like procoagulant effects.

Possible lab changes:

- May increase cholesterol levels.

Avoid or use precaution in patients with:

- Hypotension, hypertension.

Echinacea

- Most efficacious species are E. purpurea, E. angustifolia, E. pallida.

Used for:

- Reduction of common cold symptoms (possibly effective).

Common side effects:

- Nausea, vomiting, diarrhea, abdominal pain.

Possible drug interactions:

- Caffeine: may increase plasma concentrations.
- Immunosuppressants: may reduce efficacy.
- Appears to inhibit CYP1A2.
- Appears to inhibit intestinal and induce hepatic CYP3A4.

Possible lab changes:

- None known.

Avoid or use precaution in patients with:

- Autoimmune diseases including HIV/AIDS, allergies to Asteraceae/Composita family (ragweed, chrysanthemums, marigolds, many others).

Feverfew
Used for:

- Migraine.

Common side effects:

- Nervousness, insomnia, dizziness, nausea, vomiting, heartburn, sun sensitivity.

Possible drug interactions:

- Anticoagulant/antiplatelet drugs: may increase bleeding risk.
- May inhibit CYP1A2, CYP2C9, CYP2C19, and CYP3A4.

Possible lab changes:

- None known.

Avoid or use precaution in patients with:

- Allergies to Asteraceae/Composita family (ragweed, chrysanthemums, marigolds, many others).

Fish Oil (Omega-3-Fatty Acids)

- Take with meals or freeze capsules to minimize gastrointestinal (GI) side effects.
- Recommend use of brands assayed to avoid contaminants including mercury.

Used for:

- Hypertriglyceridemia.
- Cardiovascular disease risk reduction (likely effective).

Common side effects:

- Fishy aftertaste, halitosis, heartburn, loose stool, bruising, bleeding.

Possible drug interactions:

- Anticoagulant/antiplatelet drugs: may increase bleeding risk.
- Antihypertensives: may have additive effect.

Possible lab changes:

- May increase international normalized ratio (INR) and prothrombin time (PT).
- May increase low-density lipoprotein (LDL) cholesterol.

Avoid or use precaution in patients with:

- Seafood allergies, implantable defibrillators.

Garlic

Used for:

- Slow development of atherosclerosis (possibly effective).
- Hypertension (possibly effective).
- Hyperlipidemia (possibly ineffective).

Common side effects:

- Breath and body odor, mouth and GI irritation, increased bruising and bleeding.

Possible drug interactions:

- Anticoagulant/antiplatelet drugs: may increase bleeding risk.
- Contraceptive drugs: may decrease effectiveness.
- Cyclosporine: may decrease effectiveness.
- Isoniazid: may inhibit absorption across intestinal mucosa, decreasing effectiveness.
- Nonnucleoside reverse transcriptase inhibitors and protease inhibitors: may decrease plasma concentrations, decreasing effectiveness.

Possible lab changes:

- May increase INR and PT.

Avoid or use precaution in patients with:

- Bleeding disorders, GI irritation,, upcoming surgery.

Ginger

Used for:

- Morning sickness (possibly effective).
- Postoperative nausea/vomiting (possibly effective).
- Vertigo (possibly effective).

Common side effects:

- Abdominal discomfort, heartburn, diarrhea, irritation of mouth and throat, hypoglycemia.

Possible drug interactions:

- Anticoagulant/antiplatelet drugs: may increase bleeding risk.

Possible lab changes:

- None known.

Avoid or use precaution in patients with:

- Bleeding conditions, diabetes (hypoglycemia), heart conditions.

Gingko

- Avoid use of seed, which can increase seizure risk.

Used for:

- Age-related memory impairment, cognitive function, dementia, intermittent claudication (possible effective).
- Altitude sickness, antidepressant-induced sexual dysfunction (possible ineffectiveness).

Common side effects:

- GI upset, restlessness, headache, lack of muscle tone or weakness, bleeding.

Possible drug interactions:

- Anticoagulant/antiplatelet drugs, ibuprofen: may increase bleeding risk.
- Trazodone: may lead to coma due to excessive GABA-ergic activity.

Possible lab changes:

- None known.

Avoid or use precaution in patients with:

- Bleeding disorders, diabetes, epilepsy, infertility attempting to conceive, upcoming surgery.

Ginseng

- Refers to species of genus *Panax*; commonly used species Asian and American.
- Does not refer to Siberian ginseng, of genus *Eleutherococcus*.

Used for:

- Improved abstract thinking (possibly effective).
- Diabetes (possibly effective).
- Erectile dysfunction (possibly effective).

Common side effects:

- GI upset, nervousness, tachycardia, insomnia.

Possible drug interactions:

- Anticoagulant/antiplatelet drugs: may increase bleeding risk.
- Caffeine: may have additive stimulant effect.

Possible lab changes:

- Activated partial thromboplastin time (aPTT), prothrombin time (PT), and thrombin time (TT) may be prolonged.

Avoid or use precaution in patients with:

- Autoimmune disease, bleeding disorders, diabetes, insomnia, organ transplants, schizophrenia, cardiovascular disease.

Glucosamine Sulfate

- Hydrochloride salt form shown not effective for osteoarthritis.
- Sometimes used in combination with chondroitin and/or methylsulfonylmethane (MSM) but with inconsistent or modest efficacy.

Used for:

- Osteoarthritis (likely effective).

Common side effects:

- Gas, abdominal bloating or cramps, short-term increases in blood sugar levels.

Possible drug interactions:

- Antimitotic chemotherapeutic agents: theoretically might induce resistance.
- Warfarin: may change INRs when used in combination with chondroitin at higher than recommended doses.

Possible lab changes:

- May increase INRs when taken in combination with warfarin and chondroitin at higher than recommended doses.
- Little or no effect noted on blood glucose or lipid levels.

Avoid or use precaution in patients with:
- Shellfish allergies, asthma.

Green Tea
- Contains caffeine.

Used for:
- Improved alertness (likely effective).
- Mental performance (likely effective).
- Cholesterol reduction (possibly effective).
- Decreased risk of developing cardiovascular disease (insufficient reliable evidence).
- Diabetes (insufficient reliable evidence).
- Hypertension (insufficient reliable evidence).

Common side effects:
- Nausea, vomiting, abdominal pain, bloating, diuresis, CNS stimulation including dizziness, insomnia, agitation, confusion.

Possible drug interactions:
- Anticoagulant/antiplatelet drugs: may increase bleeding risk.
- Clozapine: may inhibit metabolism, increasing serum concentrations.
- Lithium: may change serum levels.
- Theophylline: may reduce clearance, increase serum levels.
- Alcohol, contraceptives, estrogen, disulfiram, fluconazole, fluvoxamine, mexiletine, nicotine, quinolone antibiotics, terbinafine, verapamil.

Possible lab changes:
- May decrease ferritin, hemoglobin, iron levels.
- May increase liver function tests.
- May interfere with dipyridamole thallium imaging.

Avoid or use precaution in patients with:
- Iron deficiency anemia, bleeding disorders, cardiac conditions, diabetes, glaucoma, hypertension, liver disease, osteoporosis.

Melatonin
- Avoid products from animal sources.

Used for:
- Insomnia (possibly effective).

- Jet lag (possibly effective).
- ADHD (insufficient reliable evidence).

Common side effects:

- Daytime drowsiness, headache, dizziness, resumption of spotting or menstrual flow in postmenopausal women, mood changes, hormonal changes.

Possible drug interactions:

- Anticoagulant/antiplatelet drugs: may increase effect, with bleeding and decreased prothrombin activity.
- Benzodiazepines, alcohol, sedatives: may have additive sedating effects.
- Immunosuppressants: may stimulate immune function and interfere with therapy.
- Nifedipine GITS: decreases effectiveness with increase in blood pressure and heart rate.

Possible lab changes:

- May increase human growth hormone levels.
- May decrease serum luteinizing hormone levels.
- May cause dose-dependent increases or decreases in oxytocin levels.
- May cause dose-dependent increases or decreases in vasopressin levels.

Avoid or use precaution in patients with:

- Depression, diabetes, hypertension, seizure disorder.

Milk Thistle

Used for:

- Treatment of liver damage and disease (insufficient reliable evidence).

Common side effects:

- Laxative effect, nausea, anorexia.

Possible drug interactions:

- May inhibit CYP2C9.
- May reduce clearance of drugs that undergo glucuronidation.

Possible lab changes:

- None known.

Avoid or use precaution in patients with:

- Allergies to Asteraceae/Composita family (ragweed, chrysanthemums, marigolds, many others).
- Hormone-sensitive cancers.

Peppermint

Used for:

- Dyspepsia (possibly effective).

Common side effects:

- Heartburn, nausea, vomiting, mouth burning and ulceration.

Possible drug interactions:

- Cyclosporine: may inhibit metabolism, increasing drug levels.
- May inhibit CYP1A2, CYP2C19, CYP2C9, and CYP3A4.
- Histamine H_2-receptor antagonists and proton pump inhibitors, may cause premature dissolution of enteric coated preparations.

Possible lab changes (observed in animal models):

- May increase follicle-stimulating hormone (FSH) levels.
- May increase luteinizing hormone (LH) levels.
- May reduce testosterone levels.

Avoid or use precaution in patients with:

- Achlorhydria, diarrhea, pregnancy, breast-feeding.

Red Clover

- Has estrogenic effects.

Used for:

- Menopausal symptoms (possibly ineffective).

Common side effects:

- Myalgia, headache, vaginal spotting, rash, nausea, breast tenderness, weight gain.

Possible drug interactions:

- Anticoagulant/antiplatelet drugs: may increase bleeding risk.
- Contraceptive drugs, estrogen, tamoxifen: may reduce efficacy.
- May inhibit CYP1A2, CYP2C19, CYP2C9, and CY3A4.

Possible lab changes:

- None known.

Avoid or use precaution in patients with:

- Breast and other hormone-sensitive cancers, coagulation disorders, pregnancy, breast-feeding.

Saw Palmetto

- Has antiestrogenic effects.

Used for:

- Benign prostatic hyperplasia (BPH) symptoms (likely effective).

Common side effects:

- Dizziness, headache, GI upset, diarrhea, increases in blood pressure.

Possible drug interactions:

- Anticoagulant/antiplatelet drugs: may increase risk of bleeding.
- Contraceptive drugs, estrogen: may interfere with hormone therapy.

Possible lab changes:

- May change INRs.
- Does not appear to significantly affect prostate-specific antigen (PSA) levels.

Avoid or use precaution in patients with:

- Planned surgery due to excessive intraoperative bleeding.

Soy

- Has estrogenic effects.

Used for:

- Reducing risk of developing breast cancer (possibly effective).
- Hyperlipidemia (possibly effective).
- Menopausal symptoms (possibly effective).

Common side effects:

- Constipation, diarrhea, bloating, nausea, acute migraine.

Possible drug interactions:

- Monoamine oxidase inhibitors (MAOI): may increase risk of hypertensive crisis when used with fermented soy products.
- Tamoxifen: may cause interference due to estrogenic effects.
- Warfarin: may decrease INRs, may inhibit platelet aggregation.

Possible lab changes:

- Parathyroid levels may be reduced in postmenopausal women.
- Prostate-specific antigen (PSA) may be reduced in men with prostate cancer.
- Thyroid stimulating hormone (TSH) may be increased.

Avoid or use precaution in patients with:

- Asthma, breast cancer, endometrial cancer, kidney stones, renal failure.

St. John's Wort
Used for:

- Mild to moderate depression (likely effective).

Common side effects:

- Insomnia, vivid dreams, agitation, irritability, GI upset, dry mouth.

Possible drug interactions:

- May increase risk of serotonin syndrome.
  - "triptans," selective serotonin reuptake inhibitors (SSRIs), monoamine oxidase inhibitors (MOAIs), nefazodone, fenfluramine, meperidine, pentazocine, tramadol.
- May induce cytochrome isoenzyme metabolism causing decreased serum concentrations and reduction in therapeutic effect.
  - Alprazolam, amitriptyline, nortriptyline, contraceptive, cyclosporine, methylphenidate, simvastatin, imatinib, irinotecan, nonnucleoside reverse transcriptase inhibitors (NNRTIs) and protease inhibitors (PIs), tacrolimus, warfarin.
- Phenobarbital, phenytoin: may increase metabolism, decreasing therapeutic levels.
- Fexofenadine: may decrease clearance, increasing serum levels.
- Clopidogrel: may increase risk of bleeding.
- Digoxin: may decrease serum levels.

Possible lab changes:

- May decrease INR and PT levels for warfarin patients.
- May increase TSH levels.

Avoid or use precaution in patients with:

- Alzheimer disease, ADHD, bipolar disease, schizophrenia, infertility attempting to conceive.

Additional Reliable Sources on Dietary Supplements:

- Natural Medicines Comprehensive Database. Available at www.naturaldatabase.com.
- The Food and Drug Administration. Available at www.fda.gov.

- National Center for Complementary and Alternative Medicine, National Institutes of Health. Available at www.nccam.nih.gov.
- Natural Standard, The Authority on Integrative Medicine. Available at www.naturalstandard.com.
- Medline Plus. Available at www.nlm.nih.gov/medlineplus/drug information.html.

References

1. Hong SH, Spadaro D, West D, et al. Patient valuation of pharmacist services for self care with OTC medications. *J Clin Pharm Ther.* 2005;30:193–199.

2. Covington TR. Nonprescription drug therapy: issues and opportunities. *Am J Pharm Educ.* 2006;70(6):137.

3. Isetts BJ, Brown LM. Patient assessment and consultation. In: Berardi RR, Kroon LA, McDermott JH, et al., eds. *Handbook of Nonprescription Drugs: An Interactive Approach to Self-Care.* 15th ed. Washington, DC: American Pharmacists Association; 2006.

4. FDA Center for Drug Evaluation and Research (CDER). Public Health Advisory—Nonprescription cough and cold medicine use in children. January 17, 2008. Available at *www.fda.gov/cder/drug/advisory/cough_cold_2008.htm.* Accessed February 5, 2008.

5. Briggs GG, Freeman RK, Yaffe SJ. *Drugs in Pregnancy and Lactation.* 7th ed. Philadelphia, PA: Lippincott Williams & Wilkins; 2005.

6. Lindbla CI, Gray SL, Guay DRP, et al., eds. *Pharmacotherapy: A Pathophysiologic Approach.* 6th ed. New York, NY: McGraw-Hill; 2005.

7. Pal S. Self-care and nonprescription pharmacotherapy. In: Berardi RR, Kroon LA, McDermott JH, et al., eds. Handbook *of Nonprescription Drugs: An Interactive Approach to Self-Care.* 15th ed. Washington, DC: American Pharmacists Association; 2006.

8. Gunn VL, Nechyba C, eds. *The Harriet Lane Handbook.* 17th ed. Philadelphia, PA: Mosby; 2005.

9. Pediatric Lex-Drugs Online 2008. Lexi-Comp, Inc. Hudson, OH. Available at *online.lexi.com.* Accessed February 7, 2008.

10. Nahata MC, Taketomo C. Pediatrics. In: DiPiro JT, Talbert RL, Yee GC, et al., eds. *Pharmacotherapy: A Pathophysiologic Approach.* 6th ed. New York, NY: McGraw-Hill; 2005.

11. American Academy of Pediatrics. Use of codeine- and dextromethorphan-containing cough remedies in children. *Pediatrics* 1997;99:918–920.

12. Scolaro KL. Disorders related to colds and allergy. In: Berardi RR, Kroon LA, McDermott JH, et al., eds. *Handbook of nonprescription Drugs: An Interactive Approach to Self-Care.* 1st ed. Washington, DC: American Pharmacists Association; 2006.

13. Tietze KJ. Cough. In: Berardi RR, Kroon LA, McDermott JH, et al., eds. *Handbook of nonprescription Drugs: An Interactive Approach to Self-Care.* 1st ed. Washington, DC: American Pharmacists Association; 2006.

14. Kennedy J. Herb and supplement use in the US adult population. *Clin Ther.* 2005;27:1847–1858.

15. National Center for Health Statistics, National Health and Nutrition Examination Survey. 2004.

16. FDA Center for Food Safety and Applied Nutrition. Dietary Supplements. Updated October 5, 2007. Available at *www.cfsan.fda.gov/~dms/supplmnt.html*. Accessed February 5, 2008.

17. FDA issues dietary supplements final rule [press release]. Rockville, MD: US Food and Drug Administration; June 22, 2007. Available at *www.fda.gov/bbs/topics/NEWS/ 2007/NEW01657.html*. Accessed January 25, 2008.

18. Kaiser Permanente Natural Products Advisory Committee (NPAC). Available at *internal.or.kp.org/Pharm/Patient-Handouts/dietarysupplement.pdf*. Accessed January 25, 2008.

19. Tindle HA, Davis RB, Phillips RS, et al. Trends in use of complementary and alternative medicine by US adults: 1997–2002. *Altern Ther Health Med.* 2005;11:42–49.

20. Barnes P, Powell-Griner E, McFann K, et al. Complementary and alternative medicine use among adults: United States, 2002. *Adv Data.* 2004 May 27;(343):1–19.

21. Consumer Reports. "Dangerous supplements, 12 supplements to avoid." May, 2004.

22. Natural Medicine Comprehensive Database. Available at *www.naturaldatabase.com*. Accessed January 25, 2008.

23. Natural Standard, The Authority on Integrative Medicine. Available at *www.naturalstandard.com*. Accessed January 25, 2008.

24. Brinker F. *Herb Contraindications & Drug Interactions.* 3rd ed. Sandy, OR: Eclectic Medical Publications; 2001.

18 Patient Consultation in the Cycle of Patient Care

Linda Garrelts MacLean

Clear communication is the foundation for effective patient consultation. This chapter will describe, highlight, and illustrate important elements of successful patient encounters, including communication techniques. To be effective during patient consultations, the pharmacist must:

- View the patient as a whole person, not just a set of symptoms.
- Be knowledgeable about diseases and medications.
- Use certain verbal and nonverbal skills relating to consultative techniques.

Pharmacist–patient consultation sessions encompass a broad range of activities including the following:

- Medication counseling.
- Medication therapy management (MTM).
- Clinical interviewing to
  ‣ Gather and evaluate information, obtain a medical history, and assess symptoms.
  ‣ Develop a care plan.
  ‣ Implement the care plan with the patient.
  ‣ Determine what follow-up and monitoring will be necessary.

An overview of the principles associated with medication counseling, MTM, and specific communication skills follows.

Getting Started

Know your patient. Maintain a broad perspective regarding the patient's involvement with the health care system.

- Patients transition between various care settings frequently, from hospital to home to nursing home to clinic and back to the hospital.
- Most patients have already been counseled by other health care practitioners.
- These experiences factor into every subsequent encounter.
- Student pharmacists must work from where the patient is, from what the patient knows and thinks about his or her medications.

Understand that patients may:

- Not be totally honest with health care providers.
- Minimize or exaggerate their needs for medication, especially analgesics.
- Have an agenda to obtain a medication they have seen on television or heard about through a friend.
- Not really want to get well.
- Not be in agreement about care.

Establish rapport between pharmacist and patient:

- Introduce yourself to the patient.
- State the purpose of the consultation.
- If not familiar with the patient, identification should be verified by either asking for identification or simply asking, "And you are . . . ?"
- Counsel the caregiver if the patient's hearing is impaired.
- Work with the interpreter if a language barrier exists.
- Use a private space for cases in which sensitive information is to be discussed.
- Face the patient and maintain the appropriate interpersonal distance (1.5–2 ft).[1]
- Verify what the patient knows.
- Do not overload or overwhelm the patient with too much information.
- Keep information brief and to the point.
- Allow the patient to openly discuss issues of concern.
- Offer your availability for further assistance.

Unique Environment Pearls: The Institutional Setting

Plan: think beyond the *acute* problem to the *chronic* care issues.

- Begin planning discharge counseling on medications at the time of the patient's admission.

- Consider compliance issues and drug use patterns that might have led to the admission.
- With the patient, determine strategies to overcome the difficulties identified.
- Pharmacists' intervention through medication review, discharge counseling, and follow-up by phone has been shown to favorably affect the rate of preventable adverse drug events 30 days after discharge.[2]

The REAP mnemonic can be used to plan discharge medication consultation in the hospital setting:

- *R*eason for admission:
  - ‣ Is it due to a drug-related problem or noncompliance?
  - ‣ How many and what kinds of diseases does the patient have?
  - ‣ What medications are currently prescribed?
  - ‣ Assess the patient's physical, emotional, and mental states in light of the patient history.
- *E*valuate current medication regimen for drug-related problems, including noncompliance:
  - ‣ Prioritize questioning, beginning with the most important medications that relate to the primary problem (e.g., insulin or hypoglycemic use in a patient who has diabetes).
  - ‣ Prioritize questioning, also focusing on those drugs with a multiple daily dosing regimen and those with special administration techniques, such as inhalers.
- *A*ssess the patient's knowledge base and skills to self-medicate; assess compliance-promoting strategies.
- *P*lan to avoid drug-related problems after discharge.

The discharge counseling session includes review of the following for each prescribed medication:

- Indication.
- Dosage.
- Administration.
- Self-monitoring.
- Follow-up laboratory tests if necessary.
- Follow-up appointments if necessary.

▮ Match Your Message to Your Patient

It is important to be aware of the Kübler-Ross stages of grief[3] and how these can relate to diagnoses that may signal the loss of one's health and proper use of medication. Once you discern where your patient is in this continuum, as a pharmacist you can be certain to frame information appropriately.

STAGES

- Denial.
  - Discussion of proper medications use is often fruitless.
- Anger.
- Depression.
- Bargaining.
- Acceptance.
  - The health care provider cannot make a patient follow a care plan or take a medication correctly.
  - The patient must have accepted the presence of an illness as warranting treatment.
  - "How do you feel about taking this medication?"

Recognize Connections

Significant information can be gleaned from a patient interview when the pharmacist understands the relationship between disease state and any associated mental and physical deficits, medication, and compliance.

- Cognitive limitations as a result of medical conditions may affect the patient's ability to self-administer and take medications correctly. Example:
  - Stroke can cause changes in mentation that preclude the patient from accurately filling a 7-day medication box.
- Physical limitations as a result of medical conditions may affect the patient's ability to apply a patch, topical medications, or eye drops. Examples:
  - Weakness associated with stroke may make it difficult to open packaging or apply topical medications.
  - Rheumatoid arthritis may prevent a patient from inserting eye drops.
- Medication actions, such as frequent urination caused by a diuretic, can deter a patient from taking medication.
- Uncover deficits in the patient's ability to self-medicate through open-ended questions and demonstration of skills such as the following:
  - What is the name of your new medicine?
  - Could you show how you will apply the patch medication that has been prescribed for you? I have a patch that does not contain any active

ingredient—we can work with it right here. Let's start by having you open up the package . . . .

Realize that patients often worry more about the bad effects from medications than dosage or even indication. Recognize this association and consider using the following guidelines on side effect consultation:

- Counsel on the most common side effects.
- Counsel on the adverse reactions that are most serious and could be life threatening.
- Advise what to do if an adverse reaction is suspected.
- Provide additional information about internet resources for the patient to access. "Web Site Review: Patient Medication Counseling" provides the pharmacist information about potential tools to recommend.[4]

Medication Counseling Techniques

The pharmacist–patient consultation program (PPCP) techniques developed by the Indian Health Service three decades ago, and further refined through pharmacists' collaboration, remains a solid practice model for medication consultation. This interactive method of consultation seeks to *verify* what the patient knows about the medication and *fill in the gaps* with only the most basic information when needed.[5] Research shows that people forget 90% of what is heard within 60 minutes of hearing it.[6] By making the patient an *active* participant in the process, learning is enhanced. Two sets of questions, one for new prescriptions (Prime Questions) and the other for refill medications (Show and Tell Questions), are used in this model to engage the patient in a dynamic, structured care session.

THE PRIME QUESTIONS FOR NEW PRESCRIPTIONS

(1) What did the doctor tell you (were you told) the medication is for?
   What problem or symptom is it supposed to help?
   What is it supposed to do?
(2) How did your doctor tell you (were you told) to take the medication?
   How often? How much? How long?
   What does X times a day mean to you?
   What did your doctor say to do if you miss a dose?
(3) What did the doctor tell you (were you told) to expect?
   What good effects? Bad effects? Precautions to take?
   What should you do if a bad reaction occurs?

SHOW-AND-TELL QUESTIONS FOR REFILL PRESCRIPTIONS

(1) What do you take this medication for?

(2) How have you been taking it?

(3) What kinds of problems are you having with it?

VERIFY THAT THE PATIENT HAS UNDERSTOOD

(1) Determine that the patient has sufficient knowledge to self-medicate.

(2) "Just to make sure I didn't leave anything out, please go over with me how you are going to use the medication."

Handling Difficulties During Counseling

Some common barriers and the skills to manage them are listed in Table 18.1. These relate to functional and/or emotional issues. Functional barriers have specific strategies for management, whereas emotional barriers require the use of active listening skills and reflecting responses.

Examples of reflecting responses include the following:

- "Sounds like you're (frustrated, mad, happy) about your visit with the doctor."
- "I can see that this is (frustrating, worrisome) for you."

Table 18.1 COMMON BARRIERS AFFECTING CONSULTATION

Barrier	Helpful Techniques
Language barrier	Identify barrier with open-ended questions. Use pictures; contact translator
Counseling a third party	Be careful regarding confidentiality; ask for identification; provide written supplements; ask patient to call
Hearing impaired	Use print material; move to a quiet space; speak more loudly Use final verification technique
Vision impaired	Use interactive dialogue, final verification Provide large-print material
Mental disorder	Identify problem early with open-ended questions Counsel caregiver; repeat information and use final verification Provide written supplements

Table 18.2 SETTING LIMITS IN THE ENCOUNTER

Example	Useful Skills for the Pharmacist
Patient is overly talkative.	Take control by piggybacking onto one of the patient's comments (e.g., "I know you don't like hospitals, so let's talk about how your medicines can keep you out of here") Interrupt the patient as gently as possible Use patient's name to register attention
Patient consistently wants lengthy encounters.	Realize patient's need for attention State clear limits on consultation (e.g., "I can only discuss this medication now with you")
Patient interrupts your daily routine.	Realize patient's need for attention Set time period for your availability (e.g., "I can meet with you for no more than 5 minutes after lunch")
Patient continues to discuss issues that cannot be resolved.	Realize patient is frustrated, wants attention, or desires control Acknowledge the differences (e.g., "We disagree on whether you should keep taking this medication") Use diverting tactics, switch to discussing something else State need to move on to next task

Table 18.2 illustrates some examples of how pharmacists can balance meeting patients' needs with their own.

What Not to Do

When dealing with patients, the pharmacy student must remember to do many things. The following list contains some things that the student must remember *not* to do:

- Do not expect the perfect patient.
  - Patients may take medications in ways different than the textbook indicates. They may take medications that are ineffective. It is the pharmacist's duty to discover if current therapies are helping and then as a pharmacist use your judgments about the drug regimen. The patient should be counseled accordingly.

- Do not expect to know everything.
  - A pharmacist must read, research, and ask for help when needed.
- Do not be afraid to make mistakes.
  - Just learn from them.
- Do not second-guess the prescriber in front of the patient.
  - Comments such as "I'm not sure why you're getting this drug when we usually use (another therapy)" should be avoided. This creates confusion and doubt in the patient's mind and can lead to conflict between medical and pharmacy staff. If the pharmacist has doubts about a prescribed drug or therapy, the physician should be consulted in a private and professional manner for clarification.
- Do not leave the patient without hope.
  - Pharmacists will counsel patients whose diseases are progressing despite maximal therapeutic efforts. These patients may be looking for answers that are not there. Statements such as "You're getting all the prescribed medications available for X condition" are not helpful and should be avoided. What patients need is support. Pharmacists should use reflecting responses such as "It must be very frustrating to feel like you're not getting any better."
- Do not judge the patient who does not adhere to the care plan.
  - Examples include patients who abuse certain substances or the patient with lung cancer who still smokes. Dealing with such patients can be frustrating to the health care provider because of the provider's *unrealistic expectations* about the patient's participation in care. Health care providers expect patients to share the same views about the need for treatment. Nevertheless, a health care practitioner should never give up on a patient. An open, honest, and sincere presence should be maintained, and information should ne provided that is appropriate to the patient's level of readiness to accept responsibility for his or her health care.

Integrate Effective Communication Skills into Patient Consultation

The specific verbal communication skills that may be incorporated into medication counseling and medication therapy management encounters are described in the following sections.

Elements to include in the patient care session:

- Open-ended questions to discover patient needs and knowledge deficiencies.

- Active listening.
- Demonstration techniques on the part of the patient and the pharmacist.
- Did learning occur? Verify and summarize what the patient knows.
- Responses that are sensitive to patient needs.
- Adherence investigation.
  - Is medication being taken correctly?
  - Is the care plan being followed?
  - Identify causes of problems.
- Work toward solutions of problems identified.
- Assess pharmacist/patient encounters: Strive for continual improvement.

Motivational interviewing is a tool that has been useful as pharmacists identify ways to encourage and empower patients to adopt change. This change could be a lifestyle modification such as increasing exercise or improving food choices or the action of taking a medication correctly every single day. This technique creates a tension or dissonance in a patient. The patient realizes that there is a conflict between personal goals and his or her behavior. An example is the patient who states that his grandkids mean everything to him, he wants to see them graduate from college, yet he continues to smoke. The pharmacist interviews the patient to help him or her recognize and resolve ambivalence in behavior. Components of motivational interviewing include the following:

- Ask open-ended questions to gather information.
  - What do you think about the changes we have discussed?
  - Tell me about what kinds of exercise you enjoy.
  - How much do you exercise?
  - Describe what kinds of activities you work into a typical week.
  - What is your view about the exercise you engage in? Do you get as much exercise as you need?
- Affirm the patient's willingness and ability to implement the care plan that has been developed.
  - What is your understanding of the consequences of not getting adequate exercise?
  - What are the positive things associated with incorporating more exercise and movement into your week? Negative?
  - Describe your goal for increasing movement and exercise.
  - How does this goal line up with where you currently are with regard to exercise?

- ‣ How might you address this discrepancy between where you are and where you want to be in the future?
- Listen actively during the patient encounter.
  - ‣ Reflect back what you have heard by paraphrasing.
  - ‣ Offer feedback.
  - ‣ Give suggestions.
- Summarize the patient's views, strategies, questions, and concerns.
  - ‣ Reiterate the pros and cons discussed.
  - ‣ Restate where the gap is between the current behavior and the target goal.
  - ‣ Reaffirm the patient's action plan and timeline.

Adherence is an arena to which the pharmacist must pay attention. Recognition of problems with adherence should be under the purview of the pharmacist. Strategies to address and improve adherence include the following:

- Use a universal statement to open the conversation. Examples include the following:
  - ‣ "Mrs J., a lot of patients have trouble fitting taking medication into their daily schedule. What's been your experience?"
  - ‣ "Many patients have trouble remembering when to take this medication, especially since it's only changed once a week. What's been your experience, Mr. K.?"
- Use a probing statement following the "I noticed/I'm concerned" formula. Examples include the following:
  - ‣ "Mr. K, I noticed this clonidine patch prescription was due to be refilled 3 weeks ago. I'm a little concerned about that."
- Listen for clues that may indicate the patient is reluctant to take the prescription. Examples include the following:
  - ‣ "Why do I have to keep taking this medicine?"
  - ‣ "My doctor *says* I should take it . . . ,"
  - ‣ "My doctor *wants* me to . . . ,"
  - ‣ "I'm *supposed* to be taking it."
- Link medication-taking to a daily activity.
- Suggest the use of pill boxes and calendars.
- Suggest that medication be kept where it is easily seen.
- The "I noticed/I'm concerned" formula should be used. For example, "Mr. K, I noticed this clonidine patch prescription was due to be refilled 3 weeks ago. I'm a little concerned about that."

- Do not assume that when a patient is doing well and has no complaints it must be because the medication is working and not causing problems.
- Do not assume that the patient is compliant with therapy.[7]
  - One third of patients do not get their original prescription filled.
  - One third of patients take the medication incorrectly.
  - One third take the medication as prescribed.

Empowering the patient is key to a successful care plan implementation or an effective medication regimen to which the patient is to adhere.

- The *patient's acceptance* that a problem exists and his or her acceptance of the value of treatment forms the essential foundation for successful treatment.
  - The *patient* controls the outcome of his or her disease by taking or not taking prescribed medications and/or implementing lifestyle changes.
    - The empowerment model shifts patients from *receiving* health care to *managing* health.
  - The practitioner's role is to facilitate the patient using medications and managing lifestyle changes to the best benefit; the pharmacist and patient form a partnership.
  - Work with the patient to identify barriers to care plan implementation, which can include the following:
    - Knowledge deficits that may prevent compliance.[8]
      - Insufficient information.
      - Insufficient skills.
      - Misinformation.
    - Practical limitations, including but not limited to the following:
      - Transportation.
      - Multiple daily doses.
      - Manual dexterity.
      - Vision and hearing difficulties.
    - Attitudinal barriers.
      - Perceived severity of risk compared with perceived benefit of treatment.[9]
      - Patient's desire to be in control.
      - Patient's belief that he or she can or cannot successfully implement the recommended treatment.[10]
      - Incorrect or inappropriate pervasive patient ideas such as:
        a. "I can develop immunity to a medication's effects."

      b. "If one pill helps, then two must be twice as good."

      c. "If I feel good, then I don't need medication."

‣ Work with the patient to prioritize barriers.

‣ Work with the patient to overcome and/or manage barriers.

 Summary

The techniques and issues discussed in this chapter contribute to good rapport with patients and success in helping patients manage chronic illnesses. Students should seek out model practitioners, observe their skills and techniques, and then practice these skills and techniques during pharmacy practice experiences.

 Acknowledgment

The author would like to acknowledge Marie Gardner on whose second edition work this current third edition has been based.

References

1. *Pharmacist-Patient Consultation Program, Unit 2: Counseling Patients in Challenging Situations.* New York, NY: Pfizer Inc.; 1993.
2. Schnipper J, Kirwin J, Cotugno M, et al. Role of pharmacist counseling in preventing adverse drug events after hospitalization. *Arch Intern Med.* 2006;166:565–571.
3. Kübler-Ross E, Wessler S, Avioli LV. On death and dying. *JAMA.* 1972;221:174–179.
4. Berry B, Kendrach M. Web site review: patient medication counseling. *Int J Pharm Educ.* 2006;1:0014–0016.
5. Boyce RW, Herrier RN, Gardner ME. *Pharmacist-Patient Consultation Program, Unit 1: An Interactive Approach to Verify Patient Understanding.* New York, NY: Pfizer Inc.; 1991.
6. Bolton R. *People Skills.* New York, NY: Simon & Schuster; 1979.
7. *Pharmacist-Patient Consultation Program, Unit 3: Counseling to Enhance Compliance.* New York, NY: Pfizer Inc.; 1995.
8. Powell MF, Burkhart VdeP, Lamy PP. Diabetic patient compliance as a function of patient counseling. *Ann Pharmacother.* 2006;40:747–752.
9. Eraker SA, Kirscht JP, Becker MH. Understanding and improving patient compliance. *Ann Intern Med.* 1984;100:258–268.
10. Viinamaki H. The patient-doctor relationship and metabolic control in patients with type 1 (insulin-dependent) diabetes mellitus. *Int J Psychiatry Med.* 1993;23:265–274.

19

Preventative Health: Vaccines and General Adult Health Screening

Kristine B. Marcus, Pauline A. Cawley, Jeffery Fortner, Kate Farthing, and Brad S. Fujisaki

Pharmacist Involvement in Immunization-Related Activities

Nearly all states now allow pharmacists and pharmacy interns under the supervision of their preceptor to administer vaccines to adults after proper training.[1] Two of the most commonly targeted and reimbursed immunizations given in pharmacies include inactivated influenza and pneumococcal polysaccharide vaccines.[2] However, pharmacists in all settings can have an impact on improving national vaccination rates for at-risk patients through participation in all three levels of vaccine practice: advocacy, facilitation, and vaccine administration (Table 19.1).

Discuss with your preceptor which of these activities you are expected to participate in while on rotation. Even if it is not a routine part of the site's practice to give immunizations, you can still contribute to the patient's preventative health by including vaccinations in your questioning when taking a medication history and recommending vaccination when appropriate.

Pharmacists as Immunizers

Pharmacy students must be aware of whether they are allowed to administer vaccines in the state where they are gaining practice experience and if there are any limitations on which vaccines may be given, if a prescription for vaccination is required, and which patient populations may be served. The requirements and restrictions on providing immunizations are usually outlined in the state's Pharmacy Practice Act that

Table 19.1 EXAMPLES OF PHARMACIST
IMMUNIZATION ACTIVITIES BY
PRACTICE SETTING

Pharmacy Practice Setting	Example Immunization Activities
Community pharmacy	• Providing vaccinations • Taking vaccination histories, screening patients, and recommending vaccination • Hosting other licensed health care providers to administer immunizations
Clinic pharmacy	• Providing vaccinations • Taking vaccination histories, screening patients, and recommending vaccination • Establishing standing orders for vaccination of eligible patients • Managing formularies to include all necessary vaccines for patient population served
Institutional pharmacy	• Taking vaccination histories, screening patients, and recommending vaccination • Establishing standing orders for vaccination of eligible patients • Managing formularies to include all necessary vaccines for patient population served
All settings	• Educating and motivating patients to obtain timely immunizations • Providing public education on vaccine-preventable diseases and the importance of immunization • Providing vaccine information to patients and other health care providers • Maintaining the cold chain and ensuring proper storage conditions of vaccines dispensed or administered

can be found in the Board of Pharmacy's Administrative Rules. These rules will generally include specifics on the training and recordkeeping that is expected when providing immunization in a pharmacy setting. Early in your rotation, review and discuss with your preceptor the rules, policies, and standard operating procedures provided by the Board of Pharmacy and your practice site.

Vaccine Administration Steps Overview

While individual site policies and procedures will be more specific, the usual steps in providing vaccination are shown in Figure 19.1. This figure

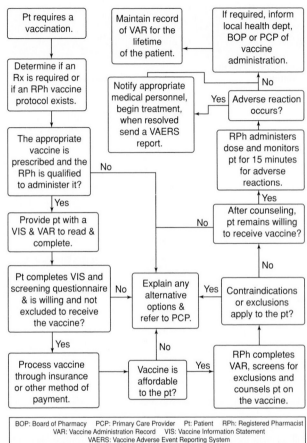

BOP: Board of Pharmacy   PCP: Primary Care Provider   Pt: Patient   RPh: Registered Pharmacist
VAR: Vaccine Administration Record   VIS: Vaccine Information Statement
VAERS: Vaccine Adverse Event Reporting System

FIGURE 19.1 Steps for administering vaccinations.

is the framework for our review on pharmacist-provided vaccinations throughout the rest of this chapter.

Identifying Who Needs Vaccination

Immunization Recommendations

Tables are available from the Centers for Disease Control and Prevention (CDC) to quickly identify patients who are recommended to receive vaccination either by age or other population target. These tables are referred to as Immunization Schedules and are updated annually. Pharmacy students administering or recommending vaccines must ensure that they are using the most current recommendations by checking the date in the upper right corner of the schedule. Due to the frequency of revision, schedules published in printed or electronic drug information references may be out of date. Changes to the Immunization Schedules are provisionally recommended by the Advisory Committee on Immunization Practices (ACIP) in February, June, and October and then are approved by the CDC and the U.S. Department of Health and Human Services. They are subsequently published in the CDC's Morbidity and Mortality Weekly Report and on the CDC's National Center for Immunization and Respiratory Diseases (NCIRD, formerly known as the National Immunization Program) Web site. Pharmacy students can stay informed of upcoming changes and refer to the most current recommendations in immunization practice through these two key sites:

- Bookmark: CDC's NCIRD web site: www.cdc.gov/vaccines/.
- Bookmark and subscribe to IAC Express news service: Immunization Action Coalition: www.immunize.org.

Using the CDC Immunization Schedules

The Immunization Schedules indicate when certain vaccines should ideally be given and how many doses are necessary to complete the primary series or to provide a booster dose. Footnotes for each vaccine provide additional detailed information and should be read in conjunction with the schedule. The user can quickly access the relevant schedule by knowing the patient's age and medical conditions. The current schedules (Table 19.2) are available in various formats (office-size poster, brochure size, pocket size, and download to PDA) at: www.cdc.gov/vaccines/recs/schedules/default.htm.

Table 19.2 CURRENT CDC IMMUNIZATION SCHEDULES

- Childhood (birth through <7 years old)
- Adolescent (7–18 years old)
- Childhood and adolescent catch-up schedule (4 months–18 years old who started late or are >1 month behind)
- Combined childhood, adolescent and catch-up schedule (0–18 years old)
- Adult (>19 years old)—includes an additional table with vaccines that might be indicated for adults based on medical and other indications

The NCIRD web site also includes links for targeted population recommendations that are subsets to the Immunization Schedules (e.g., college students; health care workers; pregnant women; patients with immune deficiencies, altered immunocompetence, or hematopoietic stem cell transplant):

- www.cdc.gov/vaccines/spec-grps/conditions.htm.

 ## Immunization General Rules and Overview

The CDC Pink Book is a frequently updated essential reference that includes chapters on principles of immunization, general recommendations for immunization and vaccine-preventable diseases, and their associated vaccines. Throughout the Pink Book the CDC highlights general rules of immunization that have been compiled in Table 19.3.

Understanding Available Vaccines

Vaccines can be distinguished from one another by several factors such as viability (live or inactive), adult versus pediatric use, inactive ingredients,

---

Table 19.3 GENERAL RULES FOR IMMUNIZATION FROM THE CDC PINK BOOK

- The more similar a vaccine is to the disease-causing form of the organism, the better the immune response to the vaccine
- Live attenuated vaccines generally produce long-lasting immunity with a single dose
- Inactivated vaccines require multiple doses and may require periodic boosting to maintain immunity
- Live attenuated vaccines may be affected by circulating antibody to the antigen
- Inactivated vaccines generally are not affected by circulating antibody to the antigen
- All vaccines can be administered at the same visit as all other vaccines
- Increasing the interval between doses of a multidose vaccine does not diminish the effectiveness of the vaccine
- Decreasing the interval between doses of a multidose vaccine may interfere with antibody response and protection

---

Adapted from Centers for Disease Control and Prevention. Principles of vaccination. In: Atkinson W, Hamborsky J, McIntyre L, Wolfe S, eds. Epidemiology and Prevention of Vaccine-Preventable Diseases (The Pink Book). 10th ed. Washington, DC: Public Health Foundation; 2007; and Centers for Disease Control and Prevention. General recommendations on immunization. In: Atkinson W, Hamborsky J, McIntyre L, Wolfe S, eds. Epidemiology and Prevention of Vaccine-Preventable Diseases (The Pink Book). 10th ed. Washington, DC: Public Health Foundation; 2007.

and methods of administration. When working with vaccines, pharmacy students will also need to be aware of vaccine nomenclature and abbreviations. Vaccines currently available in the United States are shown in Table 19.4.[5]

Viability—Why It Matters

Certain patient populations (e.g., immunocompromised, pregnant) are excluded from receiving live vaccines because of the theoretical health risk of contracting the disease from the vaccine. In these populations of patients, the risk of vaccine use (even from attenuated vaccines that contain weakened, avirulent, or altered live bacteria or viruses) generally outweighs the perceived benefit of vaccination. Inactivated vaccines that are formulated with killed whole or isolated components of bacteria or virus do not pose this same risk.

The issue of interference of immunogenecity between simultaneous administrations of a live vaccine with other vaccines or circulating antibodies has been a historical concern. Current recommendations state that live vaccines may be coadministered in eligible patients with other live vaccines or inactive vaccines at the same immunization session. However, if two parenteral live vaccines or live intranasal influenza vaccine are not administered at the same visit, then they must be separated by 4 weeks to reduce the chance that the first vaccine may result in a suboptimal response to the second vaccine.[4] Likewise, the presence of circulating antibodies contained in blood products may impair the patient's response to a live vaccine. If the live vaccine was given first, then administration of the antibody should be delayed 2 weeks. If the antibody was given first, then administration of the live vaccine is generally delayed for ≥ 3 months with notable exceptions.[4]

Adult versus Pediatric Vaccines

Confusion among available vaccines can be expected since different formulations of vaccines contain similar active ingredients but may be administered to different age groups or at different doses. The pharmacy student needs to be aware of which vaccines are indicated for which age groups and what the appropriate age-based dose is to avoid errors. One example is diphtheria, tetanus, and acellular pertussis vaccines. DTaP is used exclusively in children aged 2 months to ≤ 7 years old. Tdap is used in adolescents and adults. Adolescent patients may receive either brand of Tdap depending on age (Boostrix for 10–18 years of age vs. Adacel if 11 years or older) whereas adults can receive only the Adacel brand of Tdap.

Table 19.4 SUMMARY OF VACCINES AVAILABLE IN THE UNITED STATES

Type of Vaccine	Proprietary Names	Viability	Route	Typical Dose
Meningococcal A, C, Y, W-135				
• Polysaccharide	Menomune-A/C/Y/W-135	Inactivated	Subcutaneous	0.5 mL
• Conjugated	Menactra	Inactivated	Intramuscular (IM)	0.5 mL
Mumps	Mumpsvax	Live	Subcutaneous	0.5 mL
Papillomavirus, types 6, 11, 16, 18	Gardasil	Inactivated	IM	0.5 mL
Pneumococcal, 7-valent	Prevnar	Inactivated	IM	0.5 mL
Pneumococcal, 23-valent	Pneumovax 23	Inactivated	Subcutaneous, IM	0.5 mL
Poliovirus inactivated	IPOL	Inactivated	Subcutaneous	0.5 mL
Rabies (various culture media)	BioRad, Imovax Rabies, RabAvert	Inactivated	IM	1 mL
Rotavirus vaccine	RotaTeq	Live	Oral	0.2 mL
Rubella	Meruvax It	Live	Subcutaneous	0.5 mL
Tetanus-diphtheria with acellular pertussis (Tdap)	Boostrix, Adacel	Inactivated	IM	0.5 mL
Tetanus toxoid (absorbed) (TT)	Generic	Inactivated	IM	0.5 mL
Tetanus-diphtheria toxoids (Td)	Generic, Decavac	Inactivated	IM	0.5 mL
Typhoid (oral)	Vivotif Berna	Live	Oral	4 capsules
Typhoid Vi (parenteral, polysaccharide)	Typhim Vi	Inactivated	IM	0.5 mL
Vaccinia	Dryvax	Live	Scarification	3 or 15 punctures
Varicella	Varivax	Live	Subcutaneous	0.5 mL
Yellow fever	YF-Vax	Live	Subcutaneous	0.5 mL
Zoster	Zostavax	Live	Subcutaneous	0.65 mL

Reprinted with permission from Grabenstein JD. *Immunofacts: Vaccines and Immunologic Drugs.* 6th ed. St. Louis, MO: Wolters Kluwer Health; 2008.

Another example is inactivated influenza vaccine for which there are multiple brands indicated for different age groups and one brand that covers the full range of indicated age groups. Fluzone brand has a pediatric unit dose syringe version formulated specifically for patients 6 to 35 months of age that is thimerosal free and delivers the recommended 0.25-mL dose. Fluzone also has a multidose vial presentation that contains thimerosal and can be used for all indicated ages of patients by withdrawing the appropriate dosage amount (i.e., 0.25 mL for ages 6 to 35 months and 0.5 mL for patients 3 years old or older) from the 5-mL vial.

A final example is pneumococcal vaccine for which a polysaccharide and conjugate formulation are available. The conjugate form (Prevnar) is used in children younger than 2 years old whereas the polysaccharide version (Pneumovax 23) is used in older children and adults.

Vaccine Inactive Ingredients
Vaccines may contain excipients that may prove problematic for some patients who have allergies or sensitivities to these ingredients used in the formulation or packaging of vaccines. Some common excipients of concern are latex in the vial or syringe components, residual egg protein or antibiotic from the vaccine production process, or added pharmaceutical aids such as thimerosal as a preservative.

Vaccine Acronyms and Nomenclature
Although the use of abbreviations when ordering medications or biologicals is error prone,[6–8] the use of these short codes for different vaccines is still prevalent. Especially with the advent of combination vaccines and vaccines indicated for restricted age groups, recognition of the content differences between brand name products is necessary to avoid errors. Pharmacy students will need to be familiar with common acronyms and trade names used when ordering or documenting administration of vaccines.

Electronic flashcards and interactive matching tables to assist students in learning common vaccine names (trade/generic/abbreviation), viability, type, and route of administration are available at the following:

- Childhood and adolescent vaccines: www.studystack.com/menu-115865.
- Adult vaccines: www.studystack.com/menu-115834.

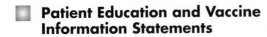 Patient Education and Vaccine Information Statements

Federal statute requires all health care providers to provide the most current edition of the CDC Vaccine Information Statements (VIS) to the patient or their proxy prior to administration of each dose of certain designated vaccines[9] (Table 19.5). State laws may be more restrictive and must also be followed. Best practice dictates providing VIS even for nondesignated vaccines. The health care provider may provide additional vaccine information materials, but these may not substitute for the CDC-produced VIS. VIS are available in multiple languages and now include a leaflet for combination vaccines and a multivaccine VIS for birth to 6 months. The most current VIS are available at www.cdc.gov/vaccines/pubs/vis/default.htm or www.immunize.org/vis/.

Vaccine Contraindications and Precautions Screening

As health care practitioners we routinely ask ourselves, "Will this patient's overall health be worse after I administer this treatment?" This primary

Table 19.5 VACCINES REQUIRING PROVISION OF VACCINE INFORMATION STATEMENTS

- Diphtheria tetanus +/− pertussis (DTaP/DT)
- *Haemophilus influenzae*, type b
- Hepatitis A
- Hepatitis B
- Human papilloma virus (HPV)
- Influenza, inactivated injectable
- Influenza, live, intranasal
- Measles, mumps, rubella (MMR)
- Meningococcal
- Pneumococcal conjugate
- Polio
- Rotavirus
- Tetanus diphtheria +/− pertussis (Td/Tdap)
- Varicella (chickenpox)
- *Or* combinations containing any of the above

Adapted from Centers for Disease Control and Prevention. Instructions for the use of Vaccine Information Statements. Atlanta, GA: Centers for Disease Control and Prevention (CDC); Feb 6, 2008, Available at www.cdc.gov/vaccines/pubs/vis/downloads/vis-Instructions.pdf.

concern can be partially addressed by always considering a treatment's contraindications and precautions. Consider the following:

- A patient with a history of egg-induced anaphylaxis receives an injection of influenza vaccine, or
- A patient with an immune deficiency receives a dose of live zoster vaccine, or
- A patient with a febrile respiratory illness receives an injection of pneumococcal vaccine.

Each of these situations could result in the vaccine administrator causing a life-threatening reaction in the patient. And each could be avoided if the administrator used a system to identify patients with contraindications. Systems to identify contraindications include the following:

- Providing the patient with a CDC-published Vaccine Information Statement that clearly lists any contraindications using terms a patient understands.
- Using a general screening questionnaire or one tailored to a specific vaccine, which identifies potential contraindications, and
- Personally counseling the patient about the vaccine and emphasizing the contraindications.

If practitioners use each of these systems, they can reasonably establish whether a patient can safely receive a vaccine.

Part of the pharmacist's role also involves clearing up patient and caregiver misconceptions about contraindications to receiving immunizations (Table 19.6). Luckily, there are few true contraindications or precautions for most vaccinations, and these are often temporary.[4]

Various screening questionnaires are available from the Immunization Action Coalition (IAC) (Table 19.7). Guides and discussions of contraindications and precautions, which can form the foundation for patient counseling, can also be found at the NCIRD Web site (Table 19.8) and in the CDC Pink Book.[4] By integrating these free resources into a vaccination routine, pharmacists can help to ensure positive patient outcomes with vaccines.

◼ Vaccine Administration

Most vaccines currently on the market are given by parenteral injection. However, there are two vaccines that are given orally and one that is given

Table 19.6 INVALID CONTRAINDICATIONS TO VACCINATION

Invalid Contraindication	Suggested Response to Misconception about Contraindication
Mild illness	• Mild acute illnesses, such as low-grade fever, upper respiratory infection, colds, and mild diarrhea do not interfere with vaccine response • ACIP has not defined a body temperature above which vaccines should not be administered. The decision to vaccinate should be based on the overall evaluation of the person rather than an arbitrary body temperature
Antimicrobial therapy	• Antibiotics do not have an effect on the immune response to most vaccines • No commonly used antimicrobial drug will inactivate a live-virus vaccine. However, antiviral drugs may affect vaccine replication in some circumstances
Disease exposure or convalescence	• There is no evidence that either disease exposure or convalescence will affect the response to a vaccine or increase the likelihood of an adverse event
Pregnant or immunosuppressed person in the household	• Vaccination of healthy contacts reduces the chance of exposure of pregnant women and immunosuppressed persons • With limited exceptions, most vaccines including live vaccines can be administered to infants or children who are household contacts
Breast-feeding	• Breast-feeding does not decrease the response to routine childhood vaccines and is not a contraindication for any vaccine except smallpox • Breast-fed infants should be vaccinated according to recommended schedules for protection against vaccine-preventable disease • The risk of transmission of vaccine virus is unknown but is probably low
Preterm birth	• Preterm infants have been shown to respond adequately to vaccines used in infancy Vaccines should be started on schedule on the basis of the child's chronologic age

Table 19.6   INVALID CONTRAINDICATIONS TO VACCINATION *(continued)*

Invalid Contraindication	Suggested Response to Misconception about Contraindication
Allergy to products not present in vaccine or allergy that is not anaphylactic	• Infants and children with nonspecific allergies, duck or feather allergy, or allergy to penicillin, children who have relatives with allergies, and children taking allergy shots can and should be immunized. No vaccine available in the United States contains duck antigen or penicillin • Anaphylactic allergy to a vaccine component (such as egg or neomycin) is a true contraindication to vaccination. If an allergy to a vaccine component is not anaphylactic, it is not a contraindication to that vaccine
Family history of adverse events	• The only family history that is relevant in the decision to vaccinate a child is immunosuppression. A family history of adverse reactions unrelated to immunosuppression or family history of seizures or sudden infant death syndrome (SIDS) is not a contraindication to vaccination
Multiple vaccines	• Administration at the same visit of all vaccines for which a person is eligible is effective and critical to reaching and maintaining high vaccination coverage • All vaccines (except smallpox) can be administered at the same visit as all other vaccines

ACIP, Advisory Committee on Immunization Practices.
Adapted from Centers for Disease Control and Prevention. General recommendations on immunization. In: Atkinson W, Hamborsky J, McIntyre L, Wolfe S, eds. *Epidemiology and prevention of vaccine-preventable diseases (The Pink Book)*. 10th ed. Washington, DC: Public Health Foundation; 2007.

intranasally. In general, live vaccines are given orally, intranasally, or by subcutaneous (SC or SQ) injection. Inactivated vaccines are generally given by intramuscular (IM) injection. A quick review of injection site location, appropriate needle length selection, and needle insertion technique is shown in Figure 19.2. Detailed instructions, photographs, and graphics of injection technique are available in the CDC Pink Book's Appendix D.[10] Refer to Table 19.4 or the product package insert for the recommended route of administration for specific vaccines.

Coadministration of the most common live and inactivated vaccines at the same immunization session results in adequate responses from the

Table 19.7	LINKS TO IMMUNIZATION ACTION COALITION (IAC) ADULT SCREENING QUESTIONNAIRES
General screening for adults	www.immunize.org/catg.d/p4065.pdf
Hepatitis A	www.immunize.org/catg.d/p2190.pdf
Hepatitis B	www.immunize.org/catg.d/p2191.pdf
Influenza, injectable	www.immunize.org/catg.d/p4066.pdf
Influenza, intranasal	www.immunize.org/catg.d/p4067.pdf
Additional languages available	www.immunize.org/printmaterials

individual vaccines and has not been associated with an increased rate of side effects.[4]

Many pharmacists will ask the patient to remain nearby for 15 minutes after administration so that the patient may be observed for the development of a life-threatening or other severe reaction to the vaccine.

 Vaccine Adverse Events

Managing and Reporting Vaccine Adverse Reactions

Although anaphylaxis from vaccine administration is rare, pharmacists providing immunizations need to be prepared to respond to these

Table 19.8	CDC LINKS TO GUIDES TO VACCINE CONTRAINDICATIONS
Guide to contraindications to vaccinations • Covers all U.S. vaccines as of Sept. 2003. Provides contraindications by condition or symptom and has vaccine content listed by vaccine	Download pdf: www.cdc.gov/vaccines/recs/vac-admin/contraindications.htm
Contraindications to vaccines chart • Presents true contraindications and precautions by vaccine as of Feb. 2004. Also includes column of invalid contraindications that should not prevent administration	Chart on web site: www.cdc.gov/vaccines/recs/vac-admin/contraindications-vacc.htm

Injection Site and Needle Size

Subcutaneous (SC) Injection
Use a 23–25 gauge needle. Choose the injection site that is appropriate to the person's age and body mass.

Age	Needle Length	Injection Site
Infants (1–12 mos)	$5/6''$	Fatty tissue over anterolateral thigh muscle
Children (≥12 mos), adolescents, & adults	$5/6''$	Fatty tissue over anterolateral thigh muscle or fatty tissue over triceps

Intramuscular (IM) Injection
Use a 22–25 gauge needle. Choose the injection site and needle length appropriate to the person's age and body mass.

Age	Needle Length	Injection Site
Newborn (1st 28 days)	$5/8''$*	Anterolateral thigh muscle
Infant (1–12 mos)	$1''$	Anterolateral thigh muscle
Toddler (1–2 yrs)	$1''–1\,1/4''$ $5/8''–1''$	Anterolateral thigh muscle or deltoid muscle of arm
Children 3–18 yrs	$5/8''$*–$1''$ $1''–1\,1/4''$	Deltoid muscle of arm or anterolateral thigh muscle
≥19 yrs (Sex/Weight)		
Male/Female less than 130 lbs	$5/8''$*–$1''$	Deltoid muscle of arm
Female (130–200 lbs) Male (130–260 lbs)	$1''–1\,1/2''$	Deltoid muscle of arm
Female (200+ lbs) Male (260+ lbs)	$1\,1/2''$	Deltoid muscle of arm

*If skin is stretched tight and subcutuneous tissue is not bunched.

FIGURE 19.2

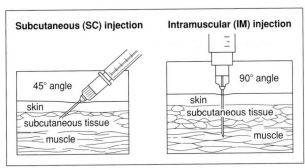

FIGURE 19.2 *(continued)* Vaccine injection basics. (From Immunization Action Coalition, www.immunize.org, with permission.)

situations until other medical help arrives (Table 19.9). All vaccine providers should have an emergency management plan in place and an adequate stock of medications and equipment necessary to respond to a severe vaccine reaction. Maintenance of basic life support (BLS) certification is also required. Appendix D of the CDC Pink Book[10] includes adult and pediatric emergency management protocols and standing order templates from the IAC that can be used by pharmacists providing vaccines.

Pharmacists are more likely to encounter patients with mild local adverse events or psychological reactions to vaccination. Appendix D of

Table 19.9 EXAMPLE MANAGEMENT OF GENERALIZED ANAPHYLACTIC REACTION TO ADULT VACCINATION

1. Have bystander call 911/EMS.
2. Administer epinephrine IM.
3. Administer diphenhydramine IM or PO.
4. Monitor vitals (HR, RR, BP).
5. Administer CPR if necessary.
6. Repeat epinephrine IM q10–20 min PRN x 3 doses until help arrives.
7. Document all vitals, medications given, and personnel providing care.
8. After event has resolved, contact protocol physician or patient's PCP to report reaction and patient condition on triage to EMS.
9. After event has resolved, document reaction and report to VAERS.

EMS, emergency medical services; IM, intramuscularly; PO, by mouth; HR, heart rate; RR, respiratory rate; BP, blood pressure; CPR cardiopulmonary resuscitation; PRN, as needed; PCP, primary care physician, VAERS, Vaccine Adverse Event Reporting System.

the CDC Pink Book also contains sections on the medical management of localized reactions, fright, and syncope.[10]

Customary practice includes documenting all vaccine reactions in the patient's pharmacy record and notifying their primary care provider so that the same information can be recorded in the patient's permanent medical record.

Health care providers and the public are encouraged to report all vaccine adverse events through the national postmarketing safety program, Vaccine Adverse Event Reporting System (VAERS). Health care providers are required by law to report certain problems listed in the Table of Reportable Events now found at www.vaers.hhs.gov/reportable.htm.[11] In general, reporting of any problem that resulted in emergency treatment, hospitalization, disability, or death is required. Causation does not need to be established before reporting of adverse events in vaccinated adults and children. Even if the reporter is uncertain if the observed reaction was related to the vaccine, he or she is encouraged to file a report. Reports can be filed online at www.vaers.hhs.gov or by calling 1-800-822-7967 or faxing 1-877-721-0366.

A federal program called the National Vaccine Injury Compensation Program exists to help pay for the care of anyone who has had a serious reaction to a routinely recommended childhood vaccine. Settlement amounts are predetermined according to the Vaccine Injury Table published in Appendix F of the CDC Pink Book.[11] More information is available at www.hrsa.gov/vaccinecompensation or 1-800-338-2382.

Vaccine Administration Documentation

Vaccine Administration Records (VARs) must be maintained by the immunization provider for all patients receiving vaccination. It is also helpful to update or issue the patient a portable vaccination record such as the yellow Adult Immunization Record pocket card (www.immunize.org/shop/). Pharmacists providing immunizations may be subject to additional or special requirements for sharing their documentation with the patient's primary care provider, health division, or licensing board. Individual state rules and standards of practice should be consulted.

Documentation required at the time of vaccination is outlined in federal law[9] (Table 19.10), but state law or insurance adjudication may

Table 19.10 MINIMUM FEDERAL REQUIREMENTS FOR VACCINE ADMINISTRATION DOCUMENTATION

(1) Edition date of the Vaccine Information Statement (VIS) distributed
(2) Date the VIS was provided to the patient or his or her proxy
(3) Name, address and title of the individual who administered the vaccine
(4) Date of administration, *and*
(5) Vaccine manufacturer and lot number of the vaccine used

Adapted from Centers for Disease Control and Prevention. Instructions for the use of Vaccine Information Statements. Atlanta, GA: Centers for Disease Control and Prevention (CDC); Feb 6, 2008, Available at www.cdc.gov/vaccines/pubs/vis/downloads/vis-Instructions.pdf.

impose further requirements. Standard practice for documenting dose administration includes the following: date and time of administration, dose/amount given, administration location, method of administration, lot number, and initials of provider (e.g., MM/DD/YYYY time Pneumovax 0.5 mL IM left deltoid, Lot ABC123, initials).

 ## Vaccination Reimbursement

Unfortunately, insurance coverage for vaccination is not universal and not all insurers recognize pharmacists as vaccination providers who are eligible for payment. Medicare Part B does recognize pharmacists as mass immunization providers who are eligible for reimbursement for both the vaccine product itself and a vaccination administration fee. Enrollment as a Medicare provider is required to bill for covered services.[12,13] Pharmacy students should check with their preceptor on the processes used at their site for billing for vaccinations.

Most pharmacists are not currently certified to administer vaccines to children but may be asked by other practitioners about the federally funded Vaccines for Children (VFC) program that provides vaccines at no cost to children who are at risk for not receiving vaccination because of inability to pay. VFC programs are required to be a part of each state's Medicaid plan and so they are often administered through state/territory health division immunization projects.

- CDC VFC homepage: www.cdc.gov/vaccines/programs/vfc/default.htm.
- State Immunization Program Web site Links are maintained by IAC at www.immunize.org/states/index.htm.

■ Recommended Key Vaccine References

Free Publications or Web Pages

General Reference

- Centers for Disease Control and Prevention. Epidemiology and Prevention of Vaccine-Preventable Diseases (The Pink Book) [book on internet]. Feb 2007 [accessed 2008 Mar]; [about 504 pp.]. Available at www.cdc.gov/vaccines/pubs/pinkbook/default.htm.
  - ‣ Essential reference for health care providers (updated annually or biannually). Chapters are presented on each vaccine-preventable disease and provide a thorough review of epidemiology, disease, transmission, vaccination recommendations, and patient selection. Also contains sections on principles of immunizations, administration technique, immunization strategies, vaccine safety, vaccine storage and handling, practice standards, and resources.
- National Center for Immunization and Respiratory Diseases. Vaccines and immunizations [home page on internet]. Atlanta, GA: Centers for Disease Control and Prevention (CDC); 2007–2008 [updated 2008; accessed 2008 Mar 10]. Available at www.cdc.gov/vaccines/.
  - ‣ Portal for national immunization program for lay and health professional target audiences. Essential for keeping up-to-date with the most current recommendations. Full of educational materials and useful links.
- Vaccination information for healthcare professionals [home page on internet]. St. Paul, MN: Immunization Action Coalition (IAC); [2008; accessed 2008 Mar 10]. Available at www.immunize.org/.
  - ‣ Portal for health professionals. This nonprofit collaborator with the CDC provides camera-ready immunization information and educational materials, copyright free. Their Ask the Experts section is particularly useful for hard-to-find information. Sign up to get their newsletters or listservs.
- Look for your local state or regional health division's immunization program web page.
  - ‣ These sites usually have a health care provider portal with useful information such as pharmacy protocols for immunization and model standing orders (e.g., www.oregon.gov/DHS/ph/imm/). These Web sites are also where local VFC vaccine program and ordering information is usually found.

Vaccine Handling and Storage

- Centers for Disease Control and Prevention (CDC). Vaccine Management:

  Recommendations for Storage and Handling of Selected Biologicals [book on internet]. Nov 2007 [accessed 2008 Mar]; [about 20 pp.]. Available at www.cdc.gov/vaccines/pubs/vac-mgt-book.htm.
  - ‣ Provides shipping requirements; condition on arrival; storage requirements; shelf life; instructions for reconstitution and use; shelf life after reconstitution, thawing. and opening; and any special instructions for all recommended vaccines.
- National Center for Immunization and Respiratory Diseases. Vaccine storage and handling toolkit [home page on internet]. Atlanta, GA: Centers for Disease Control and Prevention (CDC). 2008 [2008 Apr; accessed 2008 Oct 19]. Available at http://www.2a.cdc.gov/vaccines/ed/shtoolkit/.

Role of Pharmacists

- American Society of Health-Systems Pharmacists. ASHP guidelines on the pharmacist's role in immunization [guideline on internet]. 2003 [accessed 2008 Oct 19]; [about 6 pp.]. Available at http://www.ashp.org/Doclibrary/BestPractices/ASHPGuidelinesPharmacistsRolein-Immunization.aspx.

Establishing a Vaccine Practice

- Centers for Disease Control (CDC). Immunization practice toolkit [Web-based program]. Sept 2004 [updated 2007; accessed 2008 March 10]. Available at www.cdc.gov/vaccines/ed/self-study.htm#12.
  - ‣ This tool kit provides a compilation of resources for health care personnel who provide or are planning to provide immunization services. Includes sections such as clinic operations, client education, and quality assurance in addition to basics of immunization delivery.
- Hogue MD. Incorporating adult immunization services into community pharmacy practice. Pharmacy Times [continuing education on the internet] Princeton, NJ: Ascend Media; 2007 [updated 2008; accessed 2008 Mar 10]. Available at https://secure.pharmacytimes.com/lessons/200707-02.asp.
  - ‣ Excellent overview of key aspects for practitioners interested in beginning to offer immunization services in community pharmacy practice.

Publications for Purchase or Subscription

- Grabenstein JD. *Immunofacts: Vaccines and Immunologic Drugs*. 6th ed. St. Louis, MO: Wolters Kluwer Health; 2008.
  - Most detailed, up-to-date reference book available on immunologic drugs.
- American Pharmacists Association. Pharmacy-based immunization delivery: a certificate program for pharmacists [self-study and live seminar continuing education program]. 2008 [updated 2008; accessed 2008 March 10] Available at www.pharmacist.com/AM/Template. cfm?Section=Upcoming_Sessions&Template=/CM/HTMLDisplay. cfm&ContentID=13232.
  - National leader in pharmacist and pharmacy student vaccination certification.
  - APhA-ASP collaboratively developed the Operation Immunization Program promoting vaccination and administering vaccines at health fairs, community pharmacies, and student health–sponsored events that many students may be familiar with.

▣ Adult Preventative Health (non–vaccine-related)

Nationwide Health Promotion

- Various programs and initiatives exist to promote the importance of disease prevention and screening to individuals and health care professionals, and also to eliminate health disparities. Of those most pertinent to pharmacy professionals, two are particularly highlighted:
  - Healthy People 2010—sponsored by The Office of Disease Prevention and Health Promotion. The American College of Clinical Pharmacy (ACCP) produced a white paper calling for pharmacist support in 2004.[14]
  - Health-system Pharmacy 2015 is an initiative from the American Society of Health-system Pharmacists designed to enhance pharmacy practice in health systems, including the adoption of evidence-based health screening and pharmacotherapy.[15]

Evidence-Based Recommendations

- The Agency for Healthcare Research and Quality (AHRQ) subgroup, U.S. Preventative Services Task Force (USPSTF) publishes recommendations for preventative services[16] that are updated periodically on almost sixty different health care concerns. Major USPSTF recommendations are summarized in the tables that follow.

- It is important to note that health screening recommendations assume a patient is asymptomatic. The presence of symptoms moves a patient from the arena of health screening into disease-specific therapy, which is outside the scope of this chapter.
- The recommendations included in this section are associated with the requisite USPSTF grading classifications (A, B, C, D, I), as follows:
  - A—The USPSTF strongly recommends that clinicians provide health screening to eligible patients. The USPSTF found at least fair evidence that the screening method improves important health outcomes and concludes that benefits substantially outweigh harms.
  - B—The USPSTF recommends that clinicians provide health screening to eligible patients. The USPSTF found at least fair evidence that the screening method improves important health outcomes and concludes that benefits outweigh harms.
  - C—The USPSTF makes no recommendation for or against routine provision of health screening. The USPSTF found at least fair evidence that the screening method can improve health outcomes but concludes that the balance of benefits and harms is too close to justify a general recommendation.
  - D—The USPSTF recommends against routinely providing health screening to asymptomatic patients. The USPSTF found at least fair evidence that the screening method is ineffective or that harms outweigh benefits.
  - I—The USPSTF concludes that the evidence is insufficient to recommend for or against routinely providing health screening. Evidence that the screening method is effective is lacking, of poor quality, or conflicting, and the balance of benefits and harms cannot be determined.

General Adult Heath Screening

Table 19.11 provides a summary of the major health screening recommendations for adult males and females.

Female-Specific Health Screening

Table 19.12 summarizes the health screening recommendations for adult females. Health screening recommendations specifically for pregnant women are presented in Table 19.13.

Table 19.11 GENERAL ADULT HEALTH SCREENING RECOMMENDATIONS SUMMARY

Health Screening Area (Internet Citation(s))	Summary of Key Recommendations	Release Date

Colorectal cancer Screening for colorectal cancer, topic page. July 2002. U.S. Preventive Services Task Force. Agency for Healthcare Research and Quality, Rockville, MD www.ahrq.gov/clinic/uspstf/uspscolo.htm healthfinder: www.healthfinder.gov National Cancer Institute: National Institutes of Health; www.nci.nih.gov	• Class A Recommendation:
	  ○ Screen men and women aged 50 years or older, at average risk
	  ○ Periodic fecal occult blood testing of stool
	  ○ Sigmoidoscopy
		2002

Diabetes mellitus Screening for type 2 Diabetes mellitus in adults, topic page. February 2003. U.S. Preventive Services Task Force. Agency for Healthcare Research and Quality, Rockville, MD www.ahrq.gov/clinic/uspstf/uspsdiab.htm American Diabetes Association: care.diabetesjournals.org/cgi/content/extract/31/Supplement_1/S12	• Class B recommendation
	  ○ Screen adults with hypertension or hyperlipidemia
	• Expert opinion
	  ○ The American Diabetes Association (ADA) recommends[17]
	    • Also screening patients with a body mass index (BMI) ≥ 25 kg/m^2
	    • Using fasting plasma glucose (FPG test) with a threshold of >126 mg/dL glucose for screening, followed by confirmatory test for positive screening results using repeat FPG on a different day.
	    • Screening every 3 y (or more frequently for high-risk individuals)
		2003*

Hypertension U.S. Preventive Services Task Force. Screening for High Blood Pressure: Clinical Summary of U.S. Preventive Services Task Force Recommendation. December 2007. Agency for Healthcare Research and Quality, Rockville, MD	• Class A recommendation ○ Screen adults for hypertension (defined as: systolic blood pressure (SBP) of ≥ 140 mm Hg, or, diastolic blood pressure (DBP) of ≥ 90 mm Hg after two or more elevated readings obtained on at least two visits spanning at least 1 to several weeks	2007

(continued)

Table 19.11 GENERAL ADULT HEALTH SCREENING RECOMMENDATIONS SUMMARY *(continued)*

Health Screening Area (Internet Citation(s))	Summary of Key Recommendations	Release Date

www.ahrq.gov/clinic/uspstf07/hbp/hbpsum.htm
www.nhlbi.nih.gov/guidelines/hypertension/jnc7full.htm
	• The Seventh Report of the Joint National Committee on Prevention, Detection, Evaluation, and Treatment of High Blood Pressure[18] (JNC 7) recommends screening:
	  ○ Every 2 years with BP <120/80, or,
	  ○ Every year with SBP of 120–139 mm Hg or DBP of 80–90 mm Hg
	• Expert opinion/2003	

Lipids
Screening for lipid disorders in adults, topic page. March 2001. U.S. Preventive Services Task Force. Agency for Healthcare Research and Quality, Rockville, MD www.ahrq.gov/clinic/uspstf/uspschol.htm
Third Report of the National Cholesterol Education Program (NCEP) Expert Panel on Detection, Evaluation, and Treatment of High Blood Cholesterol in Adults (Adult Treatment Panel III). www.nhlbi.nih.gov/guidelines/cholesterol/atp3full.pdf
	• Class A recommendation
	  ○ Men aged 20–35 years and women aged 20–45 years in the presence of any of the following:
	    • Diabetes
	    • A family history of cardiovascular disease before age 50 years in male relatives or age 60 years in female relatives
	    • A family history suggestive of familial hyperlipidemia
	    • Multiple coronary heart disease risk factors
	  ○ Screen for elevated total cholesterol (TC) and decreased high-density lipoprotein cholesterol (HDLc) based on fasting or non-fasting samples
	• Expert opinion
	  ○ The National Cholesterol Education Program[19] (NCEP) Adult Treatment Panel III recommends screening every 5 years, or more frequently for patients with lipid levels approaching treatment threshold
		2001*

Table 19.11 GENERAL ADULT HEALTH
SCREENING RECOMMENDATIONS
SUMMARY *(continued)*

Health Screening Area (Internet Citation(s))	Summary of Key Recommendations	Release Date
Obesity Screening and interventions to prevent obesity in adults, topic page. December 2003. U.S. Preventive Services Task Force. Agency for Healthcare Research and Quality, Rockville, MD www.ahrq.gov/clinic/uspstf/uspsobes.htm	• Class B recommendation ○ Screen for obesity (defined as BMI ≥ 30 kg/m^2)	2003
Oral cancer Screening for oral cancer, topic page. February 2004. U.S. Preventive Services Task Force. Agency for Healthcare Research and Quality, Rockville, MD www.ahrq.gov/clinic/uspstf/uspsoral.htm	• Class I recommendation ○ No evidence to support routine screening	2004
Skin cancer Screening for skin cancer, topic page. April 2001. U.S. Preventive Services Task Force. Agency for Healthcare Research and Quality, Rockville, MD www.ahrq.gov/clinic/uspstf/uspsskca.htm	• Class I recommendation ○ No evidence to support routine screening	2001*
Thyroid cancer Screening for thyroid cancer, topic page. U.S. Preventive Services Task Force. Agency for Healthcare Research and Quality, Rockville, MD www.ahrq.gov/clinic/uspstf/uspsthca.htm	• New evidence currently under examination. Revised recommendations to be published	1996*
Tobacco use Counseling to prevent tobacco use and tobacco-caused disease, topic page. November 2003. U.S. Preventive Services Task Force. Agency for Healthcare Research and Quality, Rockville, MD www.ahrq.gov/clinic/uspstf/uspstbac.htm	• Class A recommendation ○ Screen for tobacco use	2003

*Update in progress.

Table 19.12 FEMALE-SPECIFIC HEALTH SCREENING

Health Screening Area (Internet Citation(s))	Summary of Key Recommendations	Release Date
Breast cancer Screening for breast cancer, topic page. November 2003. U.S. Preventive Services Task Force. Agency for Healthcare Research and Quality, Rockville, MD www.ahrq.gov/clinic/uspstf/uspsbrca.htm	• Class B recommendation ○ Screening mammography, with or without clinical breast examination (CBE), every 1–2 years for women aged 40 years and older	2002

Cervical cancer
Screening for cervical cancer, topic page. January 2003. U.S. Preventive Services Task Force. Agency for Healthcare Research and Quality, Rockville, MD
www.ahrq.gov/clinic/uspstf/uspscerv.htm
	• Class A recommendation
	  ○ Screen all females with a cervix who are sexually active with cervical cytology (Pap smears) at least every 3 y.
	  ○ Begin screening within 3 y. of onset of sexual activity or age 21 (whichever comes first)
		2003

Chlamydial infection
Screening for chlamydial infection, topic page. June 2007. U.S. Preventive Services Task Force. Agency for Healthcare Research and Quality, Rockville, MD
www.ahrq.gov/clinic/uspstf/uspschlm.htm
	• Class A recommendation
	  ○ Screen for chlamydial infection:
	    • All sexually active nonpregnant young women aged 24 y and younger
	    • Women 25 y or older who are not pregnant but are at increased risk (previous chlamydial infection or other sexually transmitted infections, new or multiple sexual partners, inconsistent condom use, sex work)
		2007

Osteoporosis Screening for osteoporosis, topic page. September 2002. U.S. Preventive Services Task Force. Agency for Healthcare Research and Quality, Rockville, MD www.ahrq.gov/clinic/uspstf/uspsoste.htm	• Class B recommendation ○ Screen women aged 65 y and older for osteoporosis (or age 60 y if at increased risk for osteoporotic fractures, such as body weight <70 kg, no current estrogen therapy use, use of certain medications associated with increased osteoporosis risk)	2002

Table 19.13 PREGNANCY-SPECIFIC HEALTH SCREENING

Health Screening Area (Internet Citation(s))	Summary of Key Recommendations	Release Date
Alcohol misuse Screening and behavioral counseling interventions in primary care to reduce alcohol misuse, topic page. April 2004. U.S. Preventive Services Task Force. Agency for Healthcare Research and Quality, Rockville, MD www.ahrq.gov/clinic/uspstf/uspsdrin.htm	• Class B recommendation ○ Screen for alcohol misuse and provide behavioral counseling interventions	2004
Bacteriuria Screening for asymptomatic bacteriuria, topic page. February 2004. U.S. Preventive Services Task Force. Agency for Healthcare Research and Quality, Rockville, MD www.ahrq.gov/clinic/uspstf/uspsbact.htm	• Class B recommendation ○ Screen for asymptomatic bacteriuria with urine culture at 12–16 weeks' gestation	2004
Chlamydial infection Screening for chlamydial infection, topic page. June 2007. U.S. Preventive Services Task Force. Agency for Healthcare Research and Quality, Rockville, MD www.ahrq.gov/clinic/uspstf/uspschlm.htm	• Class B recommendation ○ Screen all pregnant women aged 24 y and younger ○ Screen pregnant women aged older than 24 y if at increased risk for a chlamydial infection (previous chlamydial infection or other sexually transmitted infections, new or multiple sexual partners, inconsistent condom use, sex work) ○ The first screening should occur at the first prenatal visit. Women at continued risk or acquiring new risk factors should receive a second screening during the third trimester	2007

(continued)

Table 19.13 PREGNANCY-SPECIFIC HEALTH SCREENING *(continued)*

Health Screening Area (Internet Citation(s))	Summary of Key Recommendations	Release Date
Gonorrhea infection Screening for gonorrhea, topic page. May 2005. U.S. Preventive Services Task Force. Agency for Healthcare Research and Quality, Rockville, MD www.ahrq.gov/clinic/uspstf/uspsgono.htm	• Class B recommendation ○ Screen for gonorrhea infection in high-risk pregnant women (history of previous gonorrhea infection, other sexually transmitted infections, new or multiple sexual partners, inconsistent condom use, sex work, and drug use). The first screening should occur at the first prenatal visit. Women at continued risk or acquiring new risk factors should receive a second screening during the third trimester	2005
Hepatitis B virus infection (HBV) Screening for hepatitis B infection, topic page. February 2004. U.S. Preventive Services Task Force. Agency for Healthcare Research and Quality, Rockville, MD www.ahrq.gov/clinic/uspstf/uspshepb.htm	• Class A recommendation ○ Screen all pregnant women for HBV at first prenatal visit	2004
HIV infection Human immunodeficiency virus infection, topic page. April 2007. U.S. Preventive Services Task Force. Agency for Healthcare Research and Quality, Rockville, MD www.ahrq.gov/clinic/uspstf/uspshivi.htm	• Class A recommendation ○ Screen all pregnant women for HIV infection	2007
Rh(D) incompatibility Screening for Rh (D) incompatibility, topic page. February 2004. U.S. Preventive Services Task Force. Agency for Healthcare Research and Quality, Rockville, MD www.ahrq.gov/clinic/uspstf/uspsdrhi.htm	• Class B recommendation ○ Complete Rh(D) blood typing and antibody testing for all pregnant women during their first visit for pregnancy-related care	2004

(continued)

Table 19.13 PREGNANCY-SPECIFIC HEALTH SCREENING (continued)

Health Screening Area (Internet Citation(s))	Summary of Key Recommendations	Release Date
Iron deficiency anemia Screening for iron deficiency anemia, topic page. May 2006 U.S. Preventive Services Task Force. Agency for Healthcare Research and Quality, Rockville, MD www.ahrq.gov/clinic/uspstf/uspsiron.htm	• Class B recommendation ○ Screen all pregnant women for iron deficiency anemia	2006
Syphilis infection Screening for syphilis infection, topic page. July 2004. U.S. Preventive Services Task Force. Agency for Healthcare Research and Quality, Rockville, MD www.ahrq.gov/clinic/uspstf/uspssyph.htm	• Class A recommendation ○ Screen all pregnant women for syphilis infection	2004
Tobacco use Counseling to prevent tobacco use and tobacco-caused disease, topic page. November 2003. U.S. Preventive Services Task Force. Agency for Healthcare Research and Quality, Rockville, MD www.ahrq.gov/clinic/uspstf/uspstbac.htm	• Class A recommendation ○ Screen all pregnant women for tobacco use and provide augmented pregnancy-tailored counseling to those who smoke	2003

Table 19.14 MALE-SPECIFIC HEALTH SCREENING

Health Screening Area (Internet Citation(s))	Summary of Key Recommendations	Release Date
Prostate cancer Screening for prostate cancer, topic page. December 2002. U.S. Preventive Services Task Force. Agency for Healthcare Research and Quality, Rockville, MD www.ahrq.gov/clinic/uspstf/uspsprca.htm	• Class I recommendation ○ There is insufficient evidence to recommend for or against routine screening for prostate cancer using prostate-specific antigen (PSA) testing or digital rectal examination (DRE)	2002
Testicular cancer Screening for testicular cancer, topic page. February 2004. U.S. Preventive Services Task Force. Agency for Healthcare Research and Quality, Rockville, MD www.ahrq.gov/clinic/uspstf/uspstest.htm	• Class D recommendation ○ There is insufficient evidence to recommend routine screening	2004

Male-Specific Health Screening

Health screening recommendations specifically for adult males are covered in Table 19.14.

References

1. Goode JV, Gatewood SBS. Update on vaccines and vaccine-preventable diseases. In: Dunsworth T, Richardson M, Chant C, et al, eds. *Pharmacotherapy Self-Assessment Program.* 6th ed. Lenexa, KS: American College of Clinical Pharmacy, 2008:55–71.

2. Kamal KM, Madhavan SS, Maine LL. Impact of the American Pharmacists Association's (APhA) immunization training certification program. *Am J Pharm Educ.* 2003;67(4):1–10.

3. Centers for Disease Control and Prevention. Principles of vaccination. In: Atkinson W, Hamborsky J, McIntyre L, Wolfe S, eds. Epidemiology and Prevention of Vaccine-Preventable Diseases (The Pink Book). 10th ed. Washington, DC: Public Health Foundation; 2007.

4. Centers for Disease Control and Prevention. General recommendations on immunization. In: Atkinson W, Hamborsky J, McIntyre L, Wolfe S, eds. Epidemiology and Prevention of Vaccine-Preventable Diseases (The Pink Book). 10th ed. Washington, DC: Public Health Foundation; 2007.

5. Grabenstein JD. *Immunofacts: Vaccines and Immunologic Drugs.* 6th ed. St. Louis, MO: Wolters Kluwer Health; 2008.

6. Results for ISMP survey on vaccine abbreviation use. Oct 2003, Available at www.ismp.org/Survey/surveyresults/SurveyHosp.asp. Accessed March 10, 2008.

7. ISMP Medication Safety Alert! ISMP quarterly action agenda: July–September 2003. Oct 2003. Available at www.ismp.org/Newsletters/acutecare/articles/A4Q03Action.asp?ptr=y. Accessed March 10, 2008.

8. The Joint Commission. "Do not use list": facts about the official "do not use" list. Jan 2007. Available at www.jointcommission.org/PatientSafety/DoNotUseList/facts_dnu.htm. Accessed March 10, 2008.

9. Centers for Disease Control and Prevention. Instructions for the use of Vaccine Information Statements. Feb 6, 2008, Available at www.cdc.gov/vaccines/pubs/vis/downloads/vis-Instructions.pdf. Accessed March 15, 2008.

10. Centers for Disease Control and Prevention. Vaccine administration. In: Atkinson W, Hamborsky J, McIntyre L, Wolfe S, eds. Epidemiology and Prevention of Vaccine-Preventable Diseases (The Pink Book). 10th ed. Washington, DC: Public Health Foundation; 2007.

11. Centers for Disease Control and Prevention. Vaccine safety. In: Atkinson W, Hamborsky J, McIntyre L, Wolfe S, eds. Epidemiology and Prevention of Vaccine-Preventable Diseases (The Pink Book). 10th ed. Washington, DC: Public Health Foundation; 2007.

12. American Society of Health-System Pharmacists. ASHP guidelines on the pharmacist's role in immunization. *Am J Health-Syst Pharm.* 2003;60:1371–1377.

13. Hogue MD. Incorporating adult immunization services into community pharmacy practice. *Pharmacy Times.* Princeton, NJ: Ascend Media; 2007 [updated 2008]. Available at secure.pharmacytimes.com/lessons/200707-02.asp. Accessed March 10, 2008.

14. Calis KA, Hutchison LC, Elliott ME, et al. Healthy People 2010: challenges, opportunities, and a call to action for America's pharmacists. *Pharmacotherapy*. 2004;24(9):1241–1294.

15. American Society for Health-System Pharmacists. Health-system Pharmacy 2015. Apr 2007. Available at www.ashp.org/s_ashp/cat1c.asp?CID=218&DID=255. Accessed March 18, 2008.

16. The Agency for Healthcare Research and Quality (AHRQ), U.S. Preventive Services Task Force. Sep 2007. Available at www.ahrq.gov/clinic/uspstf/uspstopics.htm. Accessed March 21, 2008.

17. American Diabetes Association. Diagnosis and classification of diabetes mellitus. *Diabetes Care*. 2007;30:S42–47.

18. Chobanian AV, Bakris GL, Black HR, et al., and the National High Blood Pressure Education Program Coordinating Committee. The seventh report of the Joint National Committee on Prevention, Detection, Evaluation, and Treatment of High Blood Pressure: the JNC 7 report. *JAMA*. 2003 May 21;289:2560–2572.

19. Expert Panel on Detection, Evaluation, and Treatment of High Blood Cholesterol in Adults. Executive summary of the third report of the National Cholesterol Education Program (NCEP) Expert Panel on Detection, Evaluation, and Treatment of High Blood Cholesterol in Adults (Adult Treatment Panel III). *JAMA*. 2001;285:2486–2497.

20

Patient Safety

Susan M. Stein

Ensuring patient safety is the goal of all health care professionals. It is the responsibility of each health care professional to educate, review, and promote patient safety in all venues at all times. A report by the Institute of Medicine in 2000 released the following figures: An estimated 44,000 to 98,000 deaths occur per year due to medical errors, equated to a jumbo jet crashing each day. The report brought patient safety to the forefront of the public domain, and it has remained there since.[1,2] This chapter is designed to provide tools to promote patient safety.

Patient Safety

Patient safety is ensured in absence of medical error or accidental injury. Medical errors can be described as errors, misadventures, or variances or system failures. An error can be defined as an unintended act or an act that doesn't achieve its intended outcome. Harm may or may not be the result. Additionally, a close call or near miss is encouraged to be included in error analysis.[1-3]

Medication Errors

Defining types of errors can be useful in analysis and system redesign. The following is a list of types of medication errors compiled by the American Society of Health-Systems Pharmacists (ASHP):[4]

1. Prescribing error: incorrect drug, dose, route, or formulation was pre-scribed. This can include prescribing a drug the patient is allergic to

2. Omission error: missed dose
3. Wrong time error: not administered within a predetermined length of time to the intended dosing time
4. Unauthorized drug error: drug not prescribed was administered
5. Improper dose error: dose different than prescribed was administered
6. Wrong dosage form error: dosage form different than prescribed was administered
7. Wrong drug preparation error: drug preparation or compounding error
8. Wrong administration technique: route or rate different than prescribed or recommended
9. Deteriorated drug error: expired or deteriorated drug administered
10. Monitoring error: interaction or adverse event occurs due to lack of monitoring
11. Compliance error: patient adherence incorrect

Report Error, Analyze Error, and Improve the System

Report Error

Improving patient safety is dependent on sharing close calls or errors that have occurred. By sharing details with others, future errors can be prevented or a deficient device can be identified and patient safety improved. This can be done using various resources listed below:

- US Pharmacopeia (USP)-ISMP Medication Errors Reporting Program (MERP).
  - www.ismp.org/orderforms/reporterrortoISMP.asp.
  - Operated by the USP and Institute for Safe Medication Practices (ISMP), MERP is a repository of medication errors. If appropriate, the information is shared with FDA and drug manufacturers. The reporter's name and affiliation are kept confidential unless permission is granted.
- Food and Drug Administration (FDA) MedWatch.
  - www.fda.gov/medwatch/.
  - Maintained by the FDA, MedWatch provides another opportunity to report problems with medications or devices. Also links to manufacturers, provides alerts, recalls, and reports when appropriate to health care professionals and the public.

Analyze Error

The most common cause of error is in the medication process itself, and careful analysis of the process can increase safety and reliability of the system. Some tools used to analyze errors are the following:

Root Cause Analysis (RCA)

This tool is used to analyze an error after it has occurred and learn from it. The basic steps used in this process are as follows:

- Describe the event—the details (when, where, how, who was involved, etc.) of the event. Collecting the information includes a meeting with all individuals involved and a facilitator. Descriptions of the event are documented in detail. White boards, sticky sheets/notes, and visual aids help identify the order of events accurately, for example, if a patient received the wrong dose of a drug, from during the evening shift on the postsurgical floor.
- Identify the proximate cause—all the actions that occurred that led to the error and often explain why it happened. In the situation of the wrong dose mentioned above, the proximate causes could be the order was written illegibly, the order was entered incorrectly, was made incorrectly, delivered to the wrong patient, and so on.
- Identify the contributing factors—factors that increase the potential for an action to be a proximate cause. Some examples include staffing shortages, poor lighting, malfunctioning technology, incorrect spelling, and so on.
- Create an action plan—the most important step. The action plan is created to decrease the potential for proximate causes in the future. The goal is to redesign the system to avoid a recurrence.

Failure Mode Effects and Analysis (FMEA)

Another technique helpful in improving systems is a proactive tool called FMEA. What-if scenerios are analyzed to identify weak links in the system. Analysis of likely errors and steps to prevent them or limit their effects are introduced into the system. The process includes the following:[2]

- Identify each step in the process or system.
- Identify failure modes or "What could go wrong?"
- Identify failure causes or "What could cause the failure to occur?"
- Identify failure effects or "What would be the consequence of this failure?"

- Identify the likelihood of failure effects or "What is the most likely error?"
- Identify the likelihood of detection of failure.
- Modify the system to prevent the most serious and most common errors.

Improve the System

Creating systems and following step-by-step processes decrease the potential for error. This can be viewed as mistake-proofing the system.[2] Continual evaluation to improve systems to maximize efficiency and quality of care is an overarching goal. Involving all interested stakeholders in the development process results in broad support and ultimate success.

Examples of systems to increase patient safety include the following:[2,7,8]

- Patient confirmation.
    - Verbalize the patient's name, procedure to be completed, or medication to be administered when possible.
- Preprinted orders.
    - Use preprinted order sets, which provide standardized drugs and dosages, administration routes and rates, and so on.
    - Example: postsurgery orders for orthopedic patients.
- Standardization.
    - Use standardized drug concentrations, which limit variation in drug concentrations available. Dosage adjustment is obtained via altering rate of administration.
    - Examples: heparin, 25,000 units in 500 mL 0.9% sodium chloride; dopamine, 250 mg in 250 mL 0.9% sodium chloride.
    - Use standardized procedures or drugs available for use in a patient care setting.
    - Use standardized available generic companies to ensure quality drug formulation.
- Read back order confirmation.
    - Verbally read back an order received orally that has been transcribed to writing prior to completing verbal conversation.
- Use two- or three-person drug order or calculation confirmation.
    - Require double signature for all chemotherapy orders.
    - Require triple sign-off system for all surgery patients to confirm procedure type, correct patient, correct limb, and so on.

- Read three times.
  - Read the drug name three times prior to dispensing the drug to the patient.
- Use bar-coding bracelets.
  - Bar-code swipe prior to medication administration to confirm correct drug for correct patient.
- Use color-coding systems.
  - Use color-coded bracelet to identify patients with specific drug, food, or latex allergies in a health care facility.
  - Use color-coded patient slippers to identify fall-risk patients.
  - Use color-coded drug labels to delineate different drug names or concentrations.
- The five rights.
  - Right drug, right dose, right route, right time, right patient.

Culture of Safety

Establishing a culture of safety to support patient safety is critical. The culture of safety acknowledges that everyone on the health care team shares responsibility to maintain and support patient safety. It acknowledges an open environment to discuss patient safety and de-emphasizes enforcing safety through punitive tactics. The culture of safety supports open discussion and incentives for system analysis and improvement. A decrease in reporting and improvement in the system is seen in a punitive environment.[9]

Our limitations as human beings are important to recognize and acknowledge. Despite the best of intentions, we do make mistakes. Additionally, patients expect us to perform without error. These conditions work in unison to increase the pressure on health care providers to perform. The best tool to aid in preventing this vicious cycle is to embrace a culture of safety.[5]

The following are examples of expectations and limitations:

- Recognize the patient, his or her rights and expectations.
  - Be cognizant of working with patients as human beings.
  - Patients expect safety at all times.
- Recognize the limitations of our abilities as human beings to work errorfree.
  - Human beings make mistakes.

Useful Web Sites and Highlights

- Institute of Safe Medical Practices.
  - www.ismp.org/.
  - Independent nonprofit agency serving as a repository of medication alerts.
  - Resources.
    - High alert list.
    - Error-prone abbreviations.
    - Do Not Crush list.
- National Patient Safety Organization.
  - www.npsf.org/.
  - Independent nonprofit with goal of improving patient safety.
  - Resources.
    - Online patient safety resources: www.npsf.org/rc/mp/opsr/.
- Institute for Healthcare Improvement.
  - www.ihi.org/IHI/Topics/PatientSafety/.
  - Independent nonprofit agency focused on improving healthcare worldwide.
  - Resources.
    - Patient safety.
    - Reducing mortality.
- Joint Commission of Accreditation of Healthcare Organizations (JCAHO).
  - www.jointcommission.org/PatientSafety/.
  - Independent for-profit agency providing accreditation to healthcare organizations.
  - Resources.
    - National patient safety goals.
    - Infection control.
    - Speak up initiatives.
    - Universal protocol for preventing wrong site, wrong procedure, wrong person surgery.
- Agency for Healthcare Research and Quality (AHRQ).
  - www.ahrq.gov/.
  - Federal agency within the Department of Health and Human Services responsible for improving the safety and efficacy of health care.
  - Resources.
    - Patient fact sheet: five steps to safer health care www.ahrq.gov/consumer/5steps.htm.

- National Center for Patient Safety (NCPS).
  - /www.patientsafety.gov/index.html.
  - Federal organization serving the Veterans Health Administration in promoting patient safety.
  - Resources.
    - Provides links to other national and international Web resources.

Summary

Frequent monitoring of primary literature and patient safety Web sites is advised to produce a valuable collection of resources. Use them wisely and often. Remain vigilant. Do not become apathetic, overconfident, or distracted. Remember, compromises to patient safety are often the result of poorly designed systems or failure to follow procedures.

References

1. Kohn L, Corrigan J, Donaldson M, eds. *To Err Is Human: Building a Safer Health System.* Washington, DC: Committee on Quality of Health Care in America, Institute of Medicine. National Academy Press; 2000.
2. Cohen MR, ed. *Medication Errors.* Washington, DC: American Pharmacists Association (APhA); 2007. Patient Safety. Institute for Healthcare Improvement. www.ihi.org/IHI/Topics/PatientSafety/. Accessed December 26, 2007.
3. Botwinick L, Bisognano M, Haraden C. Leadership Guide to Patient Safety. IHI Innovation Series white paper. Cambridge, MA: Institute for Healthcare Improvement; 2006. Available at www.IHI.org.
4. American Society of Hospital Pharmacists. ASHP guidelines on preventing medication errors in hospitals. *Am J Hosp Pharm.* 1993;50:305–314.
5. Patient Safety. Institute for Healthcare Improvement. www.ihi.org/IHI/Topics/PatientSafety/. Accessed December 26, 2007.
6. Grout J. Mistake-Proofing the Design of Health Care Processes. (Prepared under an IPA with Berry College). AHRQ Publication No. 07-0020. Rockville, MD: Agency for Healthcare Research and Quality; May 2007.
7. Institute for Safe Medication Practices. The "five rights." 1999 Aug 17. Available at www.ismp.org/MSAarticles/FiveRights.htm.
8. Cohen MR, Smetzer JL. Lack of standard dosing methods contribute to IV errors. *Hosp Pharm.* 2007;42(12):1100–1101.
9. McIntyre N, Popper K. The critical attitude in medicine: the need for a new ethics. *Br Med J (Clin Res Ed).*1989;287:1919–1923.

21 The Law and the Clinical Practice of Pharmacy

William E. Fassett

The Law's Proper Place in Clinical Decision Making

If pharmacists think about the law at all during their daily work, many do so by asking the question, "What does the law allow me to do for this patient?" This is a good question, but it must not be the first question asked in any clinical situation. This chapter begins with the assertion that the first question to be considered in any patient clinical encounter is "What does this patient need from me at this time to ensure optimal outcomes from his or her drug therapy?"

Many pharmacists who engage in a formal evaluation of a patient's care needs do so using a structured documentation process and format developed for use in the Problem-Oriented Medical Record.[1] Known by the acronym SOAP, standing for Subjective, Objective, Assessment, and Plan, each of its elements is intended to help organize the medical record. However, SOAP also serves as a process for clinical decision making. Although it has been criticized as the ideal approach to clinical diagnosis,[2,3] it remains widely taught in U.S. doctor of pharmacy programs. So, we start by using the SOAP outline to summarize the points at which legal considerations may arise during clinical decision making in Table 21.1.

Note how late in the process it is before most legal limitations appear as possible considerations. To reiterate, pharmacists are not lawyers, but primary care providers; their first responsibility is to consider how best to meet patient needs, and then to make sure they are doing so in a legally appropriate manner.

Quite a few legal considerations arise as pharmacists are engaged in activities necessary to maintain their license to practice or for the operation

Table 21.1 SUMMARY OF LEGAL ISSUES ARISING DURING CLINICAL DECISION MAKING

SOAP Element	Typical Elements	Potential Legal Considerations
Subjective data	Chief complaint Patient's symptoms and feelings Patient's self-reported history	Does the pharmacist have permission to take or review history?
Objective data	Physical exam Laboratory data Diagnostic procedures Medication use record	Does the pharmacist have permission to examine the patient and/or permission to obtain records?
Assessment	Identify drug therapy–related problems For each problem, identify a desired outcome, expressed in measurable terms For each problem/outcome, list available therapeutic alternatives Rank available therapeutic alternatives	Has the pharmacist considered clinical, economic, and humanistic outcomes (particularly professional standards, quality of life, and moral and ethical issues) when ranking alternatives?
Plan	With patient, select preferred alternative Prepare patient to be able to adhere to plan Follow up	Has the pharmacist considered whether the plan can be legally implemented? What documentation or record-keeping requirements are essential to implementing the plan? If the pharmacist is acting as the prescribing practitioner, has he or she obtained informed consent from the patient?

of a practice site. However, this chapter focuses primarily on laws relating to the routine clinical functions needed to implement pharmaceutical care for specific patients.

How to Use This Chapter

The rest of this chapter consists primarily of summary tables. Every state must consider a set of important issues when it decides how pharmacy should be practiced within its borders. These decisions by the states interact with federal law governing drugs, devices, and controlled substances. The two most important federal laws are the Food, Drug, and Cosmetic Act (FDCA) and the Controlled Substances Act (CSA). In the following tables, federal law—where appropriate—is set out, and then typical options among the states are listed. The reader should identify those options chosen by his or her state, using the check boxes or the additional space provided.

Practice of Pharmacy

Pharmacists' Scope of Practice

State laws define the scope of practice of pharmacists. Table 21.2 summarizes the major functions of pharmacists allowed in the states. As of early 2008, 40 states allow some form of prescribing by pharmacists under protocol, and 45 permit pharmacists to administer drugs or at least some vaccines.[4]

Table 21.2 ACTIONS THE PHARMACIST MAY PERFORM

	Your State?	
	Yes	**No**
Interpreting prescription or orders for legend drugs and devices	*	
Compounding, packaging, labeling, and dispensing drugs	*	
Providing information on the hazards and uses of drugs	*	
Maintaining proper records of drugs purchased and dispensed	*	
Monitoring of drug therapy: May include ordering of laboratory tests, drug blood levels, and/or assessing vital signs. Note any special requirements:		
Administering drugs generally: "Administration" generally includes application of a drug to the body of a patient by injection, inhalation, ingestion, or other means	*	
Administering immunizations: Note any special requirements:	*	
Prescribing under protocol: Note any special requirements:	*	

*Allowed in most states.

Use of Pharmacy Technicians

Most states permit, either explicitly or implicitly, the use of ancillary personnel, such as pharmacy technicians, when under the direction of a pharmacist. Table 21.3 indicates typical activities that are allowed by pharmacy technicians.

Functions That Technicians May *Not* Perform

Many states are explicit concerning activities or decisions that must be performed by pharmacists (or interns) and may *not* be delegated to technicians. In most states, allowing a nonpharmacist to perform these functions is considered permitting the unlicensed practice of pharmacy and a cause for discipline. Table 21.4 lists functions that technicians are usually prohibited from undertaking.

Privileges of Pharmacy Interns

Intern pharmacists may generally perform any function that can be performed by pharmacists, while under a pharmacist's supervision. Some states are more restrictive than others regarding how closely interns must be supervised, and states interpret certain federal laws differently. For example, Drug Enforcement Administration (DEA) regulations governing transfer of refill information between pharmacies for Schedule III, IV, and V controlled substances specify that the transfer must be "communicated directly between two licensed pharmacists."[5] Boards of Pharmacy differ whether that phrase excludes interns from transferring controlled substances prescriptions. Table 21.5 lists some of the functions that may not be allowed in all states.

■ Dispensing or Delivering Prescription Drugs to Patients

Although distributive functions related to drug dispensing are increasingly being performed by technicians and with the aid of pharmacy automation, it remains a critical clinical responsibility of pharmacists to supervise the distribution system and to evaluate the appropriateness and correctness of every order or prescription that is processed for a patient.

Table 21.3 TYPICAL FUNCTIONS OF PHARMACY TECHNICIANS

	Your State?	
	Yes	**No**
Packaging, pouring, or placing drugs in containers for dispensing	*	
Reconstituting prescription medications subject to verification of accuracy	*	
Affixing required labels	*	
Entering information into the pharmacy computer subject to verification	*	
Prepackaging and labeling multidose and unit-dose packages, subject to verification	*	
Picking doses for unit-dose cart fill for hospital and nursing homes, subject to verification	*	
Recording patient or medication information in the computer subject to verification	*	
Bulk compounding subject to verification	*	
Reconstitution of single or multiple units that will be given to a patient as a single dose, subject to verification	*	
Addition of a single ingredient to a prepared unit of another drug, subject to verification	*	
Initiating or accepting oral or electronic refill information from prescribers that does not change the prescription in any way		
Mixing more than one ingredient into a parenteral medication, subject to verification		
Checking nursing units for nonjudgmental tasks such as sanitation and outdated medications, subject to pharmacist review of problems found		
Checking unit-dose medications in a tech-check-tech program		
Stocking of dispensing machines		
Are technicians required to pass national certifying exam?		
Are technicians required to have special training for any of the above functions?		
Is there a limit on the ratio of technicians to pharmacists in your state?		
Notes:		

*Allowed in most states.

Table 21.4 TYPICAL FUNCTIONS PROHIBITED TO BE PERFORMED BY PHARMACY TECHNICIANS

	Prohibited in Your State?	
	Yes	**No**
Receipt of a verbal prescription other than a refill authorization	*	
Receive or transfer a prescription to another pharmacy	*	
Provide a prescription or medication to a patient without a pharmacist's verification of accuracy of the prescription	*	
Deliver a prescription to the patient when the pharmacist is absent from the pharmacy	*	
Consultation with the patient regarding the prescription and/or regarding any information in the patient medication record	*	
Consultation with the prescriber regarding the patient and the patient's prescription	*	
Interpretation of the data in the patient medication record system	*	
Ultimate responsibility for the correctness of a dispensed prescription	*	
Signing of documents or registry books that require a pharmacist's signature	*	
Professional communications with physicians, dentists, nurses, and other health care practitioners	*	
Making the offer to counsel as required by OBRA-90		

*Prohibited in most states.

Requirements of a Valid Prescription

Dispensing or delivering prescription drugs in the absence of a legally valid order or prescription is prohibited by the federal Food, Drug, and Cosmetic Act, by the Controlled Substances Act, and by the laws of every state; it is called diversion. Table 21.6 summarizes the four conditions that are necessary to make a prescription valid.

Tamper-Proof Prescription Pads

Under a recent amendment to the U.S. Patriot Act, prescriptions written for Medicaid patients must be written on tamper-proof prescription pads,

Table 21.5 POSSIBLE STATE RESTRICTION OF INTERN'S ACTIVITIES

	Your State?	
	Yes	**No**
May interns transfer or receive transfers of prescriptions for controlled substances in Schedule III, IV, or V?		
May interns sign the log book for sale of OTC Schedule V drugs?		
Does the supervising pharmacist need to recheck every prescription filled by an intern?		
Are there other restrictions on what interns may do?		

effective April 1, 2008. This rule does not apply to Medicaid prescriptions that are faxed, telephoned, or electronically prescribed.

Illegible Prescriptions

Prescriptions that cannot be easily read and interpreted by pharmacists are legally invalid in several states, and in some states this rule applies to any prescription that is written in cursive handwriting. Pharmacists should always confirm with the prescriber the exact details of any prescription that is hard to read.

Table 21.6 FOUR QUESTIONS TO ASK BEFORE FILLING A PRESCRIPTION.

	Rx Checklist	
	Yes	**No**
Is it issued for a specific patient? Note: A prescription issued with "for office use" in the patient name field is not valid		
Is it issued by an authorized prescriber?		
Was it issued in the due course of the prescriber's professional practice? ↳ Did a bona fide physician–patient relationship exist? ↳ Is the prescription within the prescriber's scope of practice?		
Is it for a legitimate medical purpose?		

Note: If No for any question, then the prescription is not valid.

Legitimate Medical Purpose

In one sense, all that is needed to meet a legitimate medical purpose is that the prescriber intends the drug to treat a bona fide patient care need. If the pharmacist knows or should know that the intended use is for recreational drug use, or solely to maintain an addiction (exceptions are drugs dispensed as part of an opiod addiction treatment program), then the pharmacist cannot legally fill the prescription.

Unapproved Indications

Manufacturers may not promote drugs for any use not included in the approved package insert; however, practitioners may prescribe drugs for off-label uses for individual patients, and pharmacists may lawfully fill those prescriptions. Pharmacists may also dispense generic equivalents for uses that are indicated only in the labeling of the brand name drug (e.g., a prescription written generically for bupropion may be filled with a generic bupropion tablet for smoking cessation, even though only Zyban includes that indication in its approved labeling). Table 21.7 summarizes special situations regarding off-label use.

Required Information on Prescriptions

Certain elements must be present on a prescription at the time it is presented to a pharmacist. These generally require the date written; the name

Table 21.7 SPECIAL SITUATIONS REGARDING OFF-LABEL USE

	Rx Checklist	
	Yes	No
Is the prescription with an off-label use intended for a Medicare or Medicaid patient? ↳ If so, is the proposed use listed as a generally recognized use supported by evidence in USP-DI or AHFS? If No, don't fill. Note: if Yes, may require prior authorization		
Is the off-label use specifically prohibited by state law? If Yes, don't fill. ↳ C-II stimulants used for weight loss? Anabolic steroids used for muscle building?		
Is the prescription for a patient with third-party insurance and the intended use considered experimental? If Yes, may require prior authorization		

of the patient; the prescription itself, the name, address, and signature of the physician (if written); and, for controlled substances, the prescriber's DEA number. Other elements must be added and recorded when the prescription is filed in the pharmacy after dispensing. Table 21.8 summarizes these elements.

Table 21.8   ELEMENTS REQUIRED ON A FILLED PRESCRIPTION

	Your State?	
	Yes	**No**
Prescriber's name, address	* †††	
Patient's name	* †††	
Patient's address (on Rx or in the patient information system)	* ††	
Date written	* †††	
Name of drug, dosage form, strength, and quantity/duration of therapy	* †††	
Prescriber's directions to the patient	* †	
Signature of prescriber if it is a written Rx	* †††	
Prescriber's DEA number if it is for a controlled substance	* ††	
Specification regarding generic substitution		
Any refill information	*	
Any additional instructions	*	
A serial number placed by the pharmacist	* †	
The date filled	*	
The initials of the responsible pharmacist who filled the Rx	*	
The identity of the actual drug dispensed (e.g., NDC number)		
Other requirements in your state:		

DEA, Drug Enforcement Administration; NDC, National Drug Code.
*Required in most states,
†Required by the Food, Drug, and Cosmetic Act (FDCA).
††Required by the Controlled Substances Act (CSA).

Who May Prescribe Legend Drugs?

Under both the FDCA and the CSA, persons authorized to prescribe drugs are those individuals who are licensed by the jurisdiction in which they practice. All states license physicians, dentists, podiatrists, and veterinarians, and most states accept prescriptions written by these prescribers who practice outside the state. Midlevel practitioners, as they are called by the DEA, practice in most states, but their scope of practice varies. Therefore, out-of-state prescriptions from nurse practitioners, physician's assistants, optometrists, naturopaths, and pharmacists are not usually accepted. Table 21.9 summarizes the various health professionals who may prescribe drugs and devices in most states. The DEA maintains a summary of controlled substances prescribing privileges for midlevel practitioners on its Web site.[6]

 New and Refill Prescriptions

New Prescriptions

Many states make a distinction in their laws between "new" prescriptions and "refills." This is often especially important when interpreting the rules for patient counseling. Many pharmacists consider a new prescription to be one for a drug the patient has not received before. However, this is more properly seen as a new drug for the patient. Legally, a "new" prescription is one that requires the pharmacy to assign it a new prescription number. When prescriptions expire in accordance with the law, such as after 6 months for C-3 or C-4 drugs, they become "new" prescriptions when reauthorized by the prescriber.

Refill Prescriptions

Refills are repeated dispensing of a drug that uses the same prescription number as a previously-filled prescription. A prescription may be refilled if authorized by the prescriber, either at the time the prescription was first written, or later, as long as the prescription has not expired.

Prescription Invalidation

Prescriptions become invalid after some time period in most states. Most states set a limit on how long a prescription is valid after the date written (e.g., 1 year). Federal law limits refills on Schedule III and IV drugs to five refills within 6 months after the date written, but federal law does not

Table 21.9 PRESCRIPTIVE AUTHORITY OF VARIOUS HEALTH PROFESSIONALS

		Your State?	
		Yes	No
Physicians (MD or DO)	All drugs, all classes for human patients, regardless of where the prescriber is licensed	✓	
Dentists (DDS or DMD)	All drugs, all classes, for human patients for head and neck conditions, regardless of where the prescriber is licensed	✓	
Podiatrists (DPM or PodD)	All drugs, all classes, for human patients, for conditions of the ankles and feet, regardless of where the prescriber is licensed	✓	
Veterinarians (DVM)	All drugs, all classes, for non-human animals, regardless of where the prescriber is licensed	✓	
Midlevel Practitioners			
Nurse Practitioners (ARNP), Clinical Nurse Specialists (CNS)	Legend drugs if appropriate to the scope of specialty and practice, only in state where licensed	*	
	↳ C-II	*	
	↳ C-III, IV, V	*	
	↳ Independent practice	*	
Nurse Midwife (CNM) (An ARNP specialty in most states)	Legend if appropriate to the care of the preterm and postpartum patient, and the newborn, only in state where licensed	*	
	↳ C-II	*	
	↳ C-III, IV, V	*	
	↳ Independent practice	*	
Nurse Anesthetists (CRNA)	Most drugs if used for preanesthesia or during anesthesia, only in state where licensed	*	
	↳ C-II	*	
	↳ C-III, IV, V	*	
	↳ Independent practice		*
Physicians Assistants (PA, PA-C)	All drugs, all classes approved by supervising physician, only in state where licensed	*	
	↳ C-II	*	
	↳ C-III, IV, V	*	
	↳ Independent practice		*

(continued)

Table 21.9 PRESCRIPTIVE AUTHORITY OF VARIOUS HEALTH PROFESSIONALS (continued)

		Your State?	
		Yes	**No**
Optometrists (OD)	Legend drugs needed to screen for glaucoma, diagnosis, and treatment of minor ophthalmic conditions, only in state where licensed	*	
	↳ Topical ophthalmic drugs for diagnosis	*	
	↳ Oral and topical legend drugs used to treat ophthalmic conditions	*	
	↳ C-II within scope of practice		*
	↳ C-III within scope of practice	*	
	↳ C-IV within scope of practice	*	
	↳ C-V within scope of practice	*	
Naturopaths (ND)	Drug used in traditional naturopathic practice, which are usually limited to drugs derived from natural sources, only in state where licensed	*	
	↳ Homeopathic remedies, herbals	*	
	↳ Legend drugs		*
	↳ C-II within scope (e.g., codeine)		*
	↳ C-III or IV within scope (e.g., codeine, testosterone)		*
	↳ C-V within scope (e.g., codeine)		*
Licensed Midwife (not an ARNP)	May order and administer certain drugs used for delivery or neonatal care, may administer drugs ordered or prescribed for use in delivery, only in state where licensed	*	
	↳ May prescribe or dispense diaphragms	*	
	↳ May prescribe prenatal vitamins		*
	↳ May prescribe oral contraceptives		*
	↳ Independent practice	*	
Pharmacists	Prescribe legend under protocol, consistent with the scope of the authorizing prescriber, only in state where licensed	*	
	↳ Controlled substances within scope of authorizing prescriber		*

✓ All states.
*Most states.

Table 21.10 TIME LIMIT AFTER WHICH PRESCRIPTIONS ARE NO LONGER VALID.

	Your State's Rule?				
	1 mo	6 mo	1 y	Never expire	Other Time Period
Noncontrolled prescription drugs				**	
Schedule II				**	
Schedules III and IV		* **			
Schedule V				**	
If a prescriber dies or loses his or her license, how long are his or her prescriptions valid?				**	

*Most states.
**Federal law.

place a limit on how long a Schedule II prescription is valid (see Controlled Substances, p. 630). States may also limit the total number of allowed refills.

It is often stated that when a prescriber dies or loses his or her license, the prescriptions written by that prescriber are no longer valid. Federal law does not create such a rule—as long as the prescriber was authorized at the time the prescription was written, it is a valid prescription. Some states have dealt with this specifically, either by regulation or by a formal Board policy. Table 21.10 provides an opportunity to record your state's rules on how long prescriptions are valid.

Prescription Transfers between Pharmacies

When a prescription has refills remaining, and has not expired, you may transfer the prescription and its refill information to another pharmacy, which may dispense the remaining refills. Once transferred to another pharmacy, the prescription may not be filled in your pharmacy, unless it is transferred back, whereupon it is treated as a new prescription. Tables 21.11 and 21.12 summarize steps pharmacists must take when transferring or receiving transferred prescriptions.

Pharmacists working in chains that share a common database among all their pharmacies are able in most states and under federal law to

Table 21.11 STEPS TO TAKE WHEN TRANSFERRING A PRESCRIPTION TO ANOTHER PHARMACY	
	Rx Checklist
Record that the prescription has been transferred in the medication record system.	
Record the name and address of the pharmacy to whom it was transferred.	
Record the full name of the pharmacist or intern to whom it was transferred.	
Other requirements in your state:	
If the prescription is for a C-3, C-4, or C-5 drug, you must also:	Locate the original hard copy of the Rx and write "Void" on its face. Record the DEA number of the pharmacy to whom it was transferred.

DEA, Drug Enforcement Administration.

simply refill the prescription at their location and record the refill in the medication record system.

Drug Classifications

Legally, drugs marketed in the United States are classified as prescription-only (legend drugs), nonprescription, or "behind-the-counter"—a relatively new classification. Drugs may also be controlled substances, whether prescription (Rx)-only or over-the-counter (OTC). Finally, certain drugs that are precursors for methamphetamine are now subject to special requirements to reduce their availability for the production of methamphetamine.

Prescription Legend Drugs

Prescription-only drugs are also known as legend drugs, because their labels were formerly required to bear the legend, "Caution: Federal law prohibits dispensing without prescription." These drugs may now be labeled "only." Prescriptions may be telephoned, faxed, written, or e-prescribed and are generally refillable without limit as long as the prescription is valid.

Table 21.12 STEPS TO TAKE WHEN RECEIVING A PRESCRIPTION FROM ANOTHER PHARMACY

		Rx Checklist
Write the word "Transfer" on your copy of the prescription		
Record the name and address of the other pharmacy		
Record the full name of the pharmacist or intern who provided you with the information (obtain both first and last name)		
Record the other pharmacy's prescription number		
Record all the other information needed for the prescription (prescriber, patient, drug, strength, quantity, directions)		
Record the following dates:	Date of the transfer	
	Date Rx was first written	
	Date Rx was last refilled	
Record the number of refills originally allowed		
Record the number of refills remaining		
Other requirements in your state:		
If the prescription is for a C-3, C-4, or C-5 drug, you must also:		
	Record the DEA number of the pharmacy from whom it was received	
	Record the DEA number of the prescriber	
	Record dates and locations of all previous fillings of the Rx	
	Record the name, address, DEA number, and serial number of the original prescription and pharmacy, if it is different from the transferring pharmacy	

DEA, Drug Enforcement Administration.

OTC Drugs

Over-the-counter or nonprescription drugs are those that may be sold to the public without a prescription, and must bear a complete label as required by the FDA. They may be prescribed and dispensed with a prescription label only if this is pursuant to a valid prescription.

Methamphetamine Precursors

OTC sales of drugs containing pseudoephedrine (or ephedrine or phenylpropanolamine—which are not generally available) must be recorded in a log by the pharmacy or retailer unless they are combination products in liquid formulations. Products subject to the record requirement may not be accessible to the public. Any person selling these products must have completed an online training program. Under federal law, the log book must contain a statement to the purchaser of the penalties for violating the purchase limits set forth by federal law.

Tables 21.13 and 21.14 summarize the federal requirements for the log book and maximum purchase limits, and provide an opportunity to record your state's limits.

Controlled Substances

Controlled substances are drugs or their precursors that have a significant potential for abuse. They are divided into five schedules, depending on their medical use and potential for abuse.

Table 21.13 LIMITS ON OVER-THE-COUNTER (OTC) SALES OF METHAMPHETAMINE PRECURSORS TO A SINGLE PURCHASER		
	Federal Law	**Your State**
Sales/day	3.6 g	
Sales/month	9 g	
Possession	No limit	
Package size	3.6 g	
Package type	Blister, two units/blister	
Sales limited to 18 years or over?	No	
Other requirements in your state?		

Table 21.14 METHAMPHETAMINE PRECURSOR SALES LOG REQUIREMENTS.		
	Federal Law	**Your State**
Purchaser's name	Yes	
Purchaser's address	Yes	
Date of birth	No	
Type of ID	No	
Name of drug	Yes	
Quantity sold	Yes	
Date of purchase	Yes	
Time of purchase	Yes	
Other requirements in your state?		

Persons or firms who prescribe or dispense controlled substances must be registered with the Drug Enforcement Administration (DEA), and prescribers must place their DEA number on all prescriptions. Schedule II drugs must be ordered on special order forms.

Table 21.15 summarizes the five schedules under the Controlled Substances Act. You should also access and review the Pharmacist's Manual on the DEA web site for more information on the federal laws and regulations governing controlled substances.[7]

Is It Legitimate?

Controlled substances prescriptions are valid only if they are issued for a "legitimate medical purpose," and the pharmacist bears a "corresponding responsibility" with the prescriber to ensure that this condition is met. Thus, with each controlled substances prescription, the pharmacist must independently determine whether the prescription is legitimate. It is important, however, to remember that the pharmacist is foremost a primary care provider, not a law enforcement officer: Deciding whether to dispense or not dispense a controlled substance must be examined in light of the needs of the patient.

Red Flags Indicating a Possible Problem with a Prescription

The DEA and other authorities[7,8] recognize several characteristics that should alert a pharmacist to a possible forged or illegitimate prescription.

Table 21.15 CONTROLLED SUBSTANCES REQUIREMENTS

CSA Schedule	Basis for Inclusion	Examples	How Prescribed	Prescriptions Expire		Refill Limits	
				Federal Law	Your State	Federal Law	Your State
I	No medical use, high potential for abuse	Heroin, LSD, psilocybin, marijuana	May not be prescribed	N/A	N/A	N/A	N/A
II	High potential for abuse	Meperidine, oxycodone, methylphenidate, amphetamines	Requires written prescription	Never		No refills	
III	Moderate potential for abuse; mostly narcotic combinations	APAP with codeine; Hydrocodone with APAP	Written or oral	6 mo from date written		5 refills	
IV	Moderate potential for abuse; nonnarcotics mostly	Benzodiazepines Testosterone	Written or oral	6 mo from date written		5 refills	
V	Codeine ≤10 mg/dose plus other ingredients; antidiarrheals	Lomotil; Tylenol with codeine Elixir; codeine cough syrups	Written or oral	Never		No limit	

CSA, Controlled Substances Act; LSD, lysergic acid diethylamide; N/A, not applicable.

Table 21.16 RED FLAGS THAT SUGGEST A FORGED, ALTERED, OR OTHERWISE INVALID PRESCRIPTION

	Rx Checklist	
	Yes	**No**
Does the prescription look "too good?"		
Does the quantity, directions, or dosage differ from usual medical usage?		
Do the abbreviations differ from standard medical abbreviations?		
Are the directions written in full with no abbreviations? (Actually a desirable practice for prescribers, but still an unusual event.)		
Is the prescription written in different color inks or different handwriting?		

Note: The greater the number of Yes checks, the greater the need for pharmacist vigilance and verification of the prescription.

Table 21.16 summarizes common red flags that may appear on individual prescriptions, and Table 21.17 summarizes some common behaviors of chronic pain patients that may indicate a need for increased vigilance. These red flags are not definitive, but if present require the pharmacist to validate the order or prescription and/or promote referral of the patient to treatment for possible addiction.

White Flags Indicating a Need by the Pharmacist to Ensure Patient Care

If the pharmacist, reacting to a red flag, delays or refuses dispensing of a prescription, the patient may suffer inappropriately if the pharmacist's decision is incorrect. Therefore, pharmacists who mistakenly refuse to dispense a legitimate prescription for controlled substances may find themselves being named in a lawsuit. As a general rule, before deciding not to dispense a prescription, the pharmacist should engage in a direct conversation with the prescriber concerning his or her decision not to dispense. Table 21.18 summarizes questions a pharmacist should ask before deciding not to dispense or to contact authorities.[9]

Table 21.17 CHRONIC PAIN PATIENTS RED FLAGS

	Rx Checklist	
	Yes	**No**
Does the patient appear to be "doctor shopping" (obtaining multiple prescriptions for the same or similar drugs from multiple prescribers)?		
Does it appear that the patient is altering or forging prescriptions?		
Are you aware of the patient selling his or her prescription drugs?		
Does the patient insist on specific brand name narcotics and refuse generics in situations where the use of generics is indicated?		
Are there multiple episodes of lost, stolen, or accidently destroyed prescriptions and/or drugs?		
Are you aware of the patient taking or using another person's drugs?		

Note: The greater the number of Yes checks, the greater the need for the pharmacist to work with prescribers to ensure that the patient is not becoming addicted.

Behind-the-Counter Drugs

Behind-the-counter (BTC) drugs may be sold without a prescription but must either be sold by a pharmacist or at least not displayed to the public. Currently BTC drugs comprise only methamphetamine precursors (see above) and the Plan B emergency contraception product. Plan B may be sold without prescription to persons aged 18 or over but may be dispensed to women under 18 only on prescription. Because the pharmacist will be held responsible for the sale of Plan B to a minor, he or she should require proof of age before selling the product without a prescription. Most states prohibit technicians from making this kind of decision.

 Drug Product Selection

Drug product selection activities by pharmacists may take two forms: generic substitution or therapeutic substitution. Virtually all states permit pharmacists to substitute generic equivalent drugs for brand name

Table 21.18   WHITE FLAGS THAT SUGGEST THIS PERSON SHOULD BE TREATED AS A PATIENT, NOT A FELON

	Rx Checklist	
	Yes	No
Did the information regarding the validity of the prescription come directly from the prescriber?		
⤷ If No, did the party inform you that the prescription is unequivocally fraudulent *and* that their response is *not* just based on a lack of information in the patient record? (If No, don't call the police.)		
Did you discuss with the prescriber that you were intending to call the police?		
⤷ If Yes, did the prescriber agree that was appropriate? (If No, be careful about calling the police.)		
Has the patient previously established a relationship with you or the pharmacy?		
⤷ If Yes, did your profile review suggest that the prescription is consistent with a pattern of reasonable treatment? (If Yes, don't call the police.)		
⤷ If Yes, did you ask the patient about any discrepancies with the prescription? (If No, be careful about calling the police.)		
⤷ If Yes, did their explanation resolve issues? (If Yes, don't call the police.)		
Are you expecting the police to investigate further? (If Yes, confirm this with the police, if contacted.)		
⤷ If No, do you believe they can rely on *your* information to conclude the prescription is fraudulent? (If No, be careful about calling the police.)		
Are you prepared to defend your decision in court? (If No, don't call the police.)		

drugs under specified conditions. Therapeutic substitution is common-place in most states in hospitals and health maintenance organizations (HMOs) by use of formularies. Many states also allow for therapeutic substitution in community settings, but the mechanisms vary widely.

Generic Substitution

Pharmacists who make the effort to provide a generically equivalent drug to patients instead of a more expensive brand name drug are performing an important patient care function and fulfilling an ethical obligation to the patient, since doing so contributes to the patient's economic welfare without compromising the patient's clinical outcomes. In many states, performing a generic substitution when permitted is also mandated by state law.

In virtually all states, a generic equivalent is a drug that meets the following criteria: (i) It is the same chemical entity as the prescribed drug; (ii) it is in the same dosage form; and (iii) it is bioequivalent, which means it has statistically the same pharmacokinetic parameters of area under the curve (AUC) and time to peak concentration (T_{max}) when compared in vivo with the prescribed drug.

States generally allow the pharmacist to substitute the generic drug for the brand name drug *if* such a substitution results in a lower price to the patient, and *if* the prescriber has not determined that the brand name drug is medically necessary.

How Do States Require the Prescriber to Prevent or Allow Substitution?

The states have essentially three options for specifying how prescribers should allow or prevent generic substitution:

1. Prohibit substitution unless the prescriber specifically allows it. In these states, prescriptions often have a check box (e.g., "☑ Substitution Permitted") to allow substitution. If the box is not checked, the pharmacist must dispense the prescribed brand name or call the physician for permission to substitute. In these states, when a prescription is verbally ordered by brand name, the pharmacist must then ask about generic substitution.

2. Allow substitution unless the prescriber specifically prohibits it. In these states, the prescriber must write "Dispense as Written" or "DAW" to prohibit substitution. A check box (e.g., "☑ DAW") is often allowed. In these states, when a prescription is verbally ordered by brand name, the prescriber must also specify to dispense as ordered if he or she wants to prohibit generic substitution.

3. Require the prescriber to specifically allow or specifically prohibit substitution on each prescription. Some states use a two-line prescription blank, and the prescriber must sign on the "Dispense as Written" line

Table 21.19 OPTIONS FOR SPECIFYING
WHETHER GENERIC SUBSTITUTION
IS ALLOWED

	Rx Checklist	
	Yes	**No**
Must you dispense the brand name prescribed unless the prescriber indicates "substitution permitted?" ↳ If Yes, did you ask about substitution on a phoned Rx?		
May you substitute a lower-cost generic equivalent unless the prescriber has specified "DAW" in some way?		
Must the prescriber sign one line on a two-line blank on every written prescription? ↳ If Yes, did you ask the prescriber about his or her substitution preferences on a phoned Rx?		

"DAW, "Dispense as Written."

or the "Substitution Permitted" line. In these states, it is incumbent
on the pharmacist to determine the prescriber's wishes about generic
substitution when prescriptions are ordered by telephone.

Table 21.19 summarizes these options.

How May Pharmacists in a Given State Determine if a Drug Product May Be Substituted?

States also generally have three approaches to specifying how pharmacists
know whether a given drug may be considered a substitutable generic
equivalent to the brand name product:

1. The state may specify a list of drugs that may *never* be substituted. This
   list usually is composed of drugs with a "narrow therapeutic index."
   Such a list is termed a "negative formulary," and if the prescribed
   brand name drug is on the list, pharmacists may substitute a generic
   equivalent only by calling the prescriber to obtain prior approval.
2. The state may specify a list of drugs that are eligible for substitution, and
   any drug products not on that list are excluded unless the prescriber
   specifically approves the substitution. Such a list is called a "positive
   formulary." Some states develop their own restrictive list, but for most
   states, the FDA Orange Book is accepted.
3. The state may set the requirements for a generic equivalent and allow the pharmacist to use such information as appropriate to determine whether the proposed substitution is appropriate. In these

Table 21.20 DETERMINING WHETHER A PRODUCT IS GENERICALLY EQUIVALENT AND ELIGIBLE FOR SUBSTITUTION	Your State?	
	Yes	**No**
Does your state have a list of "narrow therapeutic index" drugs that cannot be the subject of generic substitution? ↳ If Yes, is the prescribed drug on the list? ↳ If Yes, did you obtain prior authorization from the prescriber to substitute a generic drug? (If No, dispense as written.)		
Does your state require the generic drug to be on a list of approved drugs? ↳ If Yes, is the proposed substitution on the list? ↳ If No, did you obtain prior authorization for the substitution from the prescriber? (If No, dispense as written.)		
Does your state allow the pharmacist to use judgment based on any reliable evidence for determining that the generic drug is bioequivalent to the prescribed drug? ↳ If Yes, do you have such evidence (e.g., AB rated in the Orange Book)? (If No, dispense as written or obtain prior authorization to dispense the generic drug.)		

states, the Orange Book is one recognized source that a pharmacist may rely on.

Table 21.20 provides a checklist for determining if your state allows a particular generic to be substituted.

Labeling of Drugs and Medicines

Distributing or dispensing a drug without approved labeling makes the drug misbranded—this is prohibited by both federal and state laws. The federal Food, Drug and Cosmetic Act (FDCA) and FDA regulations establish required labeling for drugs. OTC drugs must contain a drug facts label. Prescription drugs must contain approved professional labeling and, where required, informational labeling for patients (patient package inserts). FDA regulations require MedGuides that must be included when dispensing a growing number of prescription drugs. A pharmacist may deliver a drug to another practitioner or pharmacy only with its FDA approved labeling intact, or to a patient with intact OTC labeling or with a prescription label when dispensed pursuant to a prescription. Federal laws specify a minimum set of elements on the labels for outpatient prescriptions and have only a few requirements for hospital drugs. Surprisingly to most pharmacists, federal law requires only the patient name and directions for use if the prescriber includes them on the prescription. States, however, have very specific requirements for drug labels, depending on the setting.

Labeling includes not only the actual label on the bottle, but the written information supplied to the patient with the container. The tables that follow indicate only what is required on the actual container or package label.

Ambulatory Prescriptions

The clinical goal of labeling for outpatient prescriptions is to give the patient information needed to use the drug appropriately. A pharmacist must always ask which information is needed by the patient, and which is best supplied in writing. It is important to *always* provide patients with patient package inserts or other labeling beyond the prescription label that will help them use the drug effectively. Also, many pharmacies provide information on their labels regarding how many refills are left, when the prescription needs to be renewed, and how to contact a pharmacist for additional information, even if this is not required by their state law. See Table 21.21 for details.

Federal Side Effects Statement

A recent revision to the FDCA requires pharmacists to provide the following side effects statement to all patients receiving outpatient prescriptions: "Call your doctor for medical advice about side effects. You may report side effects to FDA at 1–800-FDA-1088." This may be placed on the label, the cap of the prescription container, a separate printed sheet, or in a MedGuide or patient information leaflet (PIL).[10]

Beyond-Use Date

A little fewer than half of U.S. jurisdictions require a beyond-use date be placed on the label of a prescription drug dispensed to an outpatient. As a general rule, the USP indicates that a pharmacist must put a beyond-use

Table 21.21 ELEMENTS REQUIRED ON LABEL OF AMBULATORY PATIENT PRESCRIPTIONS

	Federal Law	Your State
Pharmacy name	✓	✓
Pharmacy address	✓	✓
Prescription number (serial number)	✓	✓
Prescriber name	✓	✓
Date filled (federal law requires date prescribed or date filled)	✓	✓
Patient name	✓†	*
Prescriber's directions for use	✓†	*
"Side effects statement" (if not provided otherwise; see discussion)	✓	✓
"Caution: Federal law prohibits dispensing of this drug to any person other than the person for whom it was prescribed."	✓††	*††
Drug name and strength		*
Pharmacist's initials		*
Necessary auxiliary and/or precautionary labels (e.g., Shake well, Take with food, Take on an empty stomach, May cause drowsiness, etc.)		*
Pharmacy telephone number		
Quantity dispensed		
Beyond-use date (see discussion) ↳ If required, is the maximum ☐ 1 y ☐ Manufacturer's date ☐ Other: _____		
Other requirements in your state:		

✓ Required.
† Only if included in prescription.
†† Controlled substances only.
* Most states.

date on the prescription label, based on information from the manufacturer or from the relevant USP monograph. If stability data is lacking for a particular packaging option, the USP indicates that the beyond-use date should be no longer than 1 year from dispensing or the manufacturer's expiration date, whichever is earlier.[11]

Compliance Packaging

An important clinical service for many patients is to provide medication in custom packaging to help ensure compliance. Examples of this type of packaging include Medi-Sets, blister packs (like bingo cards), or strip packaging. When dispensed directly to patients, these must generally be labeled with the same information as required on a standard prescription vial. Because this packaging is not usually child resistant, permission to use non–child resistant containers must be obtained from the patient or patient's agent.

Long-term Care

Pharmacies serving nursing home patients typically choose from one of three types of distribution systems: unit dose, modified unit dose, and traditional prescription containers. Child-resistant containers are not required for nursing homes, except when medications are sent home with a patient for short excursions or on discharge.

Unit Dose

Unit dose systems involve individual patient cassettes (small drawers) labeled for each patient, with individual unit-dose packages placed into them. Cassettes are usually transported in carts, and one set of carts is at the nursing home while a second set is at the pharmacy being prepared for the next set of doses. Carts then are exchanged at a set interval (often 48 hours to 7 days). Most states allow unused unit doses to be redispensed.

Traditional Prescriptions and Modified Unit-Dose (MUD)

Traditional prescription containers are usually dispensed with a 30-day supply of medication. MUD packaging, often in the form of bingo card-type blister packs, may be dispensed in 1-week to 30-day supplies. Drugs dispensed in traditional containers cannot be reused if discontinued and must be destroyed. Many states allow the return and reuse of drugs in MUD packaging when the pharmacist can determine the package has not been damaged or tampered with. Table 21.22 summarizes typical requirements for nursing home labeling.

Inpatient Medications

Table 21.23 summarizes typical requirements for labeling of inpatient drugs in hospitals.

Table 21.22 LABELING AND RETURN REQUIREMENTS FOR NURSING HOME DISTRIBUTION SYSTEMS

	Your State?		
	Traditional Prescription	MUD	UD
Name and strength of medication	*	*	*
Quantity	*	*	*
Lot number			*
Expiration date	*	*	*
Patient name	*	*	†
Patient location			†
Directions for use			
Controlled substances schedule number			
May unused drugs be returned for credit and reused?		*	*
Other requirements in your state:			

MUD, modified unit dose; UD, unit dose.
*Most states.
†On individual patient cassette.

Child-Resistant Containers

The federal Poison Prevention Packaging Act requires that certain household substances be packaged in child-resistant containers (CRCs). A copy of the publication Poison Prevention Packaging: A Guide for Healthcare Professionals can be found at www.cpsc.gov/cpscpub/pubs/384.pdf.

It is important to understand that CRCs are designed so that 90% of elderly adults can open them if shown how. When you realize that one in six children younger than 4 years who are poisoned by prescription drugs have obtained them from a container belonging to a grandparent or great-grandparent,[12] it will become clear that pharmacists owe their elderly patients a chance to learn how to open CRCs before agreeing to dispense with easy-open caps.

Table 21.23 LABELING REQUIREMENTS FOR HOSPITAL INPATIENT DRUGS

	Your State?
Inpatient Oral Drugs	
Drug name	*
Strength	*
Expiration date, if applicable	*
Auxiliary labeling as applicable	*
Other requirements in your state:	
Hospital Parenteral Drugs	
Name and concentration of base solution	*
Name and amount of added drugs	*
Name and location of patient	*
Appropriate expiration dating	*
Initials of personnel who prepared the solution	
Other requirements in your state:	

*Most states.

OTC Drugs

Most OTC drugs do not require child-resistant containers. Those that do include oral drugs containing aspirin, ibuprofen, naproxen, iron salts, diphenhydramine, fluoride, lidocaine, loperamide, and newer drugs that have been switched to OTC status since 2001 (e.g., omeprazole, ranitidine, cetirizine). Caustic substances (strong acids or bases) and hydrocarbons also require CRCs.

Manufacturers may exempt one package in each product line, providing it is labeled "Not for Use in Households with Small Children."

Legend Drugs

All oral prescription drugs require CRCs when dispensed by prescription, with a small list of exceptions. The most important exceptions include nitroglycerine sublingual tablets and chewable and sublingual isosorbide tablets containing ≤10 mg per tablet.

Pharmacists may dispense prescriptions without CRCs only when authorized by (a) the patient; (b) the patient's agent—which cannot be pharmacy personnel; or (c) the prescriber, if indicated individually on each prescription. Some states require the authorization by the patient or agent to be in writing, although this is not required by federal law.

Patient Medication Records

All but eight jurisdictions (Alaska, Colorado, District of Columbia, Guam, Louisiana, Maryland, Minnesota, Puerto Rico, and Virginia)[4] mandate that pharmacies maintain patient medication records that record medications used by and dispensed to patients, along with patient information needed to properly screen prescriptions for problems and to monitor drug use. Federal law governing Medicaid (OBRA-90)[13] requires states to ensure that pharmacies maintain these records for all Medicaid patients and use the information contained in them to perform prospective drug use review.

Required Elements

Table 21.24 summarizes typical required elements for patient medication record systems.

Drug Use Review

OBRA-90 requires pharmacists to screen new orders against the patient drug history prior to dispensing, an activity known as prospective drug use review (P-DUR). This is required for all Medicaid patients, and states that require counseling for non-Medicaid patients (all but eight) generally require P-DUR for all patients as well. It is expected that a pharmacist who detects a problem through P-DUR will take an appropriate action to resolve the problem before delivering the drug to the patient. In some cases, patient interviews can resolve apparent issues, but often a call to the prescriber is necessary. Failure to carry out required P-DUR and properly resolve discovered problems is a growing cause of lawsuits against pharmacists.[14] Tables 21.25 and 21.26 summarize requirements for P-DUR and provide a checklist for P-DUR for individual prescriptions.

Privacy

Patients have an expectation of privacy in their relationships with pharmacists. Principle II of the Code of Ethics for Pharmacists states that "A pharmacist promotes the good of every patient in a caring, compassionate, and confidential manner."[15] As a general rule, health providers caring for patients are entitled to know details of the patient's conditions and therapy

Table 21.24 ELEMENTS REQUIRED IN PATIENT MEDICATION RECORDS

	Medicaid Patients	Your State?
Is a patient medication record or patient profile required?	✓	*
Patient full name	✓	*
Patient address (required on all CSA prescriptions)	†	*
Patient age or date of birth	†	*
Patient telephone number	†	
Patient gender	†	*
Clinically important medical conditions	†	*
Drug allergies or drug reactions	†	*
↳ If none, must this be indicated (e.g., "NKA")?		*
A list of drugs and devices previously used by the patient	†	
↳ OTCs used by patient		
↳ Prescription drugs obtained from other pharmacies	†	
↳ Devices obtained from other sources	†	
↳ Medications or devices dispensed by this pharmacy	✓	*
↳ Prescription number		*
↳ Date dispensed		*
Name, strength, dosage form		*
Quantity dispensed		*
Prescriber name or ID		*
Dispenser's initials		
Pharmacists' comments on the patient's drug therapy	✓	
Authorization for use of non–child-resistant containers		
Other elements in your state:		

CSA, Controlled Substances Act; NKA, no known allergies; OTC, over-the-counter.
✓Required.
†Must make reasonable attempt to obtain.
*Most states.

Table 21.25 PROSPECTIVE DRUG USE REVIEW

	Medicaid Patients	Your State?
Is P-DUR required for all patients?	✓	*
↳ New prescriptions?	✓	*
↳ Refill prescriptions?		

P-DUR, prospective drug use review.
✓ Required.
*Most states.

necessary for that provider to provide patient care, including receiving payment for services and ensuring quality of care, but for no other purposes, unless the patient has consented. This has been formalized under federal law by the Privacy Rule enacted under provisions of the Health Insurance Portability and Accountability Act of 1996 (HIPAA).[16] Under these rules, pharmacists may use protected health information (PHI)—information about the patient's health care that identifies the patient—for providing treatment, for obtaining payment, or for health care operations (TPHCO). Any other release of PHI requires written authorization of the patient, the patient's guardian, or the patient's agent.

Prior to use of PHI, a pharmacist must provide the patient with a Notice of Privacy Practices (NOPP), which explains how the pharmacy will use PHI and gives patients information about their rights under HIPAA or applicable state law. The patient must acknowledge receipt of the NOPP in writing. Provision of the NOPP must be done on the first visit.

Each provider must appoint a Privacy Officer who deals with requests from patients for access to their records and requests for modification of their records. Pharmacists must know the identity of their pharmacy's Privacy Officer and be able to refer patients to that person.

Special considerations exist for patient records for minors. Normally, parents or legal guardians may have access to a minor's records and may consent to care for the minor. However, when state law provides the minor with the right to consent to a given type of care, the minor then gains control over his or her PHI, and parents may not see such information without the minor's consent. In many states, minors may consent to emergency treatment or treatment for sexually transmitted diseases, reproductive health (including contraception), substance abuse, or mental health, often at age 13 or older. Also, minors who are considered emancipated as the result of court action, or are minors married to an adult, usually control

Table 21.26 ELEMENTS SPECIFIED BY OBRA-90 WHEN P-DUR IS REQUIRED

	Rx Checklist	
	Yes	**No**
Is the drug in this order contraindicated in this patient? ⤷ If Yes, the product should *not* be dispensed.		
Is this prescription or order for a drug which duplicates therapy the patient is already receiving? ⤷ If Yes, did you determine that the other therapy has been discontinued? ⤷ Or, did you determine that the other therapy is appropriate and desired?		
Does the drug in this order potentially react adversely with any of the patient's medical conditions? ⤷ If Yes, did you determine that the physician is aware and believes the benefits outweigh the risk?		
Does the drug in this order pose possible adverse drug interactions? ⤷ If Yes, have you ruled out the possibility based on dose, separation of doses, order of dosing, or other basis? ⤷ Or, did you determine that the prescriber is aware of the interaction and believes the benefits outweigh the risk?		
Does the dose or duration of treatment prescribed in this order appear to be too high or too low? ⤷ If Yes, have you contacted the prescriber to correct the dose or duration? ⤷ Or, have you determined that the prescriber is aware of the normal dose and has confirmed this particular dose or duration?		
Is there information suggesting the patient may be allergic or cross-allergic to the drug in this order? ⤷ If Yes, have you ruled out the possibility based on patient history, interview, or confirmation with the prescriber? ⤷ Or, did you determine that the prescriber is aware of the possibility and believes the benefits outweigh the risks?		

(continued)

Table 21.26 ELEMENTS SPECIFIED BY OBRA-90 WHEN P-DUR IS REQUIRED *(continued)*

	Rx Checklist	
	Yes	No
Does the patient's drug use history suggest that he or she is underusing or overusing the drug in this order, or otherwise misusing the drug?		
⤷ If Yes, have you identified a documented reason that explains the apparent abuse/misuse and determined that it is not an actual problem?		
⤷ Or, have you educated the patient on the proper use and believe that he or she is equipped to take the drug properly in the future?		
⤷ Or, have you confirmed with the prescriber the apparent misuse or abuse and the prescriber has confirmed that the prescription should be filled at this time?		

OBRA-90, Omnibus Budget Reconciliation Act of 1990; P-DUR, prospective drug use review.

their own PHI. Table 21.27 provides a checklist for the most common factors affecting a release of information about a given patient.

Providing Information and Counseling to Patients

OBRA-90 requires states to ensure that pharmacists make an "offer to counsel" all Medicaid patients with each new prescription. Most states extend the requirement to counsel patients to all patients. Most states also require pharmacists to provide additional written material that may be necessary to ensure proper medication use, and federal law requires certain written information to be provided with specific drug products.

Required Patient Counseling

Most states allow the pharmacist to use judgment in determining which information to provide to a patient concerning his or her drug therapy.

Offer to Counsel

All states permit patients or their agents to decline counseling, and most require that the pharmacist at least make an offer on new prescriptions. Some states allow the offer to be made by a technician, and a few allow the

Table 21.27 PRIVACY CHECKLIST, PRIOR TO RELEASE OF PATIENT PHI TO ANOTHER PERSON OR ENTITY	Yes	No
Has the patient received and acknowledged the NOPP?		
Treatment (if Yes to any of the following, release is allowed) Is the release to another provider known to be caring for the patient?		
Is this a prescription transfer to another pharmacy at the patient's request?		
Is the release to a caregiver or patient's agent?		
Is the release to a person specifically listed by the patient as eligible to receive information?		
Is the release to a former provider, *and* the patient has not specifically requested that information not be provided to that provider?		
Has the patient specifically requested the release in writing?		
Payment (if Yes to any of the following, release is allowed) Is the release to a third-party payer to determine eligibility for payment?		
Is the release a finished claim to a third-party payer?		
Is the release to a credit card company used by the patient to pay for a professional service, in response to a justification of the charge, and contains the minimum information necessary?		
Is the release to a collection agency of the minimum information necessary to collect patient debts to the provider?		
Has the patient specifically allowed the release in writing (e.g., on a claim form or release to a third party)?		
Release of information concerning minors		
Does the minor control the information? If Yes Is it for treatment that the minor was allowed to consent to?		
↳ Or, is the minor emancipated or married to an adult, and thus allowed to consent to health care in your state?		
If Yes Does it meet the criteria for release for TPHCO?		
↳ Or, did the minor specifically allow the release in writing?		
If No Does it meet the criteria for release for TPHCO?		
↳ Or, has a parent or legal guardian specifically allowed the release in writing?		

PHI, protected health information; NOPP, Notice of Privacy Practices; TPHCO, treatment, payment, health care operations.

Table 21.28 PATIENT COUNSELING REQUIREMENTS

	Medicaid Patients	Your State?
Is patient counseling required for Medicaid patients?	✓	✓
All other patients?		*
New prescriptions?	✓	*
Refill prescriptions?		*
May the pharmacist use judgment in deciding to counsel?		*
The offer to counsel Is not allowed, but counseling must be done		
May only be made by the pharmacist face-to-face	*	*
May be made by a technician		
May be made by a sign in the pharmacy		
Documentation of counseling Is required when counseling is given and/or when it is refused		
Is required only if patient or agent refuses counseling		
Is not required	*	*

✓ Required.
*Most states.

offer to be made by a sign in the pharmacy. A few states mandate counseling and do not allow counseling to be satisfied by an "offer." Table 21.28 summarizes these options for advising patients that there is information available from the pharmacist.

Elements of Counseling

The goal of patient counseling is to ensure that the patient has the information and understanding necessary to properly use his or her medication. OBRA-90 provides guidelines for the content of counseling. Dr. Bruce Berger has provided a detailed checklist for the patient counseling session, with suggestions for pharmacist actions at each step of the process;[17] Table 21.29 is an example Rx checklist that could be used to record completion of such counseling for a given prescription on a given visit. The pharmacist can record that a given element was completed at that visit, that the patient was already aware of the information, that the element

Table 21.29 RX COUNSELING CHECKLIST

Pt: Rx No: Pharm:	Date of Visit:			
	Com- pleted	Pt. Aware	Defer	N/A
Name and description of medication				
Route of administration				
Dose and regimen				
Maximum daily dose				
Dosage form				
Duration of therapy				
Special directions and precautions for preparing or taking				
Commonly experienced: ↳ Side effects ↳ Adverse effects ↳ Drug interactions ↳ Contraindications ↳ How to avoid the above ↳ What to do if the above are encountered				
Techniques for self-monitoring				
Proper storage				
Refill information and how to obtain refills				
What to do if a dose is missed				
☐ Counseling declined: "The pharmacist advised me of an opportunity to learn more about my medication, but I have chosen to decline this offer"	Patient or agent signature:			

is deferred for a future visit, or that the element is not applicable for this medication.

Written Drug Information

Most pharmacies' computer systems produce patient information leaflets (PILs) with new prescriptions for outpatients. This is a required element of many state laws. Certain drug products have product information for patients that is mandated by federal law in one of three ways: (i) particular

Table 21.30 RX CHECKLIST FOR WRITTEN INFORMATION

	Yes	No
Do any of the following conditions apply to this drug?		
Is the product an oral contraceptive or estrogen?		
Is there a required MedGuide for this product? (www.fda.gov/cder/offices/ods/medication_guides.htm)		
Is there a patient package insert included with the product labeling (e.g., inhalers, injectables)?		
If Yes		
↳ Provide to patient with each dispensing of the drug		
Does your pharmacy produce a patient information leaflet for this product?		
If Yes		
↳ Provide to patient as required by state law or as indicated by patient need		

regulations governing a class of drugs (e.g., oral contraceptives and estrogens); (ii) patient information specified in the official product labeling that was agreed to by the manufacturer when the drug was approved; or (iii) MedGuides for specific products required by FDA regulations. Whenever federal law specifies specific patient information, the pharmacist is required to provide this information to the patient with every prescription (new or refill) and on request.

Always remember, too, that most states require the labels of prescription containers to contain appropriate caution labels (e.g., "Take with Food" or "May Cause Drowsiness") to alert patients to critical information on proper use or storage of the drug. Table 21.30 is a checklist for determining when written information should be provided.

▮ Concluding Comment

State and federal laws and regulations have evolved over the last 100 years in response to real problems in the manufacture, promotion, dispensing, prescribing, and use of medications. They set a minimum standard of behavior for producers, prescribers, and dispensers and provide patients with important rights regarding their medical records and the information they should be provided by providers. However, strict adherence to the letter of the law, and doing nothing more, will neither ensure optimum patient care nor continue to earn for pharmacists their respect as a trusted profession. Only competent and consistent provision of pharmaceutical care to every patient can continue to assure our profession's high esteem.

References

1. Wood LL. *Medical Records, Medical Education, and Patient Care*. Chicago, IL: Year Book Medical; 1971.
2. Delitto A, Snyder-Mackler L. The diagnostic process: examples in orthopedic physical therapy. *Phys Ther*. 1995 Mar;73(3):203–211.
3. Bossen C. Evaluation of a computerized problem-oriented medical record in a hospital department: does it support daily clinical practice? *Int J Med Inform*. 2007 Aug;76(8):592–600.
4. *Survey of State Pharmacy Laws, 2008*. Chicago, IL: National Association of Boards of Pharmacy; 2008.
5. Title 21 Code of Federal Regulations (CFR) Section 1306.25(a)(1).
6. www.deadiversion.usdoj.gov/drugreg/practitioners/index.html. Accessed January 13, 2008.
7. www.deadiversion.usdoj.gov/pubs/manuals/pharm2/index.htm. Accessed February 27, 2008.
8. Seeger VB. Is it legitimate? Strategies for assessing questionable prescriptions and DEA considerations. APHA annual mtg., Orlando, FL; 2005; April 4th.
9. Fassett WE. Is it legitimate? Accessing controlled substances prescriptions. APHA annual mtg., Orlando, FL; 2005; April 4th.
10. Title21 CFR Section 209.1–209.11; 73 FR 404, January 3, 2008.
11. USP Pharmacist's Pharmacopeia. 1st ed. Rockville, MD: The United States Pharmacopeial Convention; 2005:12.
12. Safe Kids, USA. Available at www.usa.safekids.org/tier3_cd.cfm?folder_id=540& content_item_id=1152. Accessed
13. Omnibus Budget Reconciliation Act of 1990, Pub. L. 101–508.
14. Pharmacists Mutual Claims Study 2007. Available at www.phmic.com/web.nsf/ pages/DrugReview.html. Accessed March 22, 2008.
15. APhA. Code of Ethics for Pharmacists. Washington, DC: American Pharmacists Association. Available at www.pharmacist.com/AM/Template.cfm?Section=Search1 &template=/CM/HTMLDisplay.cfm&ContentID=2903.
16. Pub. L. 104–191.
17. Berger B. Effective patient counseling. *US Pharm*. 1999;24(2):, Available at www. uspharmacist.com/oldformat.asp?url=newlook/files/Phar/ACF59D.cfm&pub_ id=8&article_id=157.

Index

Note: Page numbers followed by *b*, *f*, or *t* indicate boxed, figures, or tables material.